Atlas of Pulmonary Cytopathology

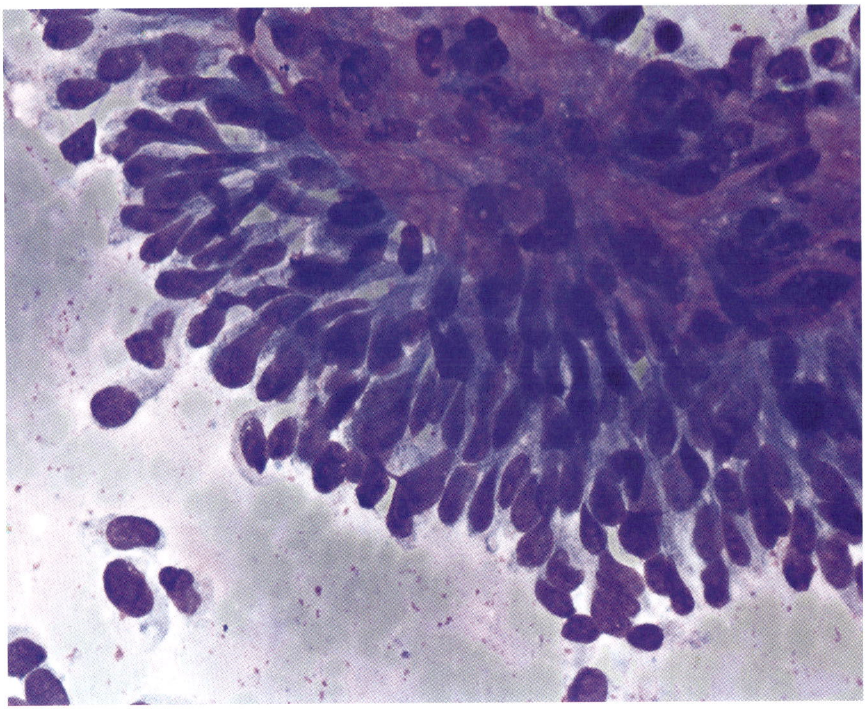

Christopher J. VandenBussche, MD, PhD
Assistant Professor of Pathology and Cytopathology Fellowship Director
The Johns Hopkins University School of Medicine
Baltimore, Maryland

Syed Z. Ali, MD, FRCPath, FIAC
Professor of Pathology and Radiology and Director of Cytopathology
The Johns Hopkins University School of Medicine
Baltimore, Maryland

Morgan L. Cowan, MD
Assistant of Pathology
The Johns Hopkins University School of Medicine
Baltimore, Maryland

Paul E. Wakely, Jr., MD
Professor of Pathology
Ohio State University Medical Center
Columbus, Ohio

Joyce E. Johnson, MD
Professor of Pathology, Microbiology, and Immunology
Director, Anatomic Pathology, VA Medical Center
Vanderbilt University School of Medicine
Nashville, Tennessee

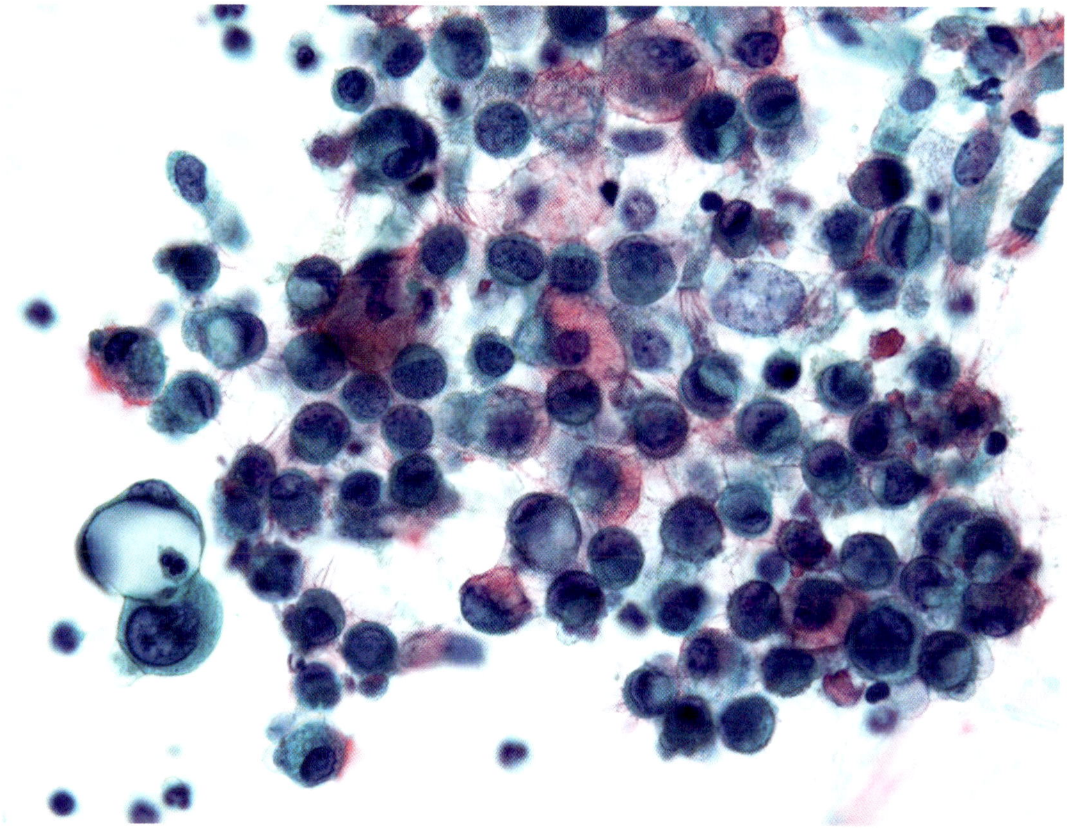

Atlas of Pulmonary Cytopathology

With Histopathologic Correlations

demosMEDICAL
An Imprint of Springer Publishing

Visit our website at www.demosmedical.com

ISBN: 9781936287161
ebook ISBN: 9781617050459

Acquisitions Editor: David D'Addona
Compositor: diacriTech

Library of Congress Cataloging-in-Publication Data
Names: VandenBussche, Christopher J., author. | Ali, Syed Z., author. | Cowan, Morgan L., author. | Wakely, Paul E., Jr., 1949- author. | Johnson, Joyce E., 1958- author.
Title: Atlas of pulmonary cytopathology with histopathologic correlations / Christopher J. VandenBussche, Syed Z. Ali, Morgan L. Cowan, Paul E. Wakely, Jr., Joyce E. Johnson.
Description: New York: Demos Medical Publishing, [2017] | Includes bibliographical references and index.
Identifiers: LCCN 2017016470| ISBN 9781936287161 | ISBN 9781617050459 (e-ISBN)
Subjects: | MESH: Lung Diseases—pathology | Lung Diseases—diagnosis | Cytodiagnosis | Atlases
Classification: LCC RC756 | NLM WF 17 | DDC 616.2/4—dc23
LC record available at https://lccn.loc.gov/2017016470

Printed in the United States of America by Bang Printing.
17 18 19 20 21 / 5 4 3 2 1

To my mother, Carol, and her parents, William and Katharine ("Vicki"). –CJV

To my parents, Bano and Mazhar. –SZA

To my first microscope, monocular and mirror-illuminated, passed on to my childhood self by my mother (and from Dr. E. L. Caudil of Elizabethton, Tennessee, before her), by which the animated cellular mysteries of the otherwise still and muddy pond behind my childhood home were first illuminated. And always, for Travis. –MLC

To my former cytopathology fellows in appreciation of the knowledge and stimulation I have received from them. –PEW

To residents and fellows, who are the future; and to patients with lung diseases, who are the reason. –JEJ

Contents

Foreword

The practice of cytopathology has undergone significant evolution in the last 50 years. Cytopathology is a diagnostic method, not simply a screening method, in most of the areas in which it is applied and has become an integral part of pathology. The importance of cytological techniques for the investigation of respiratory conditions has been recognized since the earliest days of clinical cytology. The study of cellular specimens from the respiratory tract is established as a vital diagnostic procedure in the evaluation of patients with suspected lung inflammatory/infectious or neoplastic diseases. The study of sputum, bronchial washings, bronchial aspirates, bronchial brushings, bronchoalveolar lavage specimens, and fine needle aspirates (FNAs) provides the morphologic basis for these diagnoses. With the advent of targeted therapy for lung cancer, ancillary testing of specimens derived from the lower respiratory tract has obtained greater importance. Traditionally, ancillary testing was confined to culture techniques for microbiologic organisms, flow cytometry for lymphoid proliferations, and immunohistochemical stains for the classification of pulmonary neoplasms. Targeted therapy has expanded the need for ancillary and, in particular, molecular testing to document the presence or absence of certain mutations, amplifications, inversions, and translocations that indicate a carcinoma susceptibility to specific targeted therapies. In fact, in lung cancer, small biopsies and cytologic specimens are the primary materials for establishing the diagnosis in most cases, as well as for studying markers driving tumor classification and providing prognostic and predictive information. Despite all of these new advances, the foundation of cytopathology is based in a correct and precise morphologic interpretation.

This *Atlas of Pulmonary Cytopathology* is an outstanding work with more than 500 high-quality images documenting a full range of nonneoplastic and neoplastic lung diseases. In addition, there is excellent documentation of the histopathology and gross examination in some cases, providing morphologic correlations useful for cytopathologists and surgical pathologists. The inclusion of a chapter dedicated to radiology is of paramount importance. In the era where clinical-pathologic correlation is becoming more and more important in the management of patients, the knowledge of how an expert radiologist deals with these correlations brings an additional value to the *Atlas* that will be very well recognized and accepted for the readers. From the cytopathology perspective, knowing the imaging characteristics of lung lesions is extremely valuable in the interpretation of specimens.

The richness of the *Atlas* content will be very helpful for general pathologists, lung pathologists, cytopathologists, and trainees in their daily practice. Moreover, the work reflects the extensive practice of cytopathology at Johns Hopkins, especially by Drs. VandenBussche and Ali, internationally recognized experts and respected cytopathologists. I am confident that this book will aid pathologists in their routine by providing essential information for better diagnosis and management of patients. Now it is time to enjoy the text and the illustrations of this *Atlas* that presents, in a didactic way, up-to-date knowledge in lung cytopathology.

Fernando Schmitt, MD, PhD, FIAC
Professor of Pathology at Medical Faculty of Porto University
Head of the Molecular Laboratory and Senior Researcher
Instituto de Patologia e Imunologia Molecular da
Universidade do Porto, Porto, Portugal
General Secretary of the International Academy of Cytology

1

Lung Radiology

INTRODUCTION

Radiologic evaluation of lung lesions can serve many roles including primary detection, narrowing of the differential diagnosis, treatment or surgical planning, and posttreatment surveillance. Plain radiographs are often the first-line modality for evaluation of symptomatic individuals and may be the source of detection of a lung lesion incidentally discovered during the course of other medical work-up. Nevertheless, CT remains as the mainstay of imaging characterization of lung disease due to its widespread access and excellent spatial resolution. CT is also often used as a rapid method of assessing the entire body for metastatic disease in the setting of lung malignancy. CT has a significant advantage over MRI in avoiding motion-related artifacts from breathing, due to the short image acquisition times possible with CT. MRI, on the other hand, is very useful in certain specific situations where its superior contrast resolution can better delineate soft tissue anatomy, such as in the evaluation of mediastinal or superior sulcus invasion by tumor. More recently, F-18 fluorodeoxyglucose-PET has become another widely used tool in diagnostic imaging of lung disease. Fluorodeoxyglucose-PET imaging utilizes the hypermetabolism of most tumors as a method of tumor localization and can be a very powerful tool in detection and assessment of tumor location and activity, sometimes revealing malignancy in places that would otherwise be overlooked by anatomic imaging alone.

In spite of all the technical advances in imaging, clinical and pathologic correlation are often necessary for accurate diagnosis. Image guidance with fluoroscopy, CT, ultrasound, and MRI is commonly used for minimally invasive tissue sampling in the hopes of avoiding or better preparing for a more extensive surgical approach.

This chapter presents the radiologic imaging of a sample of lung pathologies presented in the following order: malignant primary lung carcinoma, benign primary lung neoplasms, metastatic disease, infections, and other miscellaneous lung lesions, some of which can mimic neoplasm on imaging. The goal of this chapter is to provide some insight into the strengths of imaging in diagnosis of lung pathology and to highlight the crucial role that patient history and pathologic correlation often play in overcoming the limitations of imaging alone in order to arrive at a final diagnosis.

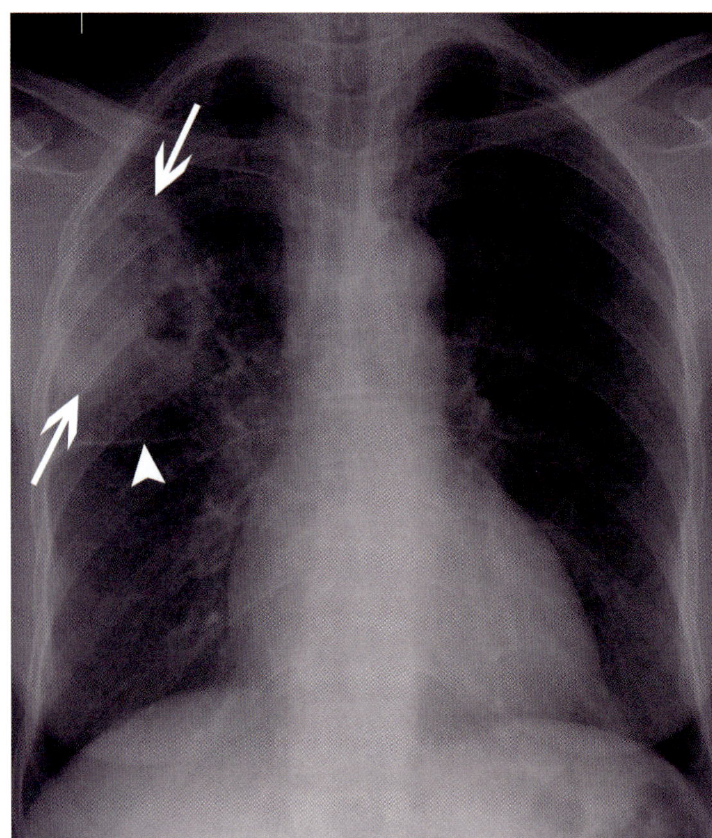

Figure 1.1a — Squamous Cell Carcinoma. Chest radiograph shows a cavitary lesion in the right upper lobe (*between arrows*). Right minor fissure thickening is also noted (*arrowhead*).

Chapter 1 was prepared by Rohan Piyasena, MD: Northside Radiology Associates, Atlanta, Georgia.

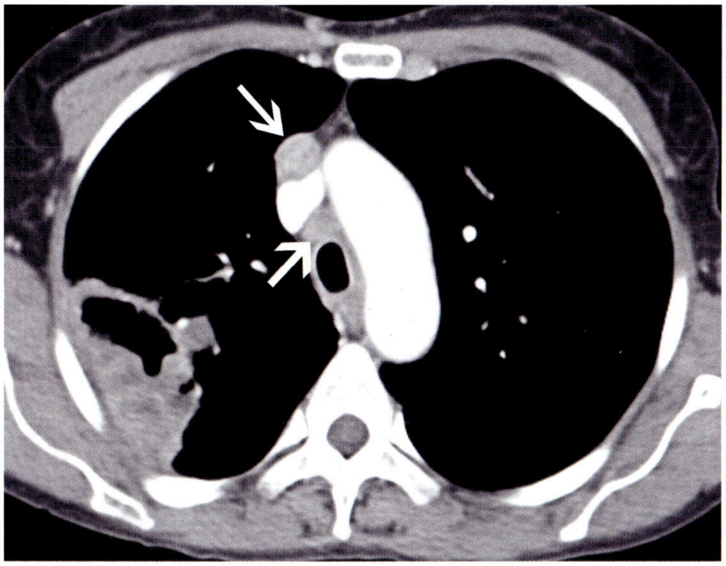

Figure 1.1b — Squamous Cell Carcinoma. Axial CT with contrast in soft tissue windows shows an irregular, enhancing nodular component within the cavitary mass. Mediastinal lymphadenopathy is also noted (*arrows*).

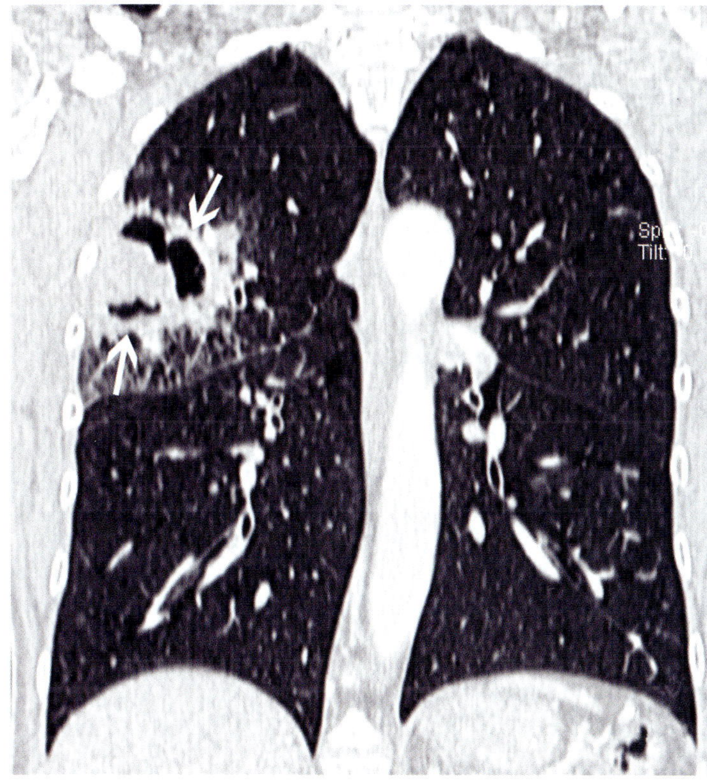

Figure 1.1c — Squamous Cell Carcinoma. Coronal CT in lung windows demonstrates the thick wall of the cavitary lesion (*arrows*). Differential considerations include *Aspergillus* colonization of a preexisting cavity (mycetoma), tuberculosis, or Wegener's granulomatosis, although the irregular enhancing nodular component highly suggests lung carcinoma. Cavitation is more common with squamous cell lung cancer than other types.

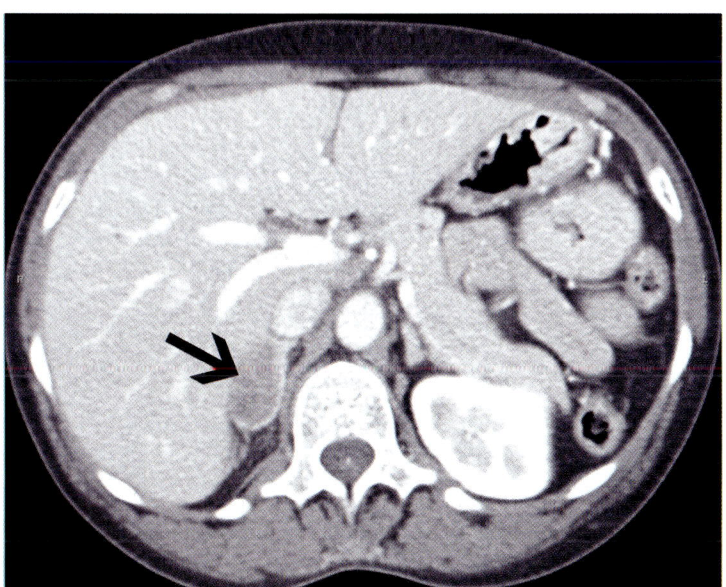

Figure 1.1d — Squamous Cell Carcinoma. Axial postcontrast image through the upper abdomen shows an enhancing right adrenal nodule (*arrow*) compatible with metastatic disease.

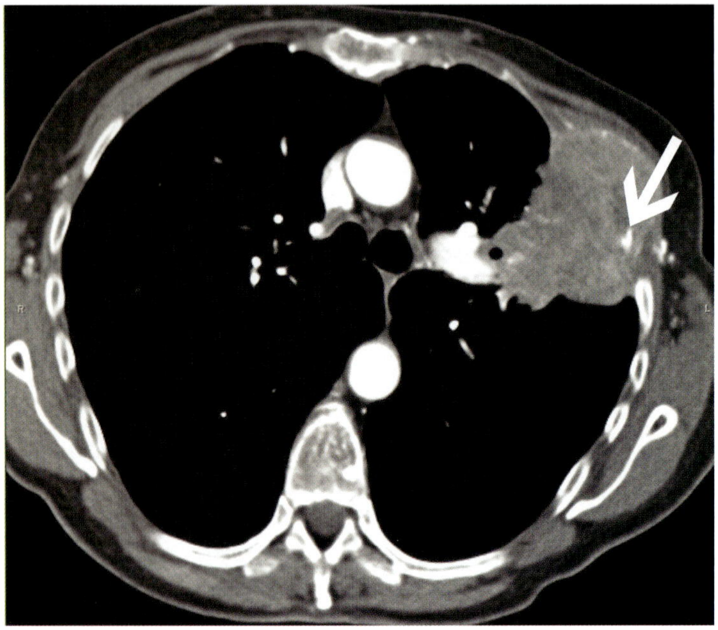

Figure 1.2a — Squamous Cell Carcinoma. Axial CT image showing a large, enhancing mass in the left upper lobe invading the chest wall with associated rib destruction (*arrow*).

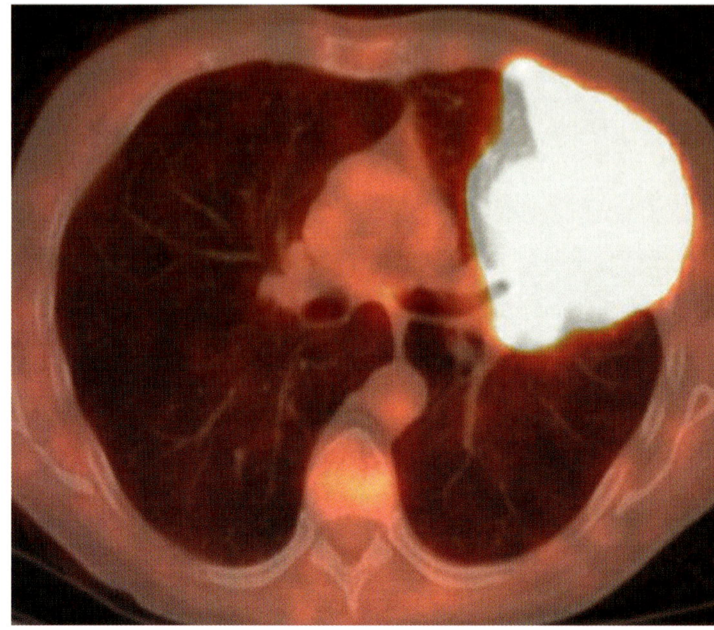

Figure 1.2b — Squamous Cell Carcinoma. PET-CT fusion image shows marked hypermetabolism in the mass consistent with the history of carcinoma. Chest wall invasion would make this lesion at least T3 using the tumor node metastasis staging system.

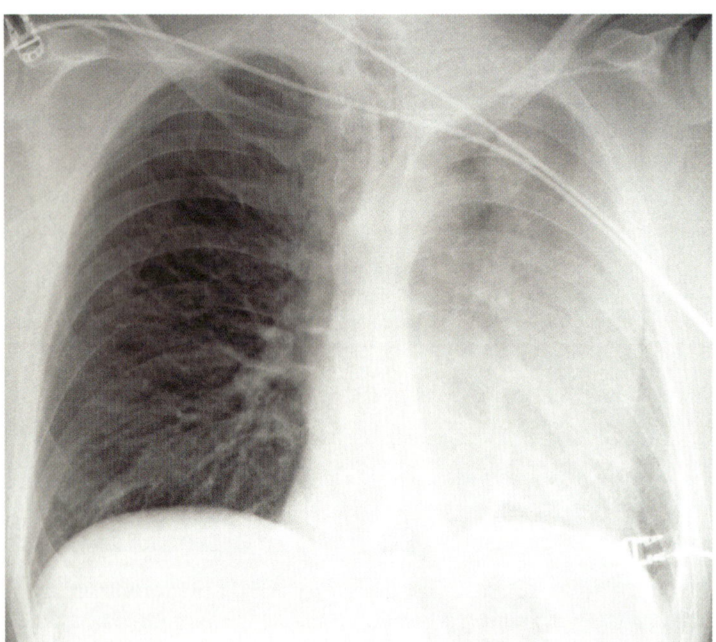

Figure 1.3a — Squamous Cell Carcinoma With Postobstructive Pneumonia. Frontal chest radiograph with asymmetric increased opacification of the left lung and nonvisualization of the left heart border, suggesting a left upper lobe process.

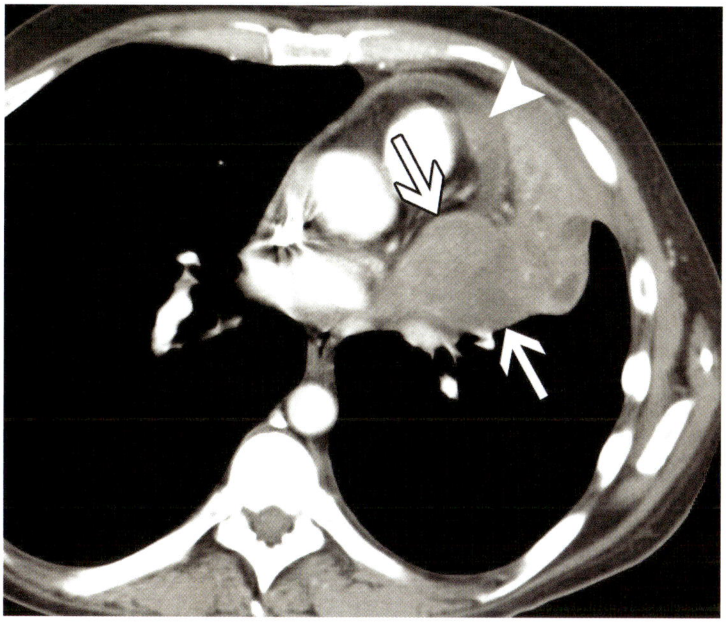

Figure 1.3b — Squamous Cell Carcinoma With Postobstructive Pneumonia. Axial CT with contrast confirms complete loss of aeration of the left upper lobe secondary to an obstructing mass (*between arrows*). The mass invades the visceral pleura and pericardium. There is a small, malignant pericardial effusion present (*arrowhead*).

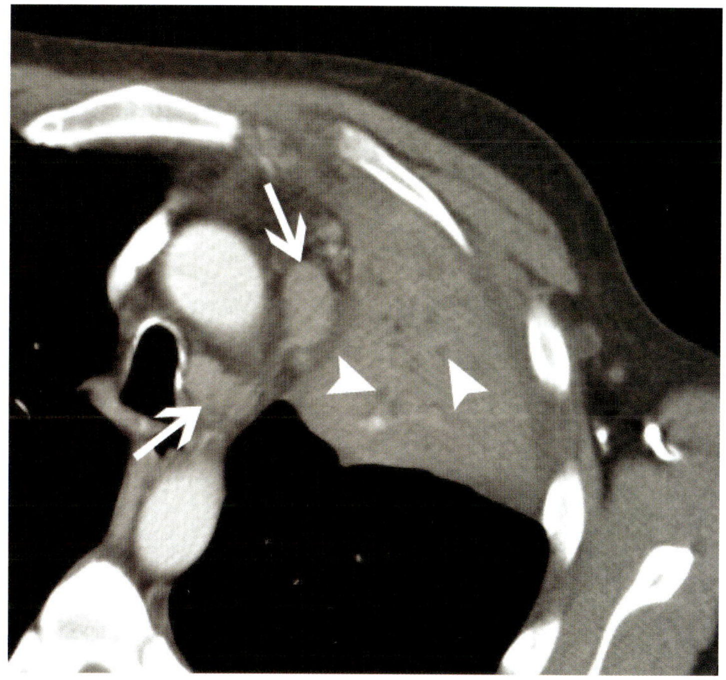

Figure 1.3c — Squamous Cell Carcinoma With Postobstructive Pneumonia. CT image obtained more superior shows obstructive atelectasis of the left upper lobe and dilated bronchi filled with low density mucus and inflammatory cells (*arrowheads*). Mediastinal adenopathy is also noted (*arrows*).

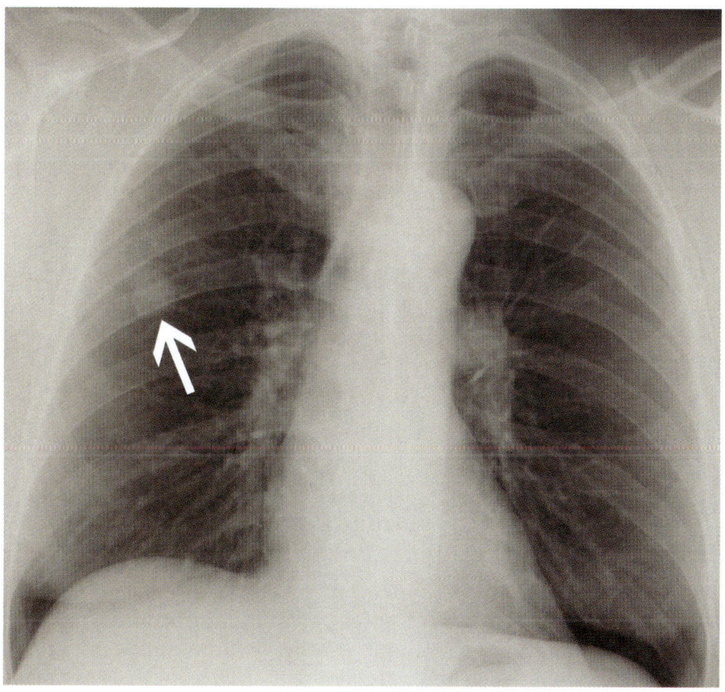

Figure 1.4a — Adenocarcinoma. Chest radiograph showing a right lung pulmonary nodule with ill-defined margins (*arrow*).

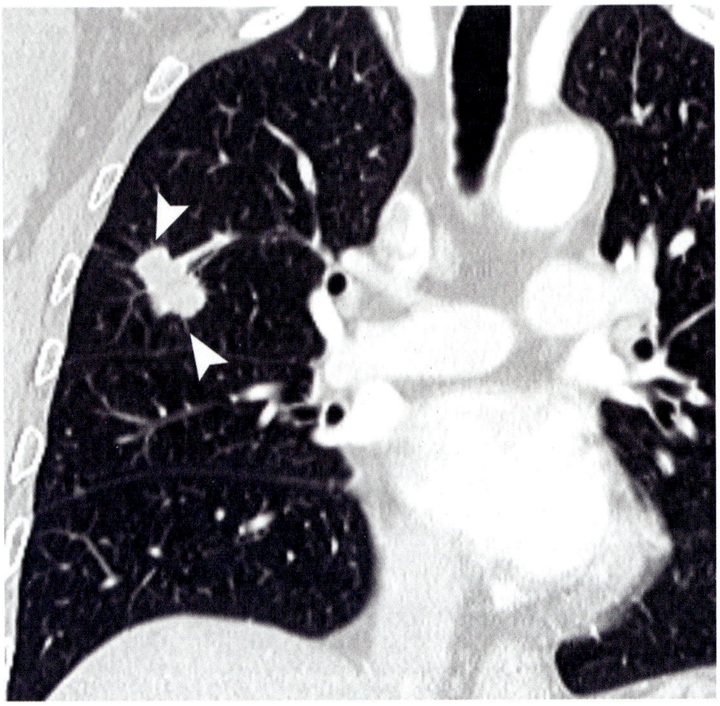

Figure 1.4b — Adenocarcinoma. Coronal CT in lung windows shows the nodule in the right upper lobe with spiculated margins (*arrowheads*), often seen with adenocarcinoma. Adenocarcinoma is the most common primary lung cancer to present as a solitary pulmonary nodule, as in this case.

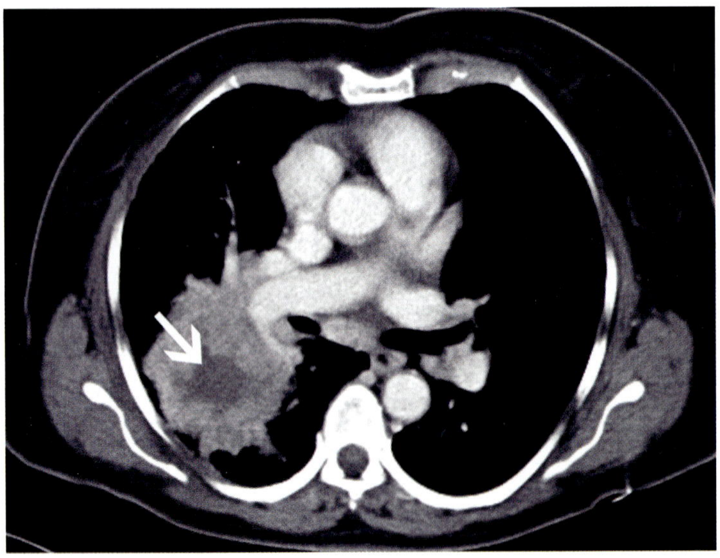

Figure 1.5a — Adenocarcinoma. Large, heterogeneous right lower lobe mass seen on contrast enhanced chest CT. The mass shows enhancement, with central low density (*arrow*) compatible with central necrosis.

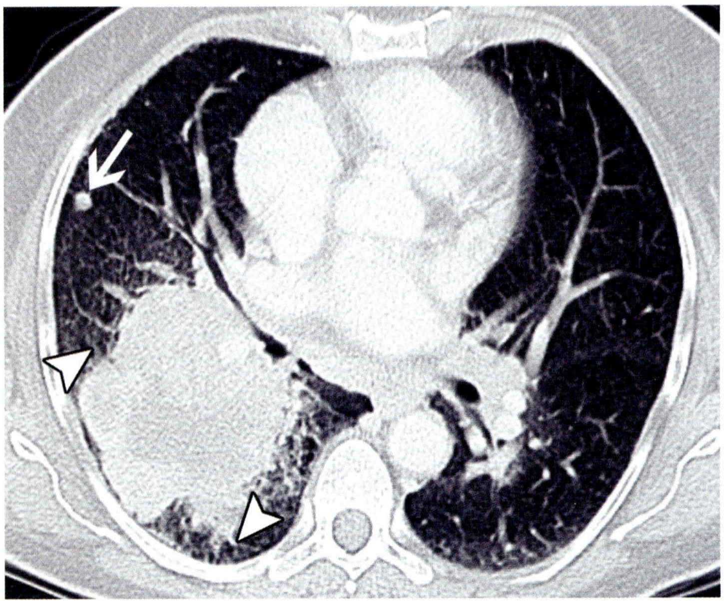

Figure 1.5b — Adenocarcinoma. Lung window shows thickening of the adjacent lung interstitium (*arrowheads*) representing lymphangitic spread of the tumor. A small satellite tumor nodule is also noted (*arrow*).

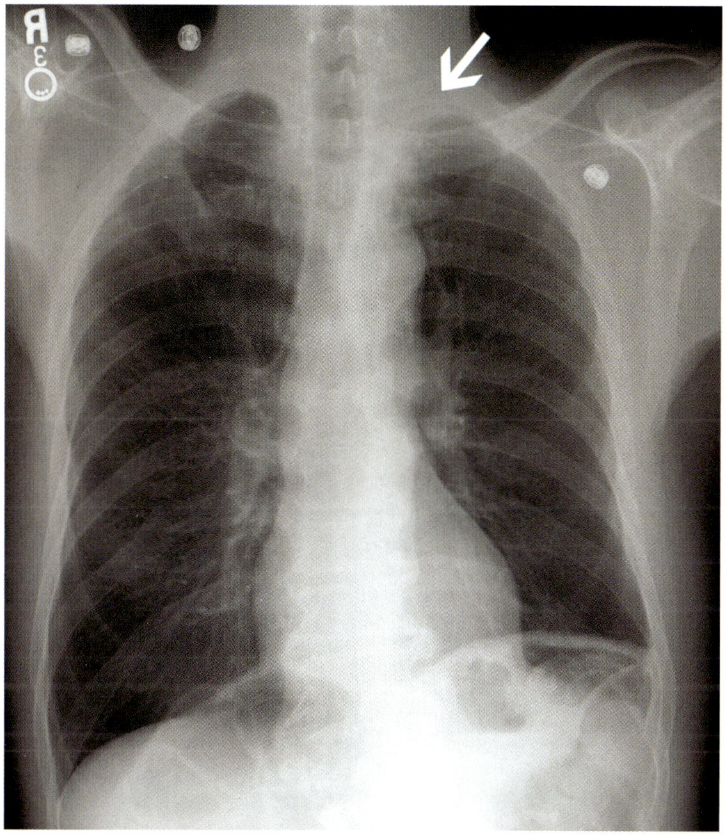

Figure 1.6a — Adenocarcinoma, Pancoast Tumor. Fifty-nine-year-old male smoker presenting with left shoulder pain. Frontal radiograph shows asymmetric left apical fullness (*arrow*) and mild left hemidiaphragm elevation.

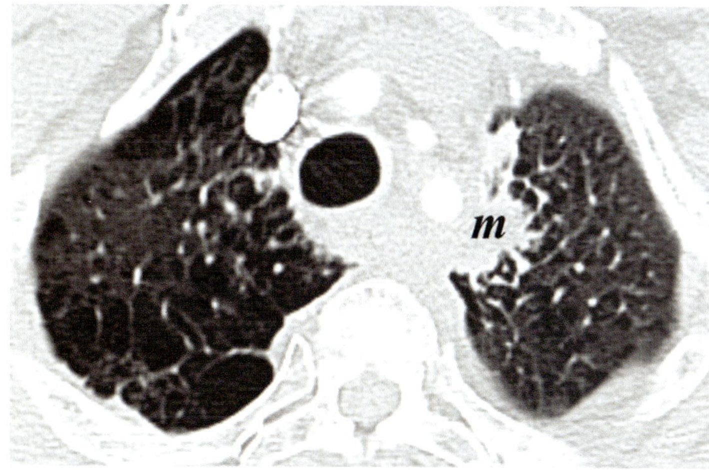

Figure 1.6b — Adenocarcinoma, Pancoast Tumor. Fifty-nine-year-old male smoker presenting with left shoulder pain. CT shows a medial left apex mass (*m*) with large amount of pleural contact suggesting invasion. Note the severe emphysema in the lung apices.

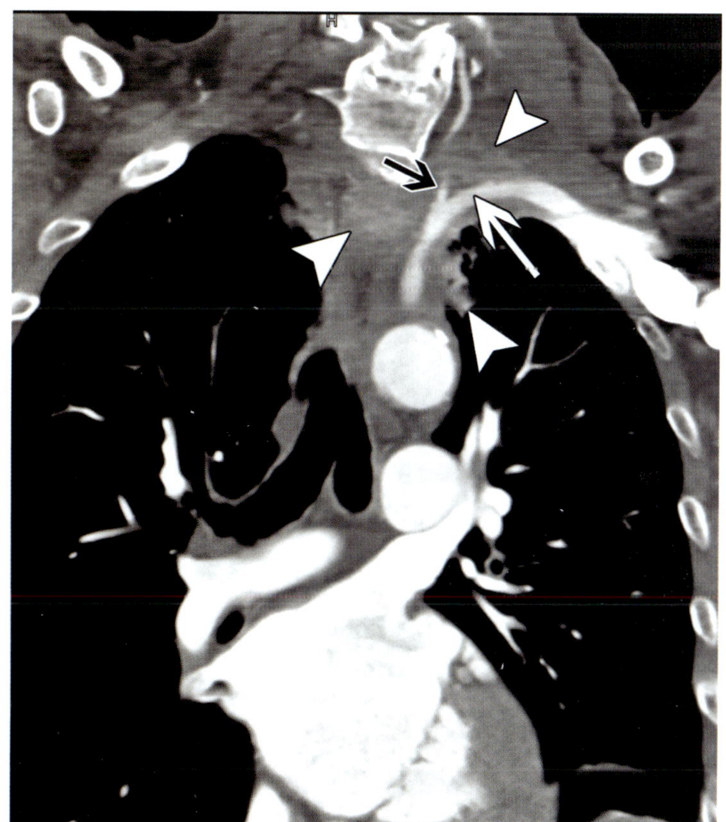

Figure 1.6c — Adenocarcinoma, Pancoast Tumor. Fifty-nine-year-old male smoker presenting with left shoulder pain. Coronal postcontrast CT image shows the mass (*between the arrowheads*) encasing the left subclavian artery (*arrow*) and left vertebral artery origin (*black arrow*).

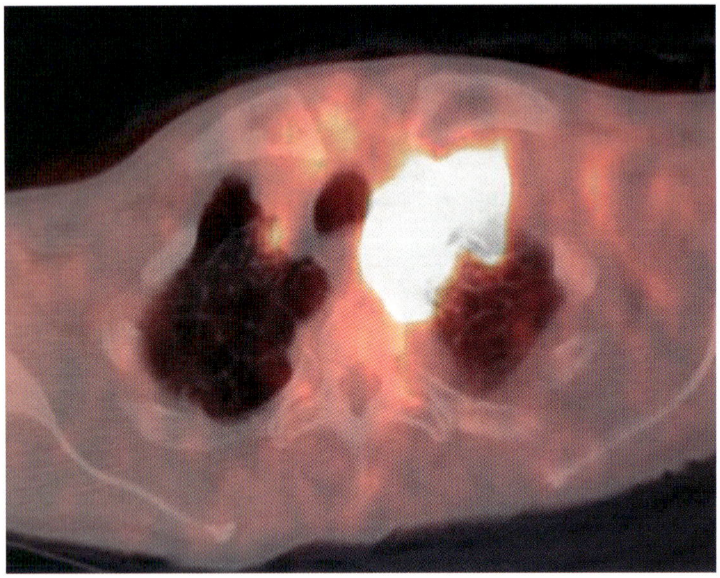

Figure 1.6d — Adenocarcinoma, Pancoast Tumor. Fifty-nine-year-old male smoker presenting with left shoulder pain. PET-CT clearly shows the hypermetabolic tumor at the left apex. In cases of superior sulcus tumor, MRI is superior to CT for evaluation of the extent of involvement of adjacent structures including the great vessels, brachial plexus, ribs, and vertebral column.

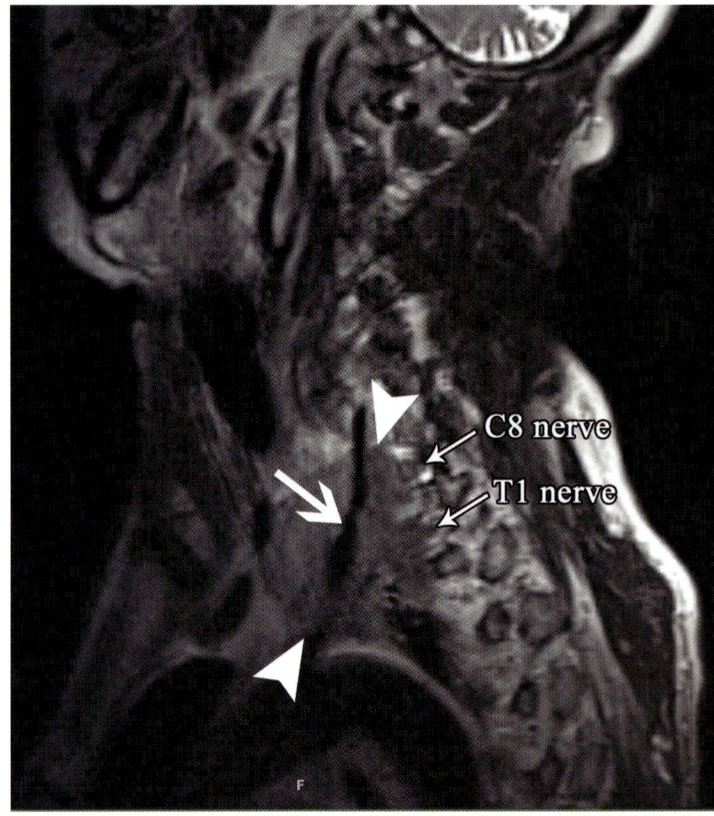

Figure 1.6e — Adenocarcinoma, Pancoast Tumor. Fifty-nine-year-old male smoker presenting with left shoulder pain. Sagittal T2 weighted MRI through the left lung apex shows encasement of the left subclavian artery and left vertebral artery origin (*arrow*) by tumor. The tumor (*between arrowheads*) also extends posteriorly to involve the brachial plexus, specifically nerve roots C8 and T1 (*labelled*).

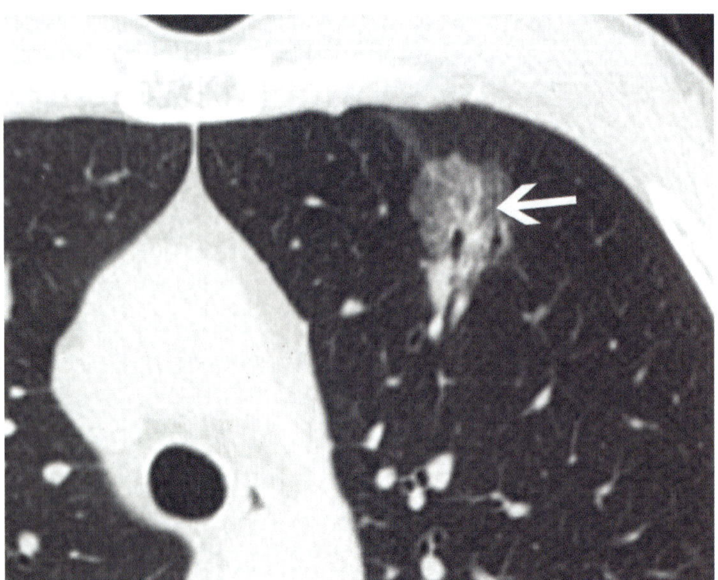

Figure 1.7 — Adenocarcinoma in Situ, Nonmucinous Subtype. CT image in lung windows shows the classic appearance of nonmucinous adenocarcinoma in situ with a left upper lobe ground glass nodule containing air bronchograms (*arrow*). PET is often of limited value as bronchoalveolar carcinomas often show only mild fluorodeoxyglucose uptake. Other differential considerations for a ground glass nodule include hypersensitivity pneumonitis, pneumonias (particularly *Pneumocystis*, viral), pulmonary edema, pulmonary hemorrhage, and bronchiolitis obliterans organizing pneumonia.

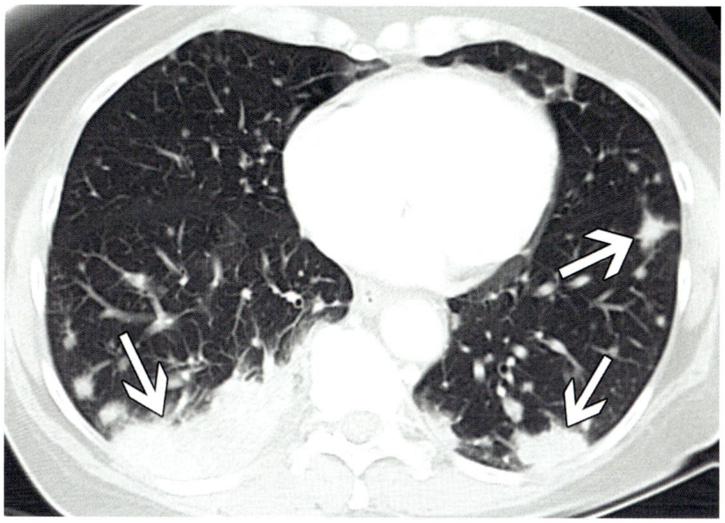

Figure 1.8a — Bronchoalveolar Carcinomas, Mucinous Subtype. Axial CT through the lung bases shows bilateral multifocal consolidation (*arrows*).

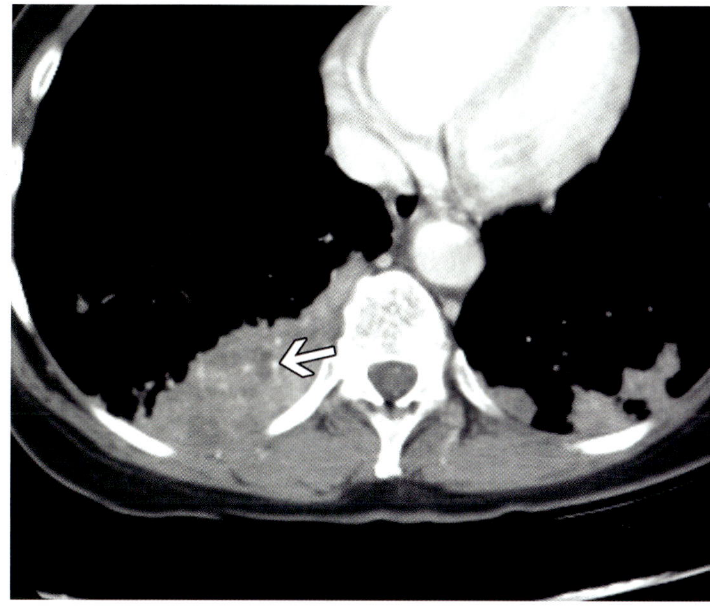

Figure 1.8b — Bronchoalveolar Carcinomas, Mucinous Subtype. Postcontrast images show vessels coursing through the area of consolidation in the right lower lobe (CT angiogram sign, *arrow*), confirming that this is an area of alveolar filling, rather than a large mass. The differential for such consolidation is large and includes pulmonary edema, pneumonia, and hemorrhage, among several others. This case proved to be bronchoalveolar carcinomas. The mucin produced by the tumor can cause consolidation and can demonstrate endobronchial spread.

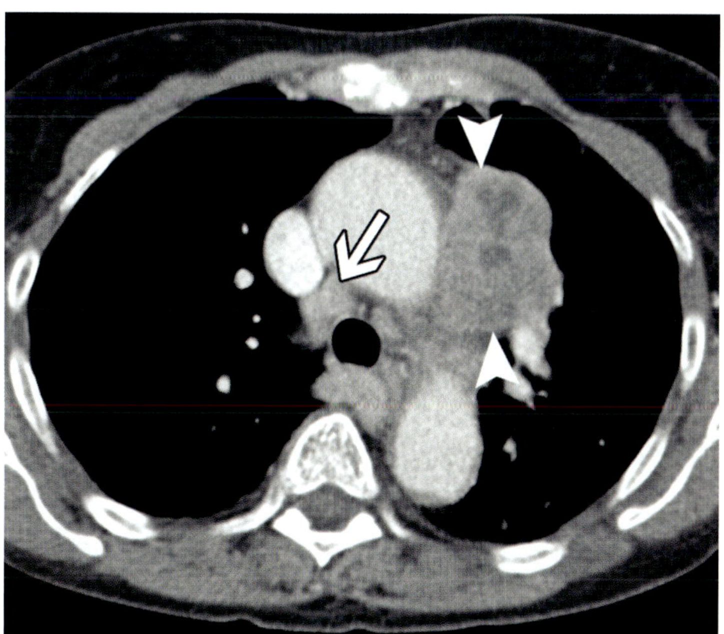

Figure 1.9a — Small Cell Carcinoma. Left superior parahilar mass (*between arrowheads*) with enhancement and probable areas of necrosis. Mediastinal adenopathy (*arrow*) is present.

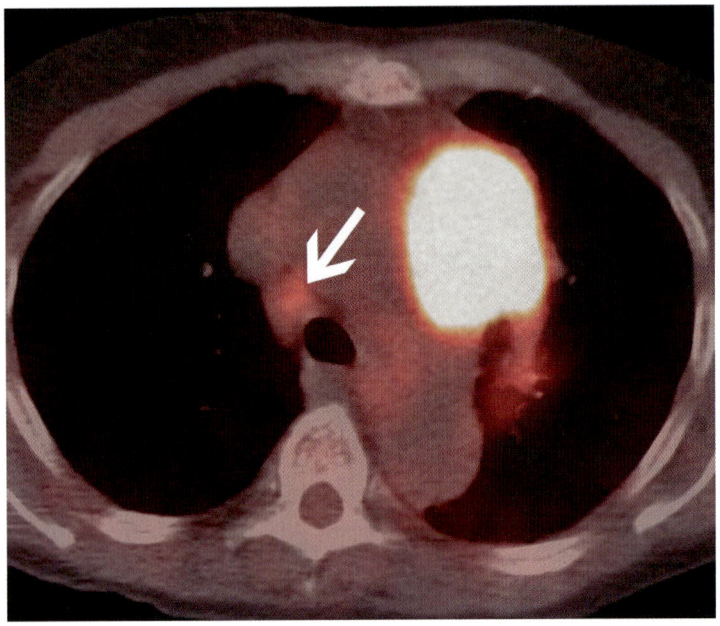

Figure 1.9b — Small Cell Carcinoma. The mass shows marked fluorodeoxyglucose (FGD) uptake. Some increased uptake is also seen in the mediastinal lymph node (*arrow*).

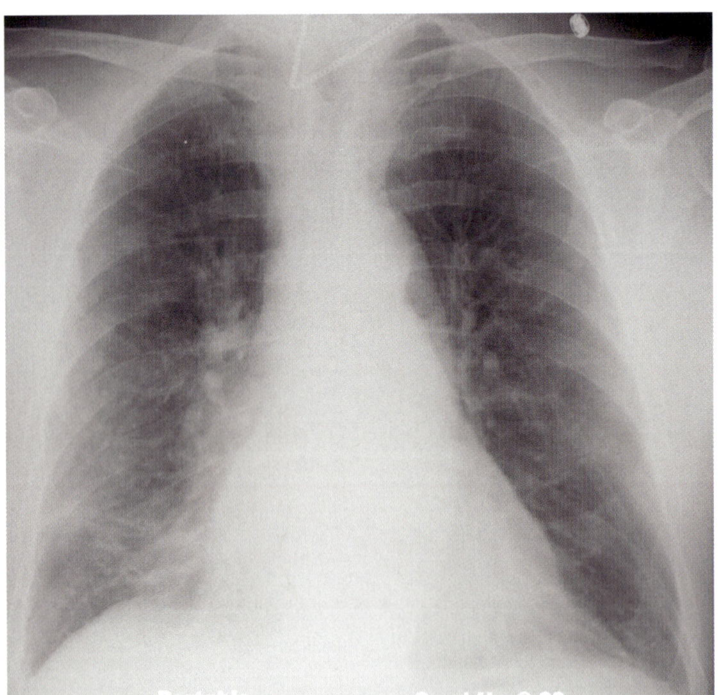

Figure 1.10a — Small Cell Carcinoma. Chest radiograph shows a right infrahilar mass (*arrows*) and blunting of the right costophrenic angle, suggesting a pleural effusion.

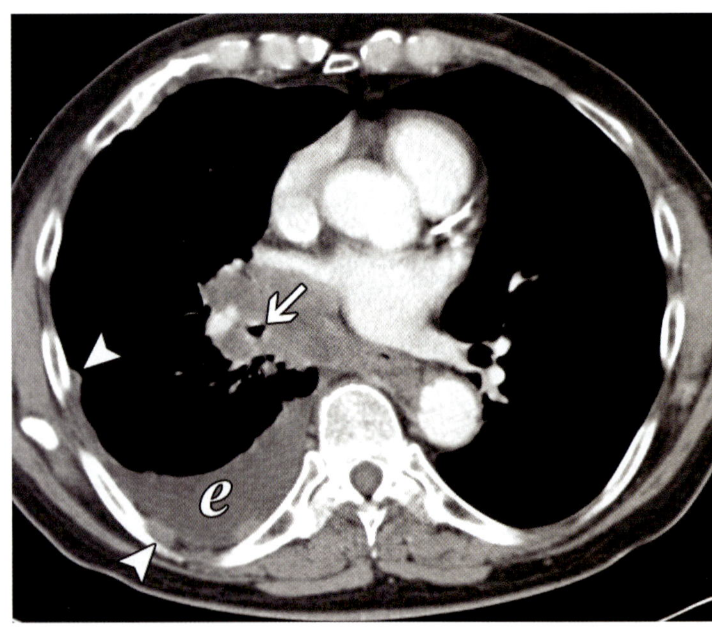

Figure 1.10b — Small Cell Carcinoma. Contrast-enhanced CT shows the right hilar mass narrowing the bronchus intermedius (*arrow*). Enhancing pleural metastases (*arrowheads*) and a malignant pleural effusion (*e*) are present. Pleural tumor nodules, as well as malignant pleural or pericardial effusion, are all considered M1 in the 2009 tumor node metastasis staging system.

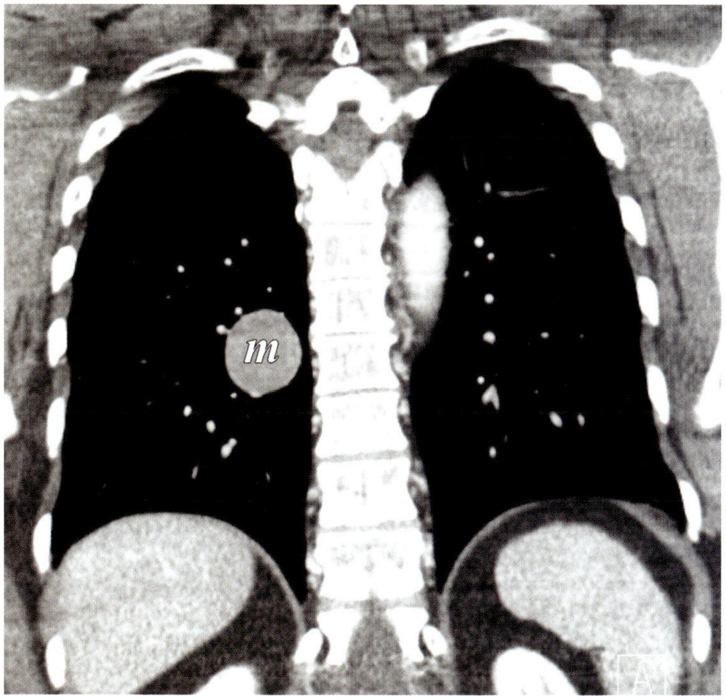

Figure 1.11a — Carcinoid Tumor. Coronal image from CT with contrast shows a well-defined, enhancing mass (*m*) in the central right lower lobe.

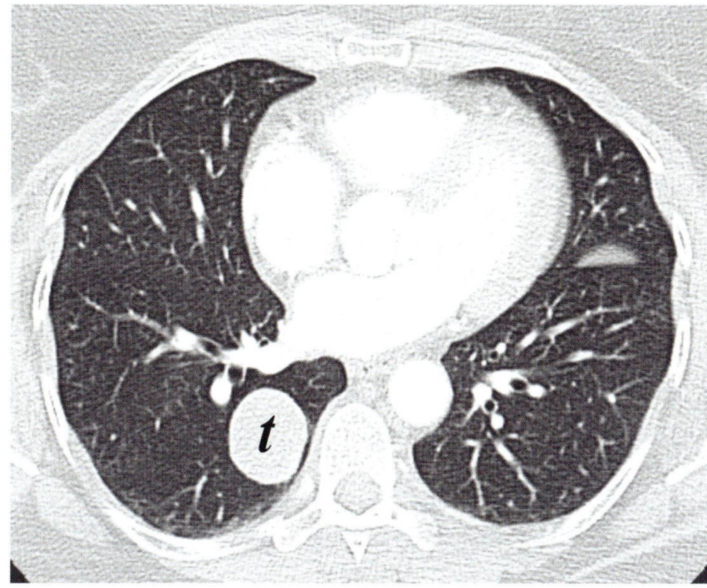

Figure 1.11b — Carcinoid Tumor. Axial image in the lung windows show the well-defined, smooth margins of the tumor (*t*) consistent with a low-grade malignancy. Carcinoids often involve the central bronchi and are often highly vascular.

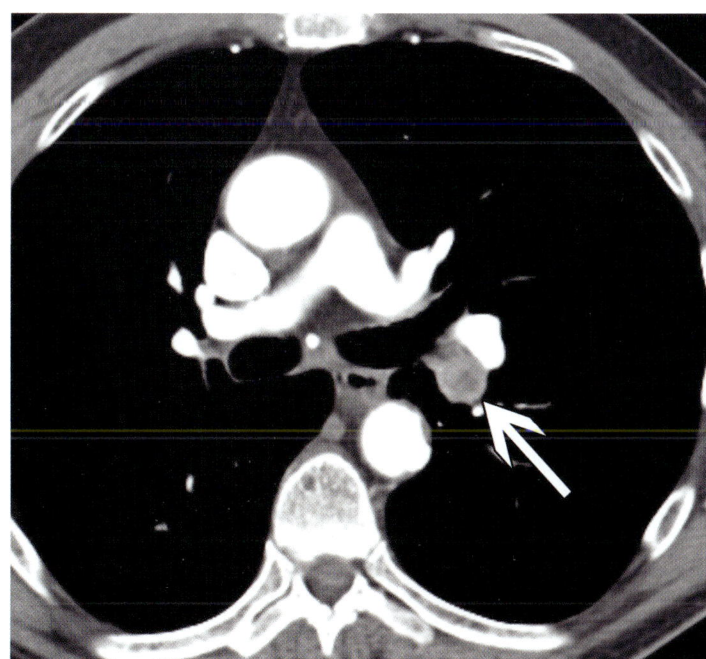

Figure 1.12a — Mucoepidermoid Carcinoma. Contrast CT shows an enhancing mass in the left hilum (*arrow*).

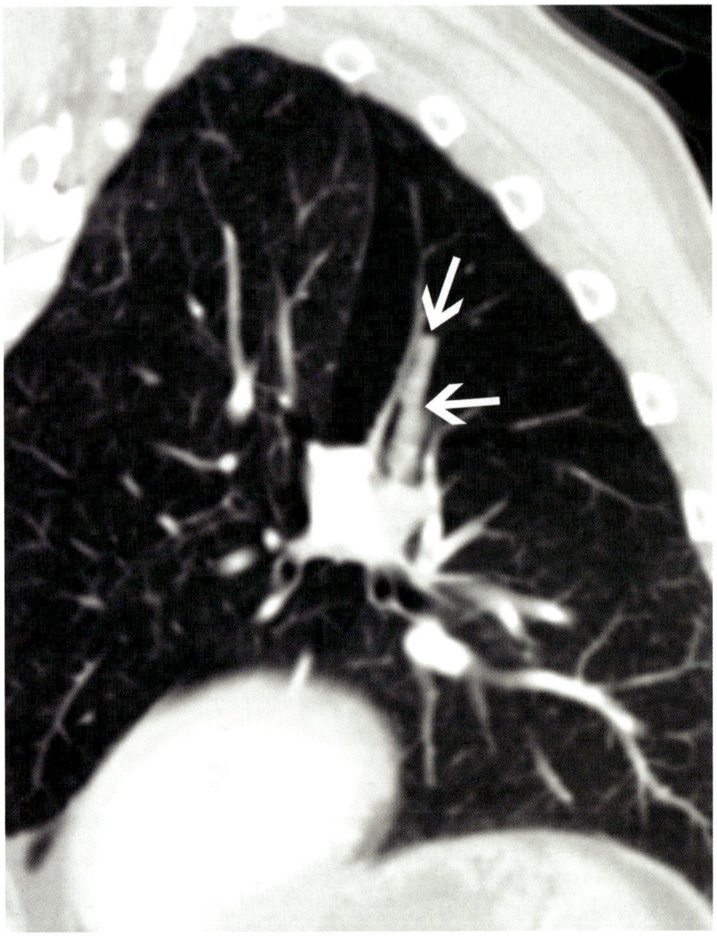

Figure 1.12b — Mucoepidermoid Carcinoma. Sagittal image through the mass shows finger-like endobronchial extension of the tumor into the superior segment of the left lower lobe (*arrows*). There is evidence of decreased lung attenuation in the obstructed segment of the lung from decreased ventilation, causing decreased perfusion. Differential considerations include carcinoid, adenoid cystic carcinoma, lung cancer, or metastatic disease.

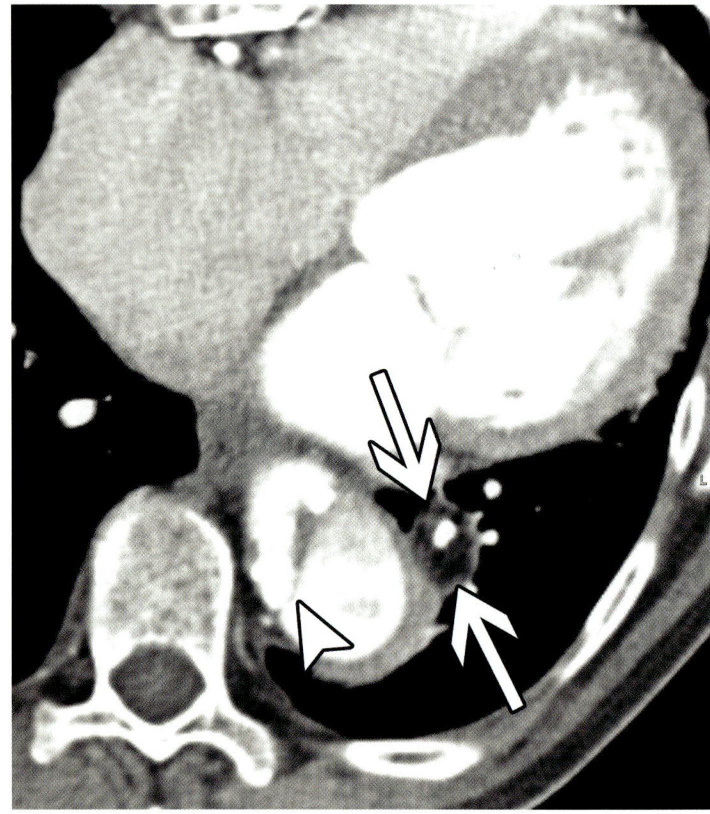

Figure 1.13a — Pulmonary Hamartoma. Axial contrast enhanced CT shows a nodule in the left lower lobe (*between arrows*) predominantly of fat density. Also noted on the image is an aortic dissection (*dissection flap indicated by arrowhead*).

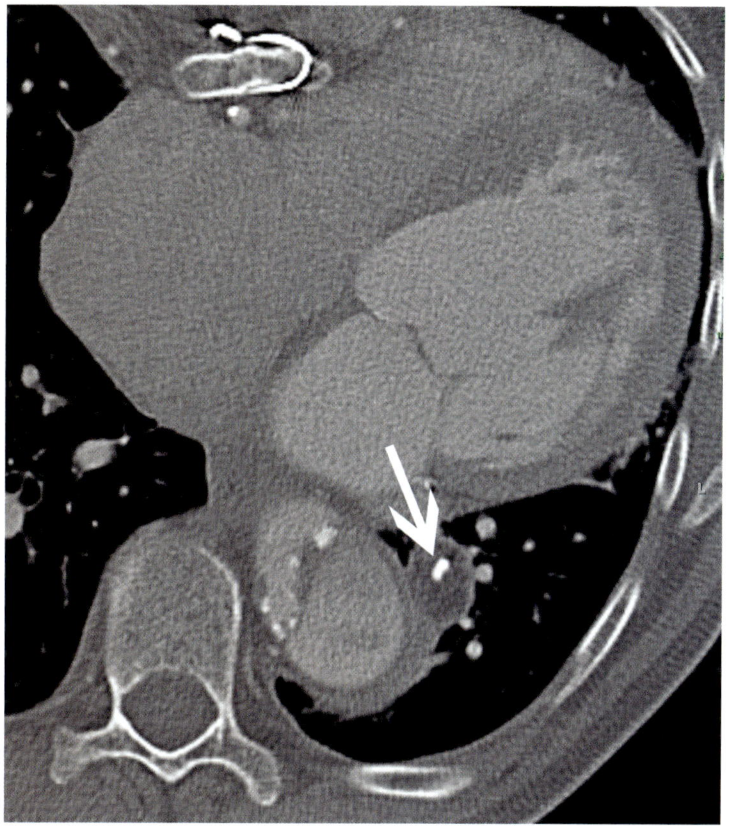

Figure 1.13b — Pulmonary Hamartoma. Bone windows nicely show the course calcification in the mass (*arrow*). The combination of fat and calcification make this pathognomonic for a hamartoma.

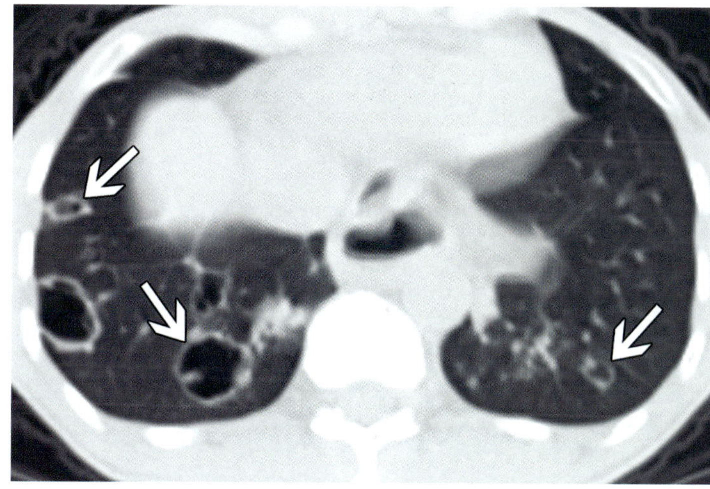

Figure 1.14 — Laryngeal Papillomatosis. CT image shows multiple bilateral cavitary lesions in the lungs (*arrows*) in this patient with a history of laryngeal papillomas. Metastatic disease (particularly squamous cell metastases), bland and septic pulmonary emboli, Wegener's granulomatosis, and fungal infections can have a similar appearance.

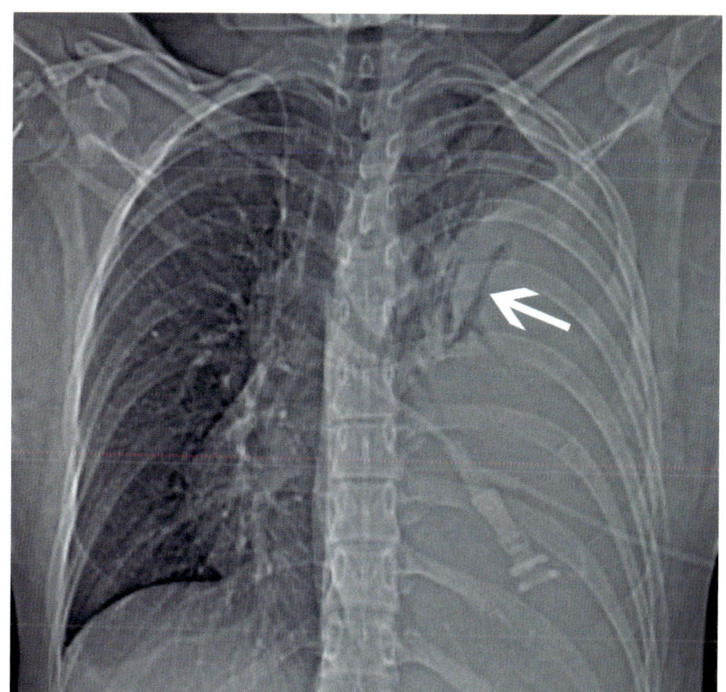

Figure 1.15a — Ewing's Family Tumor of the Chest Wall and Pleural Space. Scout image from a CT shows a large mass occupying the mid and lower left pleural cavity with mass effect on the heart and a few air bronchograms (*arrow*).

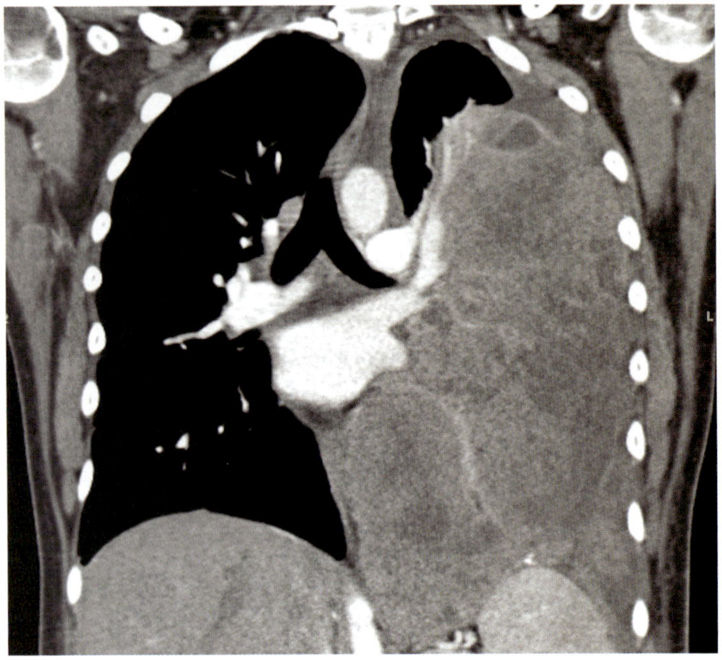

Figure 1.15b — Ewing's Family Tumor of the Chest Wall and Pleural Space. Coronal CT shows the massive tumor with heterogeneous enhancement.

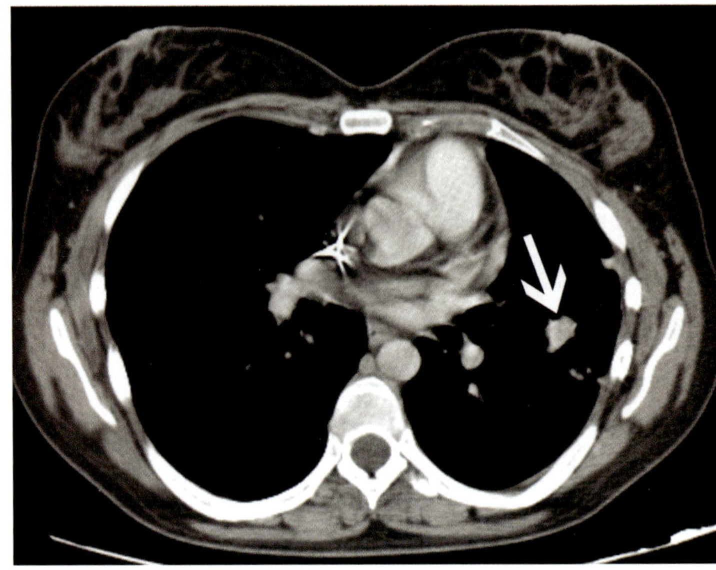

Figure 1.15c — Ewing's Family Tumor of the Chest Wall and Pleural Space. Axial CT obtained 3 months after initiation of chemotherapy shows dramatic response with only minimal residual disease (*arrow*).

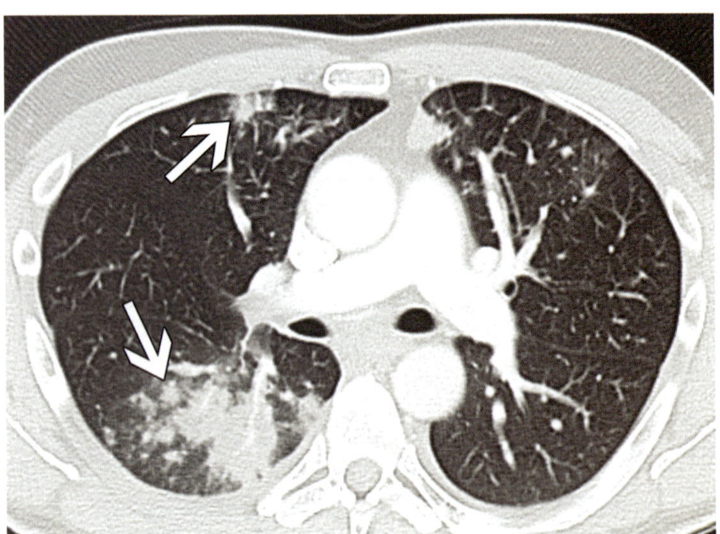

Figure 1.16a — Pulmonary Kaposi Sarcoma. Thirty-nine-year-old male with AIDS and known cutaneous Kaposi sarcoma. CT image of the lungs shows bilateral, poorly defined, spiculated or "flame-shaped" nodules (*arrows*) in a bronchovascular distribution compatible with pulmonary Kaposi sarcoma.

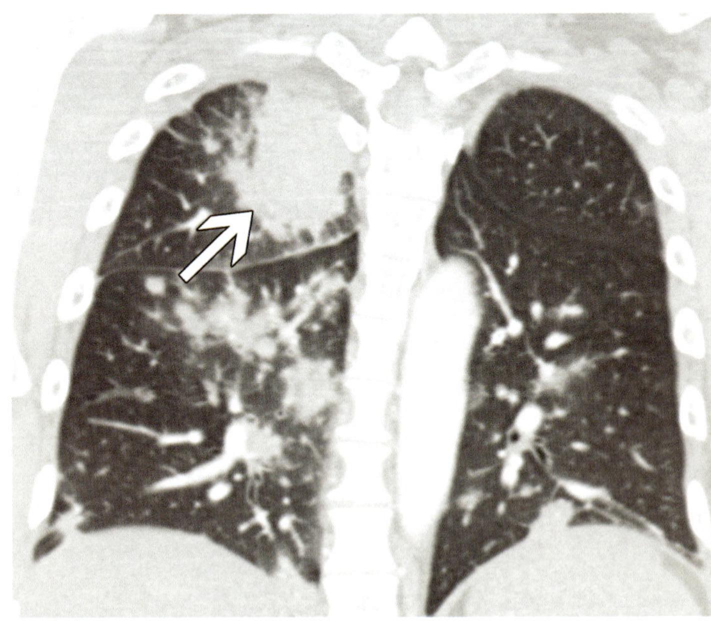

Figure 1.16b — Pulmonary Kaposi Sarcoma. Thirty-nine-year-old male with AIDS and known cutaneous Kaposi sarcoma. Ill-defined mass is identified at the right apex (*arrow*) on the coronal CT image. Reddish purple patches were seen in the airways on bronchoscopy.

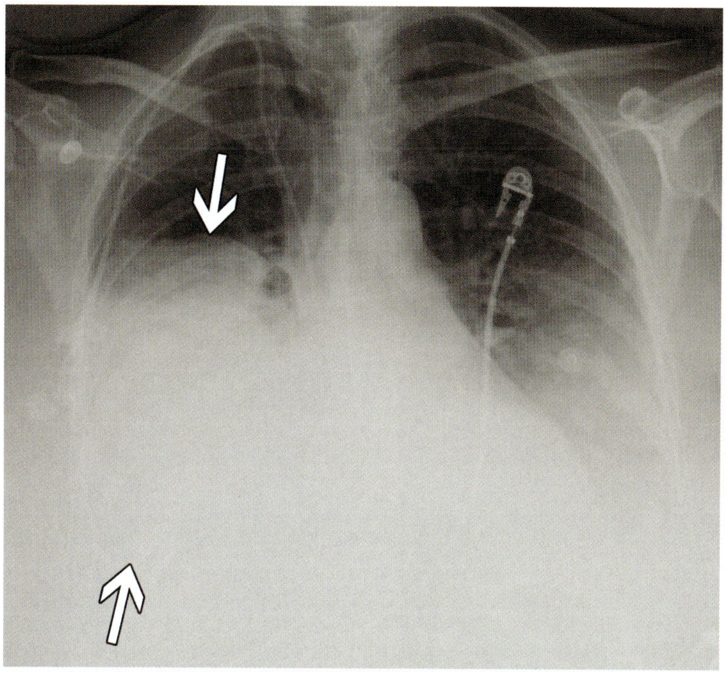

Figure 1.17a — Melanoma Metastasis. Frontal radiograph demonstrates a large mass in the right mid/lower lung (*between arrows*). Left pleural effusion is also noted.

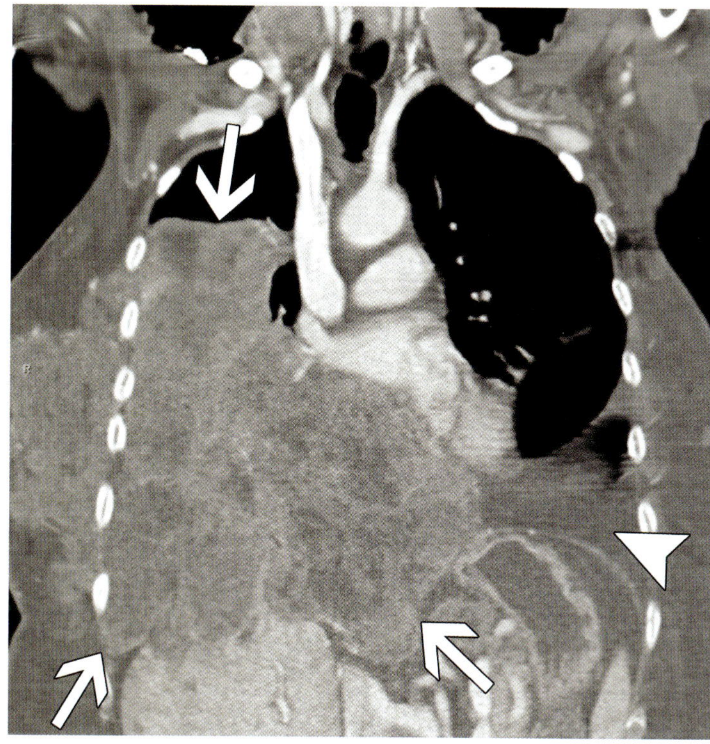

Figure 1.17b — Melanoma Metastasis. Coronal maximum intensity projection image from contrast-enhanced CT shows the extent of the tumor (*between arrows*). There is extension into the chest wall and significant mass effect on the heart. The left pleural effusion is also seen (*arrowhead*).

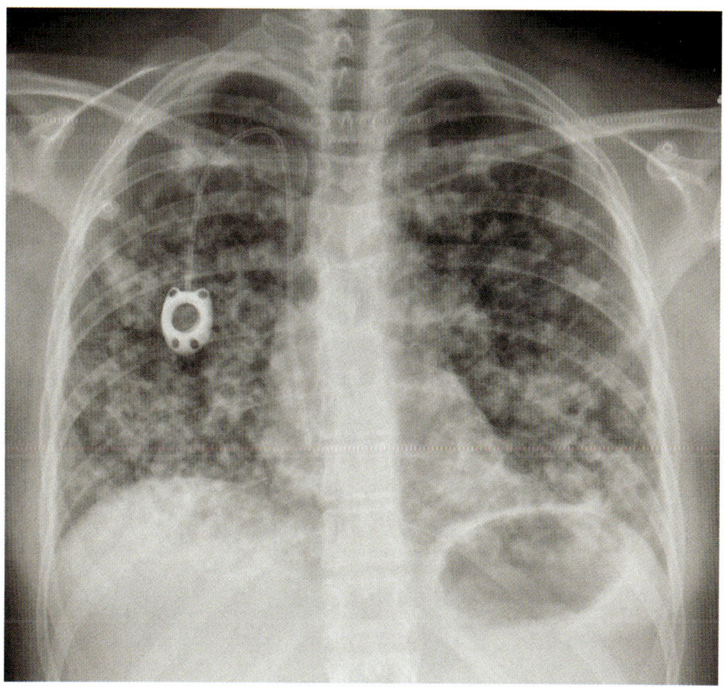

Figure 1.18a — Colon Cancer Metastases, Cavitary. Frontal radiograph showing numerous bilateral cavitary pulmonary nodules.

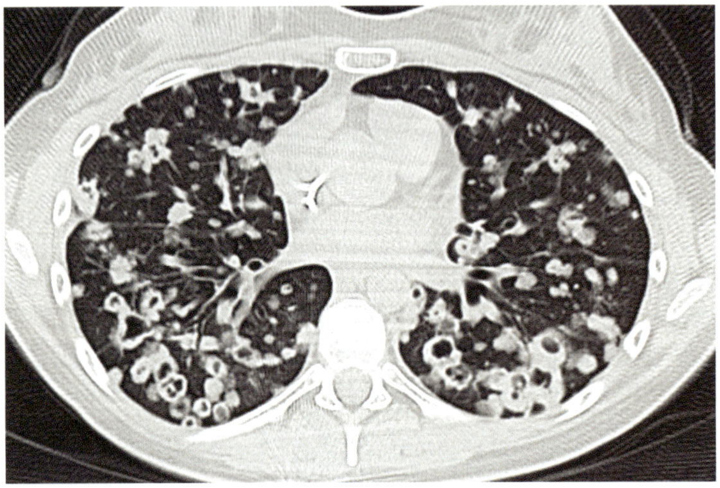

Figure 1.18b — Colon Cancer Metastases, Cavitary. Axial CT confirms the presence of bilateral pulmonary nodules, the majority of which are cavitary. Cavitary metastases can be seen with adenocarcinoma, squamous cell carcinoma, and transitional cell carcinoma.

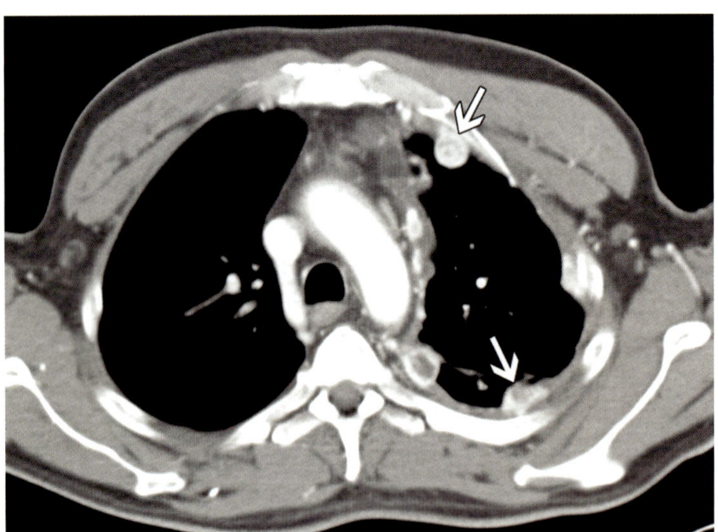

Figure 1.19a — Metastatic Renal Cell Carcinoma, Pleural. CT with contrast shows multiple avidly enhancing nodules in the left pleural space (*arrows*).

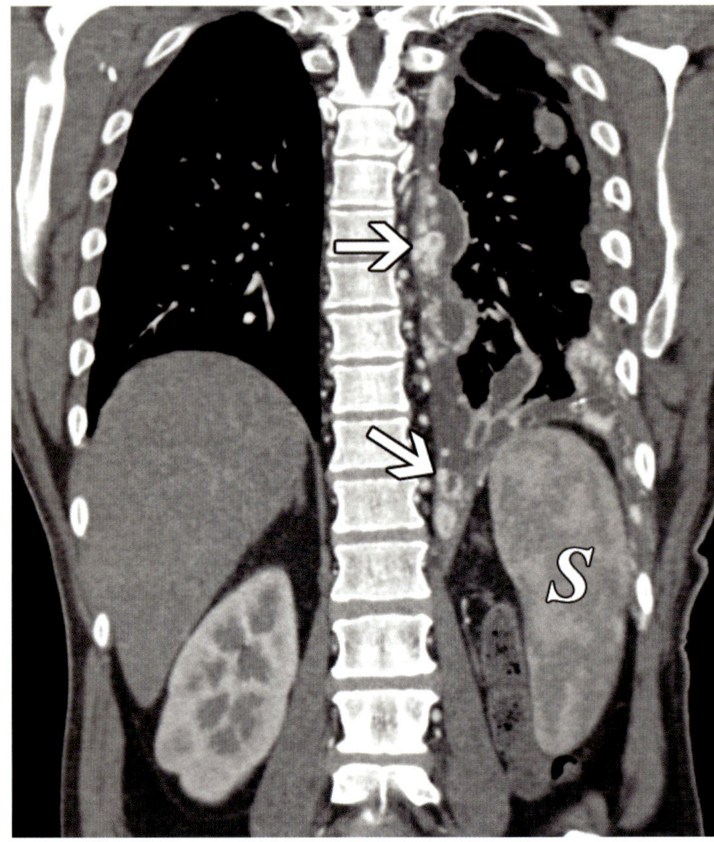

Figure 1.19b — Metastatic Renal Cell Carcinoma, Pleural. Coronal CT image shows additional enhancing nodules in the medial left pleural space (*arrows*). The patient has had a left nephrectomy for renal cell carcinoma. *S = spleen.*

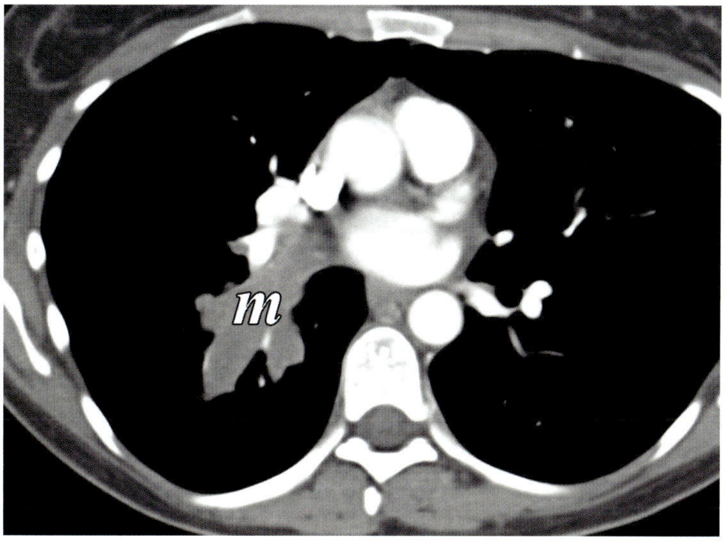

Figure 1.20a — Metastatic Melanoma, Endobronchial. Thirty-six-year-old female lifeguard with history of melanoma of the shoulder. Contrast-enhanced CT shows a branching endobronchial mass (*m*) extending into and expanding the right lower lobe bronchi.

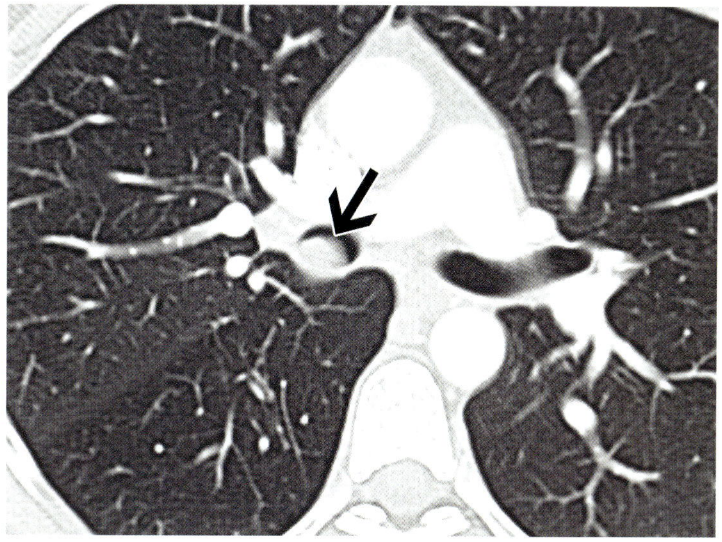

Figure 1.20b — Metastatic Melanoma, Endobronchial. Thirty-six-year-old female lifeguard with history of melanoma of the shoulder. CT image at a more superior level shows the convex leading edge of the endobronchial mass in the bronchus intermedius (*arrow*). Other primary neoplasms that can have endobronchial metastases include thyroid, renal cell, and breast carcinomas.

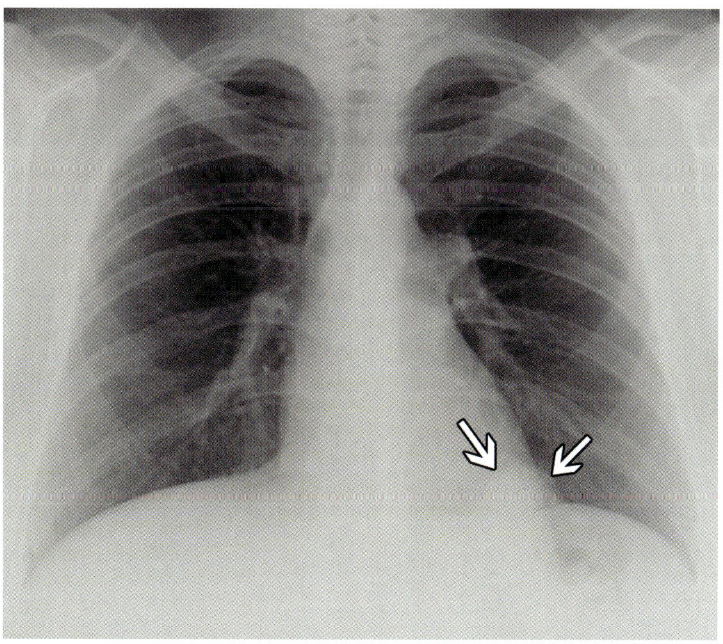

Figure 1.21a — Benign Metastasizing Leiomyoma Metastases. Frontal chest radiograph shows a mass at the base of the left lung (*arrows*).

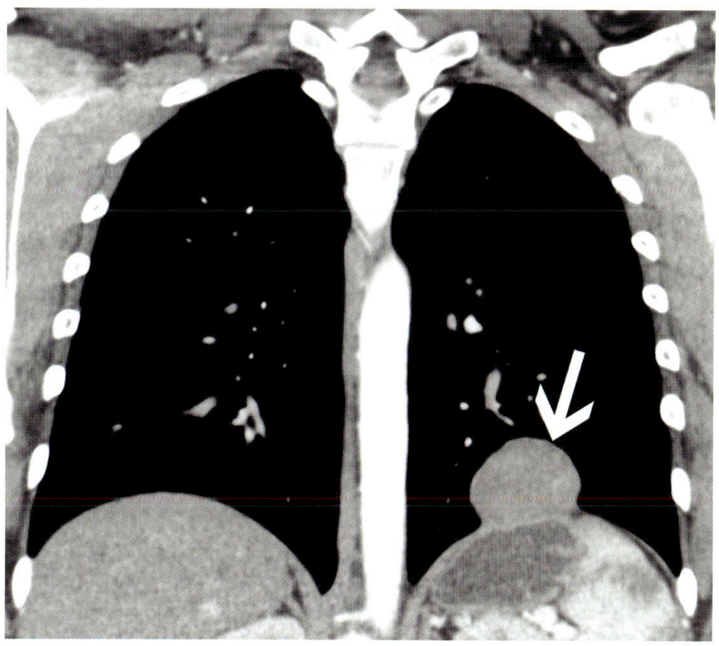

Figure 1.21b — Benign Metastasizing Leiomyoma Metastases. Coronal CT confirms the presence of a left lower lobe enhancing mass (*arrow*).

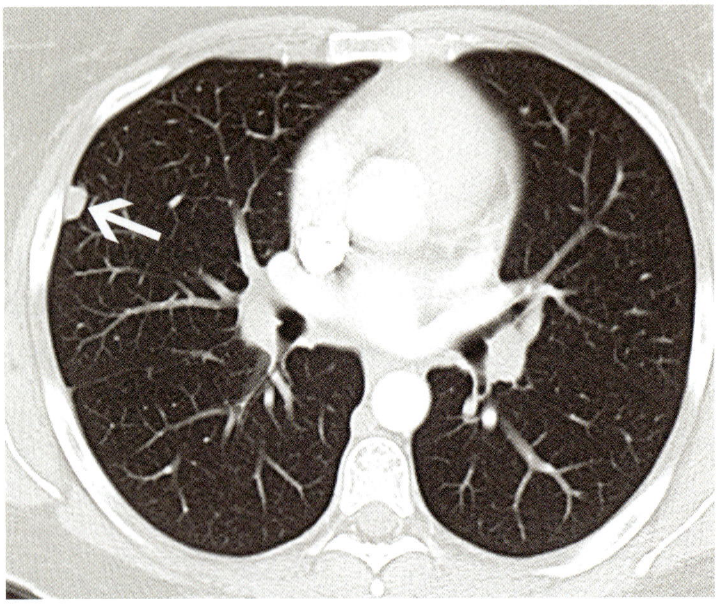

Figure 1.21c — Benign Metastasizing Leiomyoma Metastases. CT in lung windows shows additional lung nodules (*arrow*), which are too small to be seen on the chest radiograph.

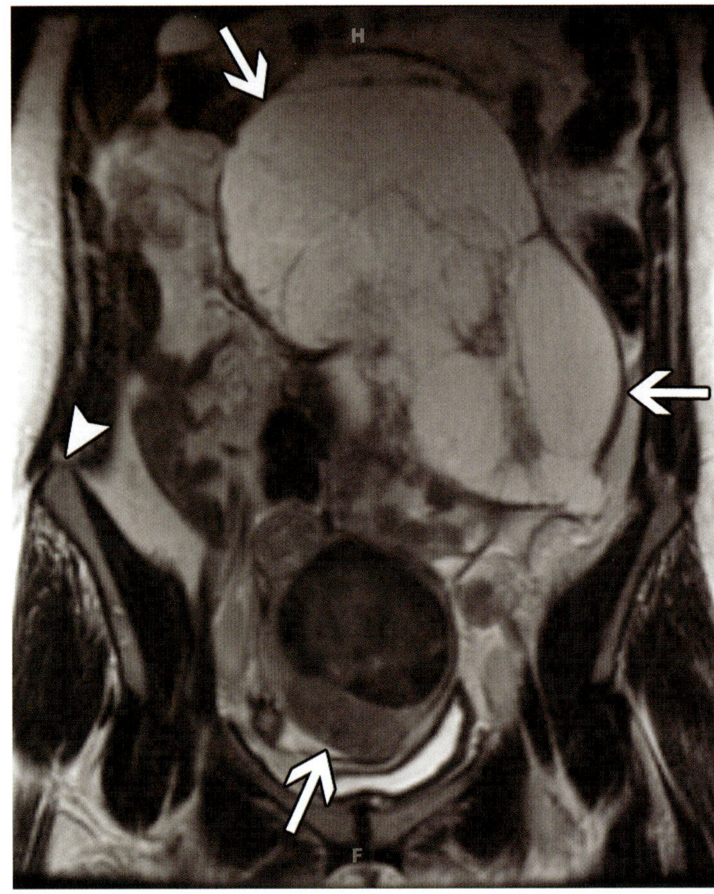

Figure 1.21d — Benign Metastasizing Leiomyoma Metastases. Coronal T2 weighted MRI image through the pelvis shows massive enlargement of the uterus (*between arrows*) containing several heterogeneous masses, some with large cystic components. The right iliac crest (*arrowhead*) is labeled for scale. Pathology from resection of the left lower lobe lung mass confirmed the diagnosis.

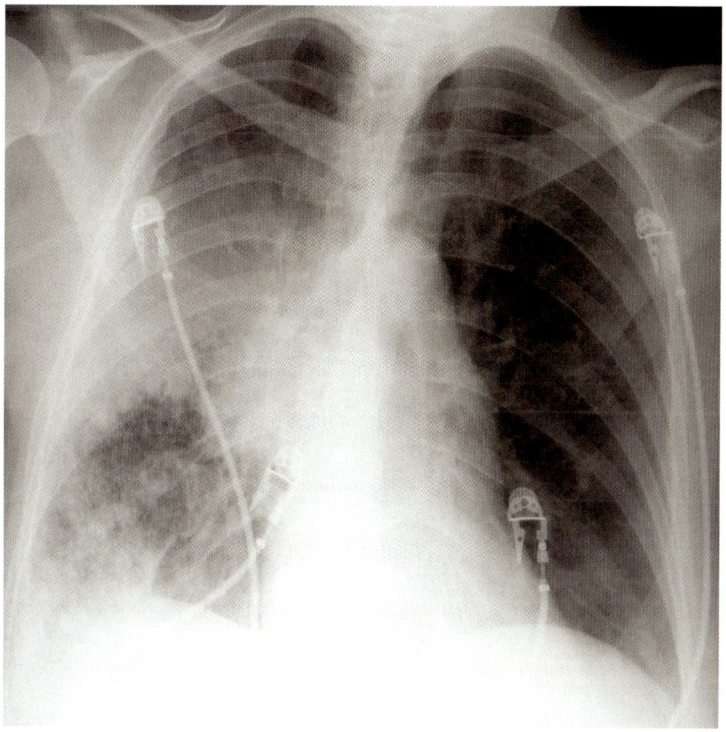

Figure 1.22a — Lobar Pneumonia, Methicillin-Resistant *Staphylococcus aureus*. Frontal radiograph shows consolidation in the mid right lung.

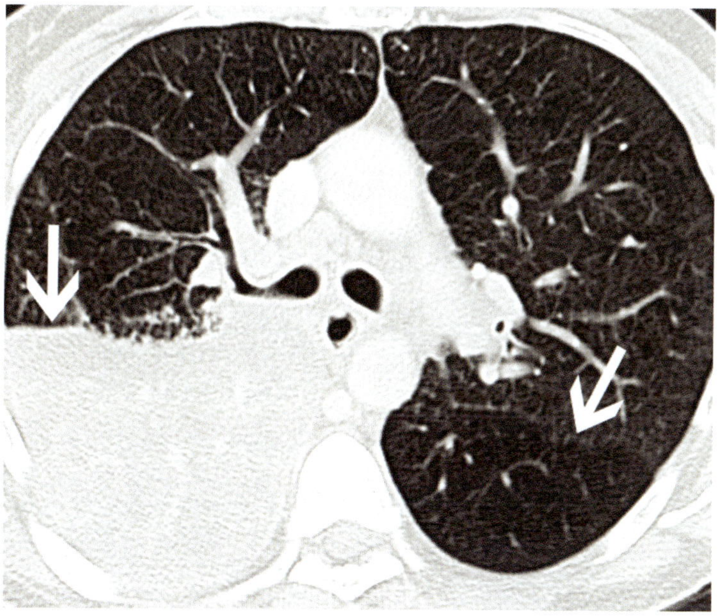

Figure 1.22b — Lobar Pneumonia, Methicillin-Resistant *Staphylococcus aureus*. CT in lung windows shows dense consolidation of the right lower lobe with expansion of the involved lung and resultant relative elevation of the right major fissure compared with the left (*arrows*).

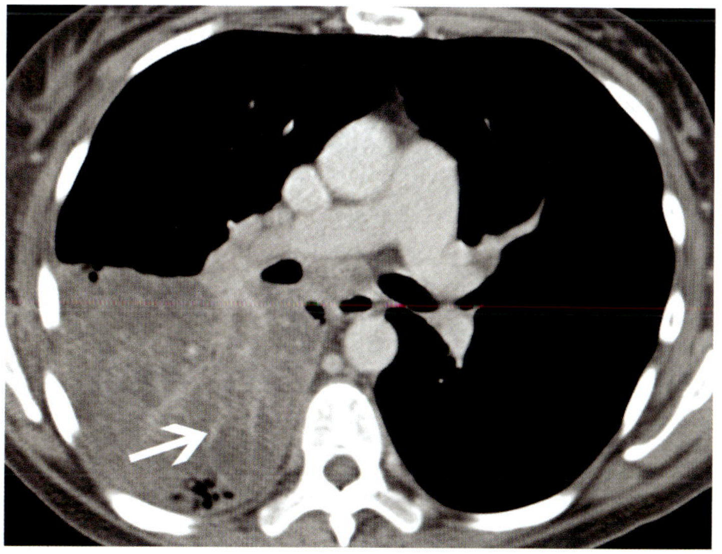

Figure 1.22c — Lobar Pneumonia, Methicillin-Resistant *Staphylococcus aureus*. CT with contrast shows normally opacified pulmonary vessels coursing through the area of consolidation (*arrow*). A mass would result in distortion of or mass effect on the vessels. *Klebsiella* and *Pneumococcus* are other possible causes of consolidation with lobar expansion.

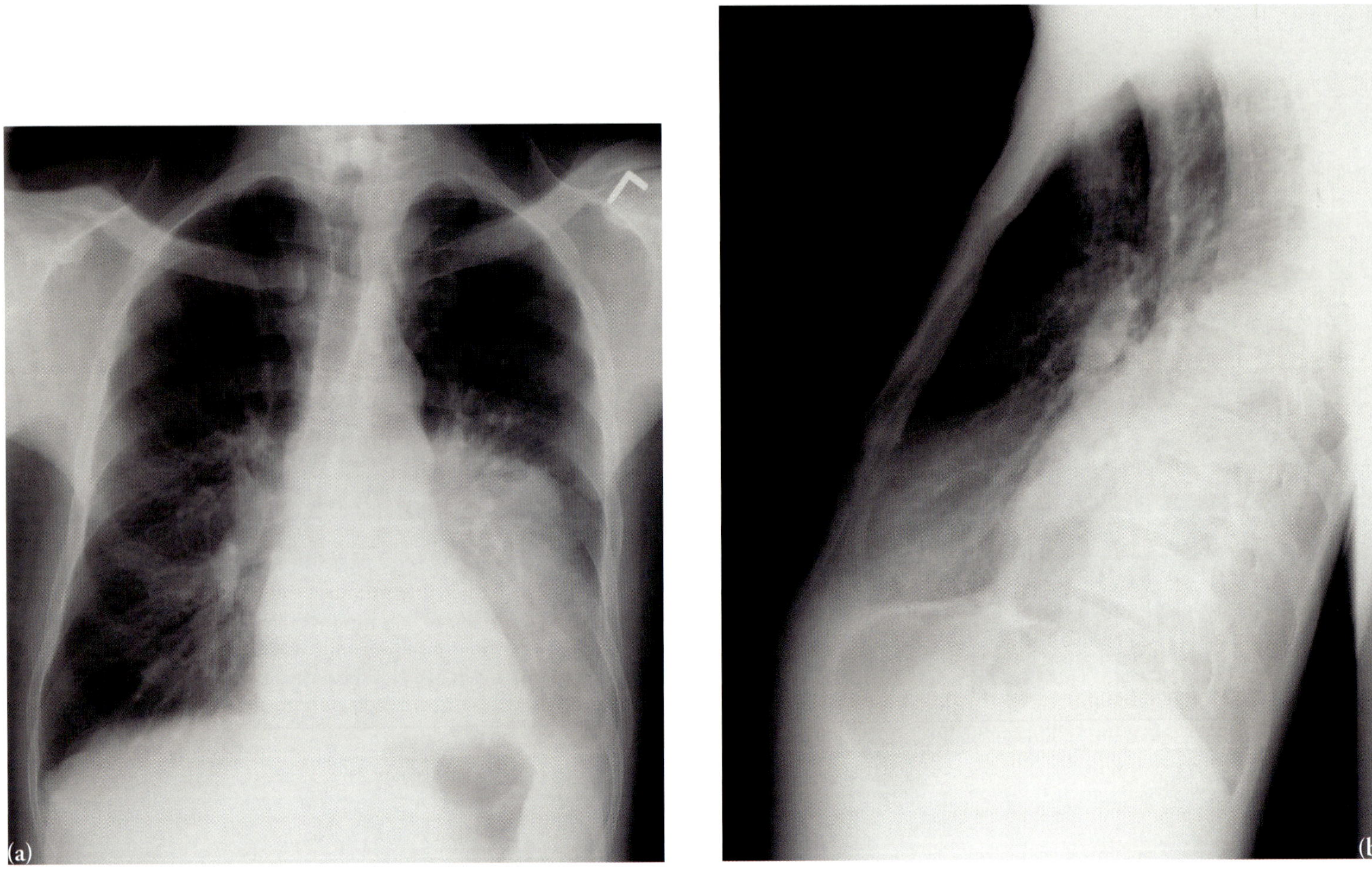

Figure 1.23(a, b) — Intrapulmonary Abscess, Klebsiella, and Enterobacter. (a) Frontal and (b) lateral radiographs demonstrate dense consolidation in the left lower lobe, which obscures visualization of the left hemidiaphragm.

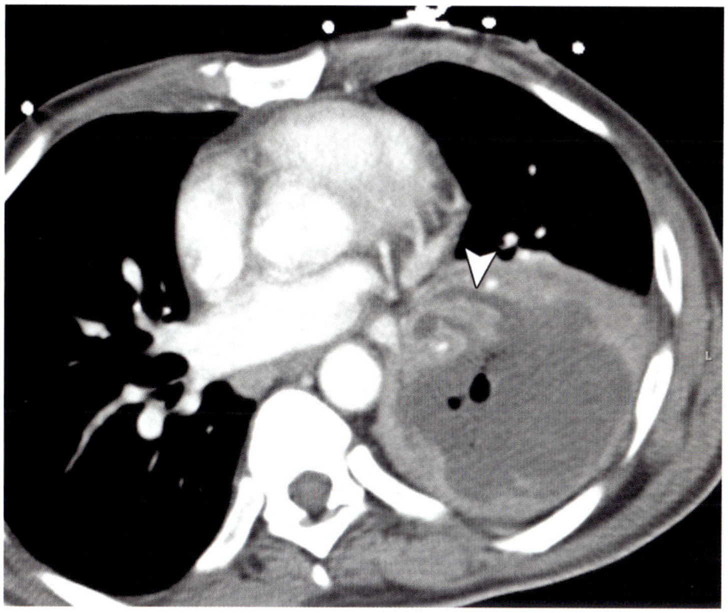

Figure 1.23c — Intrapulmonary Abscess, Klebsiella, and Enterobacter. CT with contrast shows a large low-density collection surrounded by lung parenchyma containing a small foci of gas compatible with an intrapulmonary abscess. Linear communication with the bronchial tree is noted (*arrowhead*).

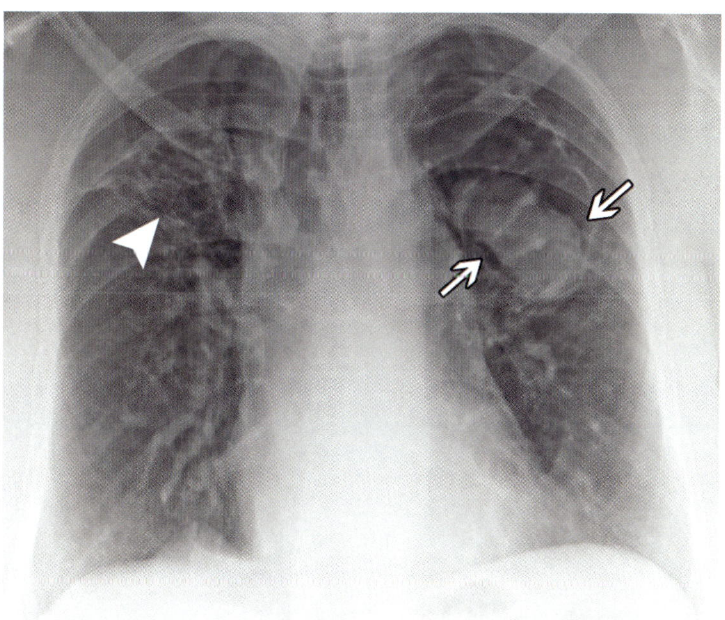

Figure 1.24a — Sarcoid Cavity With *Aspergillus* Fungus Ball (Mycetoma). Chest radiograph shows a large cavity in the left upper lobe containing a large soft tissue nodule separated from the cavity wall by a crescent of air ("air crescent" sign, *arrows*). There is evidence of scarring in the right upper lobe with bronchiectasis (*arrowhead*) and right hilar elevation.

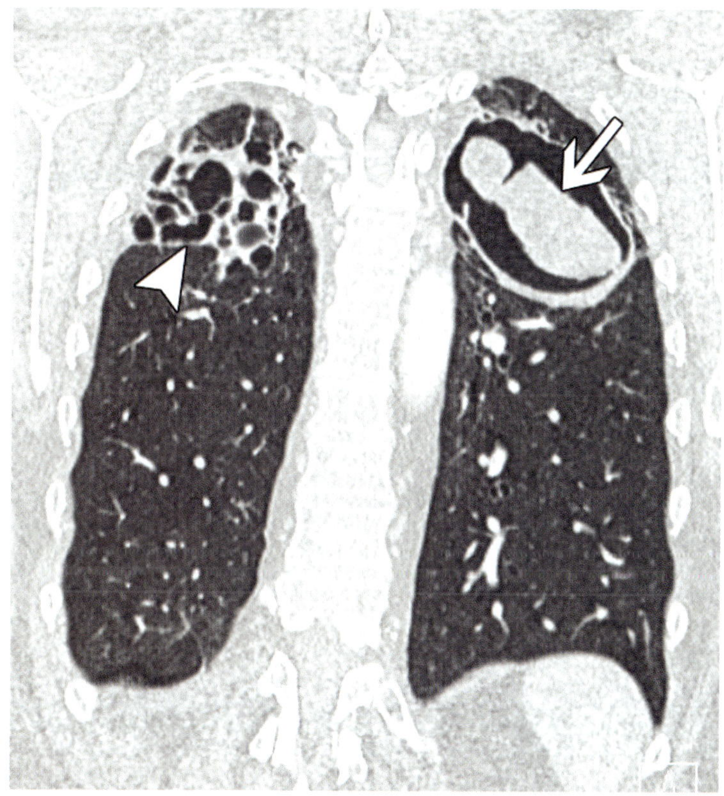

Figure 1.24b — Sarcoid Cavity With *Aspergillus* Fungus Ball (Mycetoma). Coronal CT shows a mass in the left upper lobe cavity representing the mycetoma (*arrow*) and right upper lobe fibrosis with traction bronchiectasis (*arrowhead*) compatible with the patient's history of sarcoidosis. The air crescent sign is characteristic of *Aspergillus* colonization of a preexisting cavity, but can also be seen with angioinvasive aspergillosis, tuberculosis, and lung cancer, as shown earlier. The presence of a preexisting sarcoid cavity; the lack of an irregular, thick rim to the cavity; and the lack of enhancement of the intra-cavitary mass (not shown) all suggest a benign etiology.

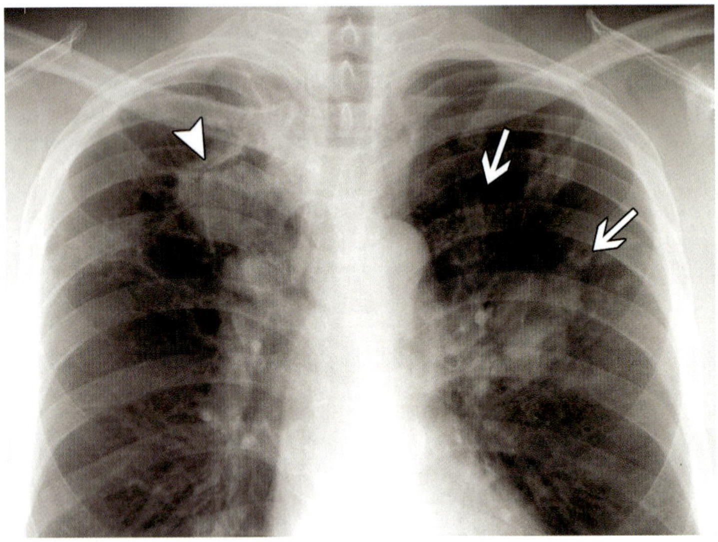

Figure 1.25a — Allergic Bronchopulmonary Aspergillosis.
Forty-six-year-old male with asthma. Chest radiograph shows a branching pattern of dilated bronchi extending from the central left upper lobe (*arrows*). Incidental note is also made of the right upper lobe mycetoma (*arrowhead*).

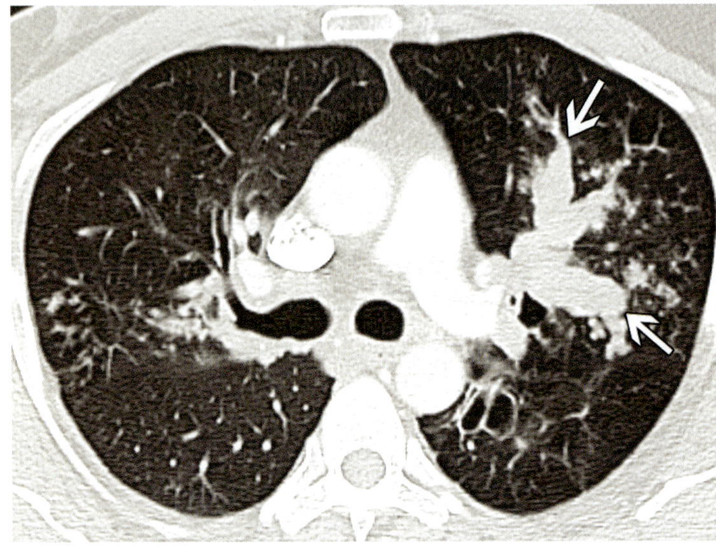

Figure 1.25b — Allergic Bronchopulmonary Aspergillosis.
Forty-six-year-old male with asthma. CT also shows the dilated, branching central bronchi ("finger-in-glove" appearance, *arrows*) associated with mucous plugs containing inflammatory cells and fungus. This appearance is classic for allergic bronchopulmonary aspergillosis, particularly in a patient with asthma or atopy. Cystic fibrosis can also appear similarly.

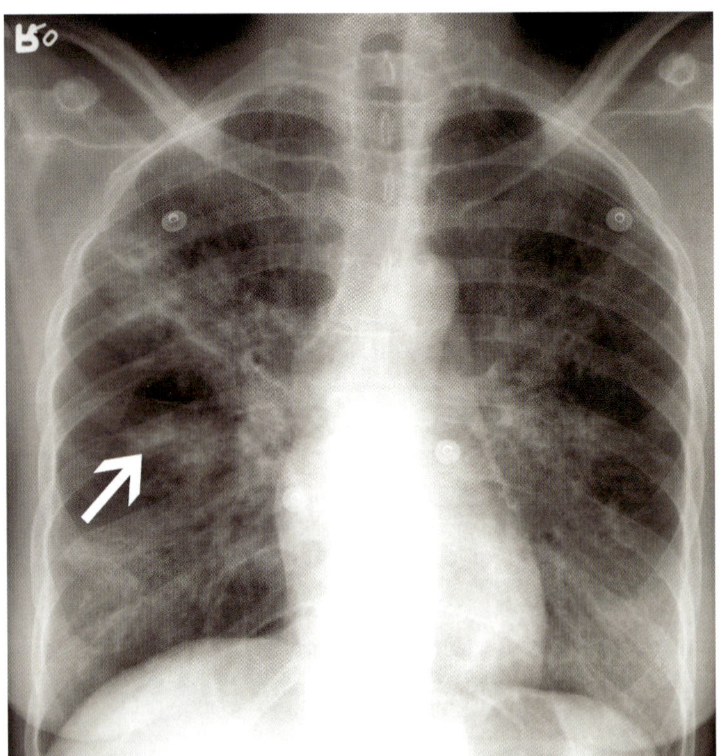

Figure 1.26a — *Pneumocystis jirovecii* Pneumonia (PJP).
Fifty-four-year-old female with AIDS. Frontal radiograph shows diffuse interstitial thickening and patchy consolidation (*arrow*).

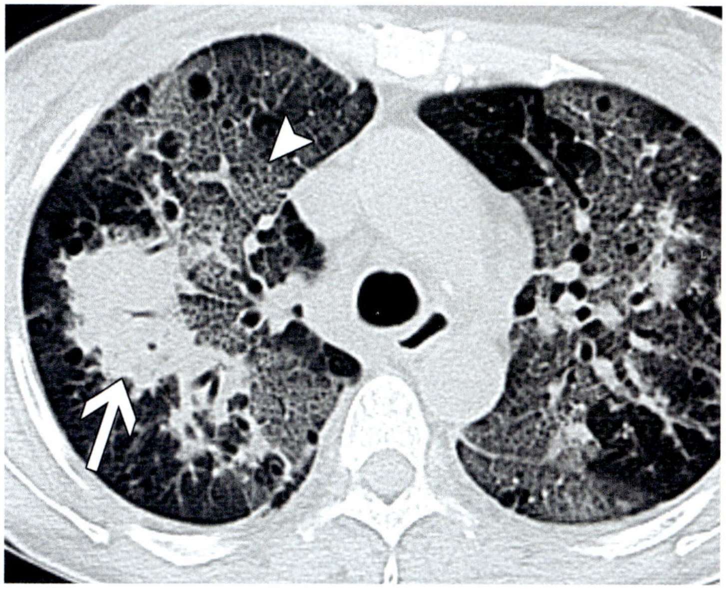

Figure 1.26b — *Pneumocystis jirovecii* Pneumonia (PJP). Fifty-four-year-old female with AIDS. CT shows patchy ground glass opacification with interlobular septal thickening ("crazy paving," *arrowhead*) and additional right upper lobe consolidation (*arrow*). Crazy paving is classically seen in pulmonary alveolar proteinosis, but can also be seen with edema, hemorrhage, viral pneumonia, and *Pneumocystis jirovecii* pneumonia.

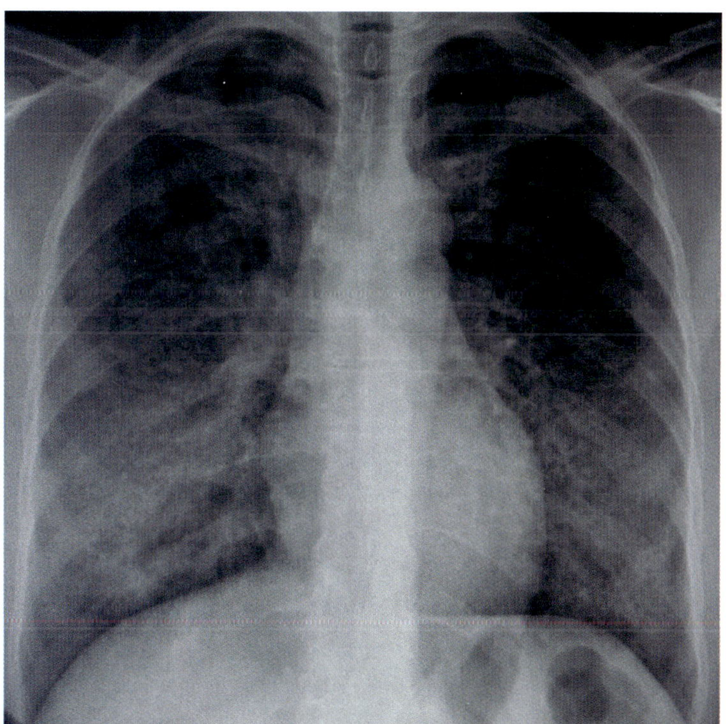

Figure 1.27a — Pulmonary Alveolar Proteinosis. Fifty-four-year-old female nonsmoker with 2- to 3-month history of cough. Biopsy confirmed the diagnosis. Chest radiographs show somewhat reticular, ill-defined opacities in the lungs, which are worse in the lower lungs.

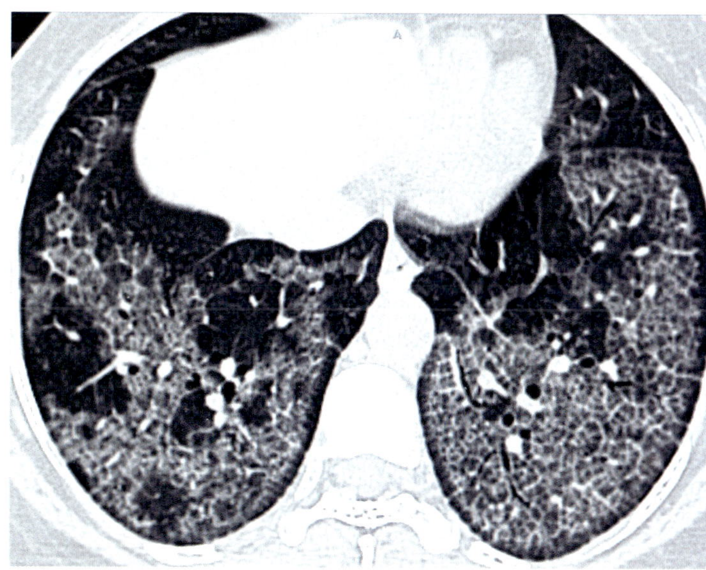

Figure 1.27b — Pulmonary Alveolar Proteinosis. Fifty-four-year-old female nonsmoker with 2- to 3-month history of cough. Biopsy confirmed the diagnosis. CT through the lower lungs shows geographic areas of ground glass opacification with interlobular septal thickening ("crazy paving") and areas of spared, normal lung. Again, this appearance is nonspecific, but is classically seen with pulmonary alveolar proteinosis. The ground glass in this case represents alveolar filling with PAS-positive proteinaceous material. Treatment usually involves bronchoalveolar lavage.

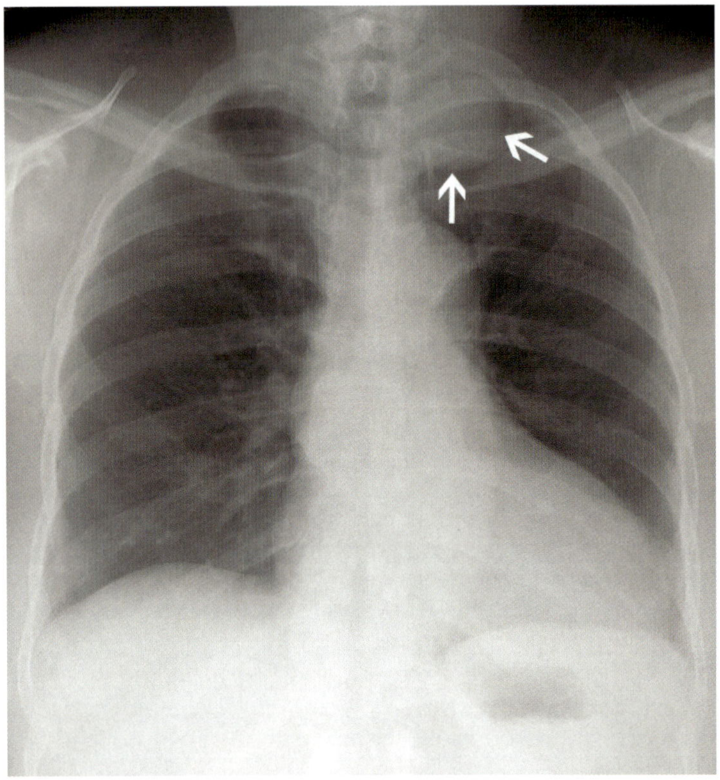

Figure 1.28a — Apical Schwannoma. Frontal chest radiograph shows a mass at the medial left lung apex with a portion of the mass demonstrating a sharp, well-defined border (*arrows*).

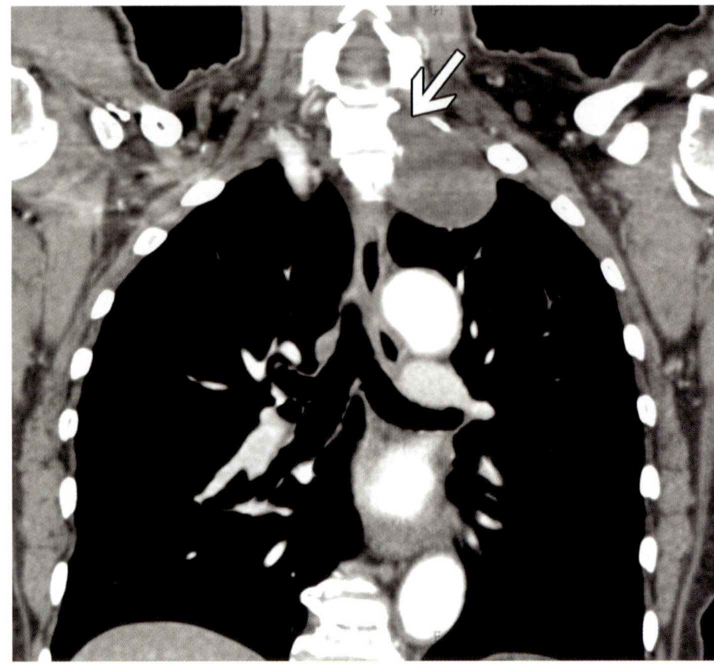

Figure 1.28b — Apical Schwannoma. Coronal CT confirms the presence of an enhancing mass at the left apex with a tail of soft tissue extending toward the neural foramen (*arrow*).

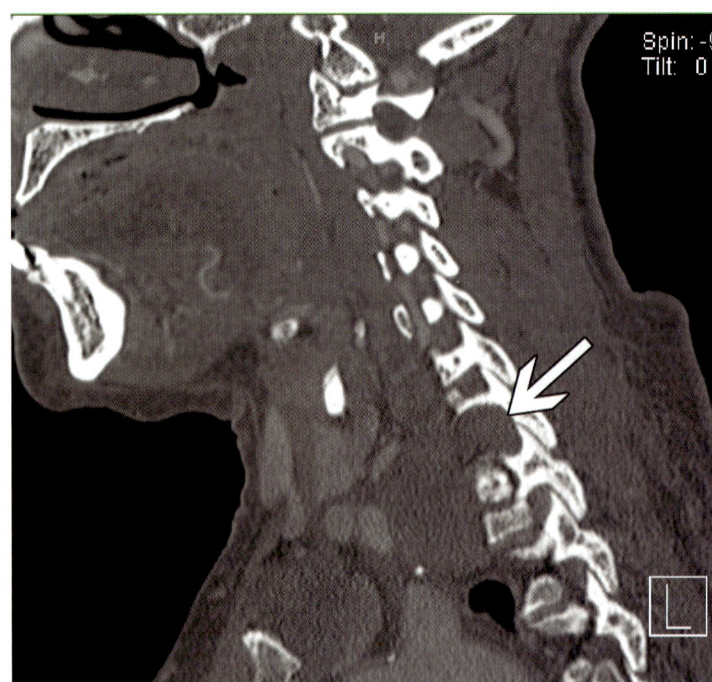

Figure 1.28c — Apical Schwannoma. Sagittal CT image in bone windows shows expansion of the involved neural foramen (*arrow*).

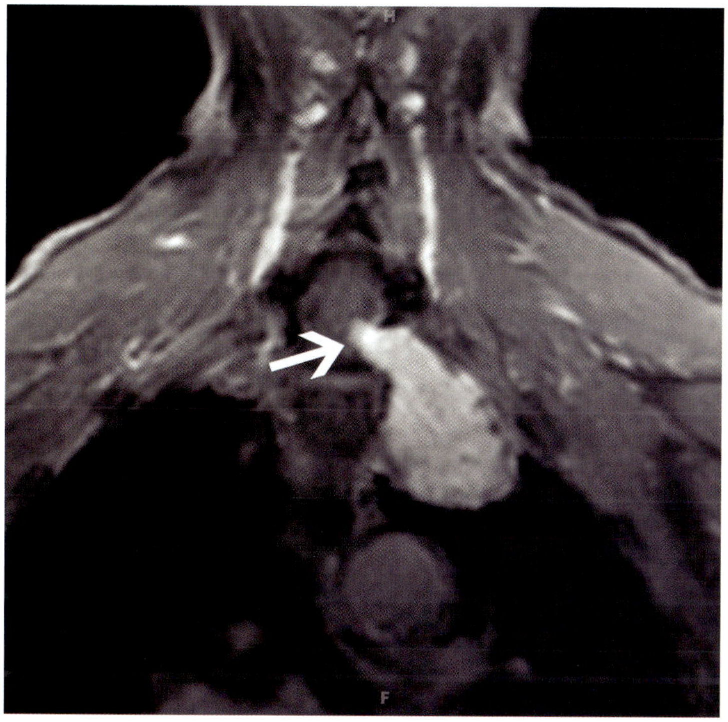

Figure 1.28d — Apical Schwannoma. Post contrast T1 MRI image with fat saturation shows homogeneous enhancement of the lesion, with the tail of tissue extending toward the neural foramen well defined (*arrow*). The other major differential consideration would be a neurofibroma. Based on the radiographic appearance alone, the differential would include a superior sulcus tumor, mesothelioma, or pleural extension of a mediastinal hematoma.

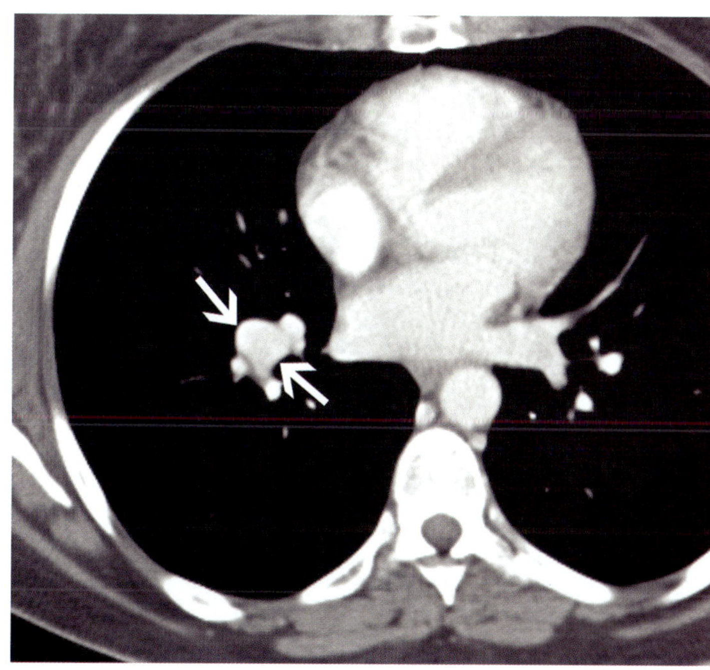

Figure 1.29a — Bronchial Artery Arteriovenous Malformation. Axial contrast CT shows a right hilar mass (*between arrows*) with homogeneous enhancement similar to the adjacent pulmonary vessels.

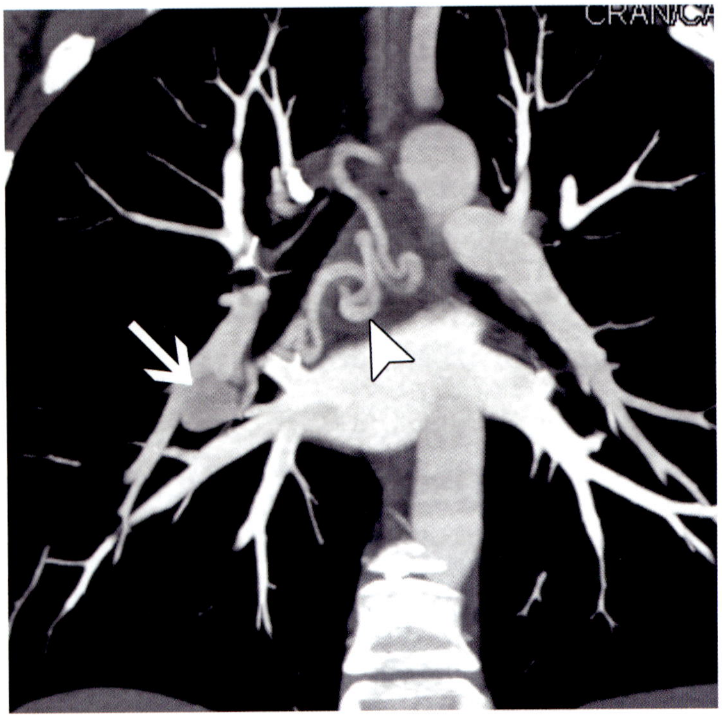

Figure 1.29b — Bronchial Artery Arteriovenous Malformation. Coronal maximum intensity projection CT image shows the right hilar mass (*arrow*) and a large feeding bronchial artery (*arrowhead*) arising from the aorta.

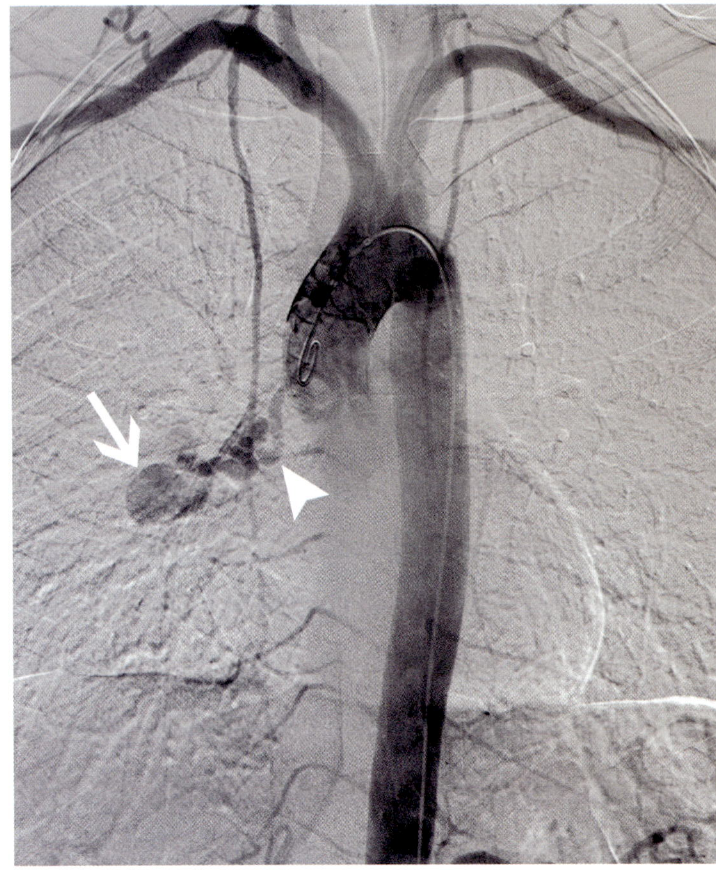

Figure 1.29c — Bronchial Artery Arteriovenous Malformation. Digital subtraction angiogram image after injection of contrast at the level of the ascending aorta confirms the presence of a large bronchial artery feeder (*arrowhead*) to the right hilar arteriovenous malformation (*arrow*).

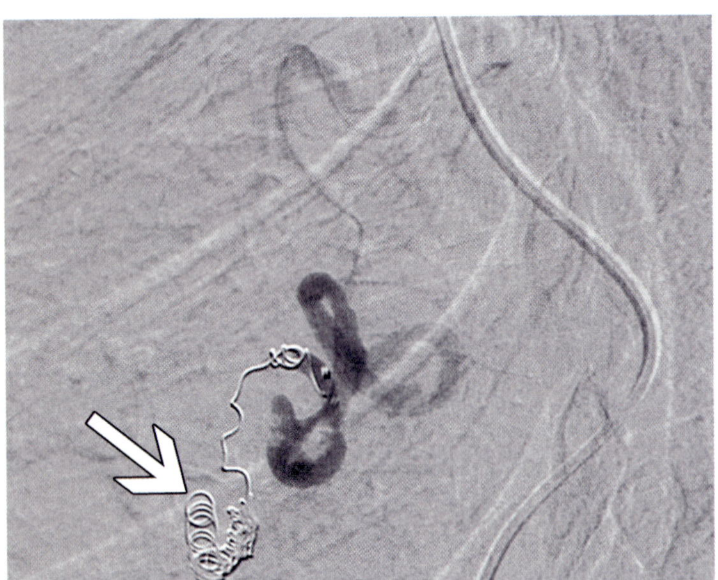

Figure 1.29d — Bronchial Artery Arteriovenous Malformation. Digital subtraction angiogram image after coil (*arrow*) embolization of the bronchial artery supplying the arteriovenous malformation shows nonopacification of the arteriovenous malformation compatible with successful embolization.

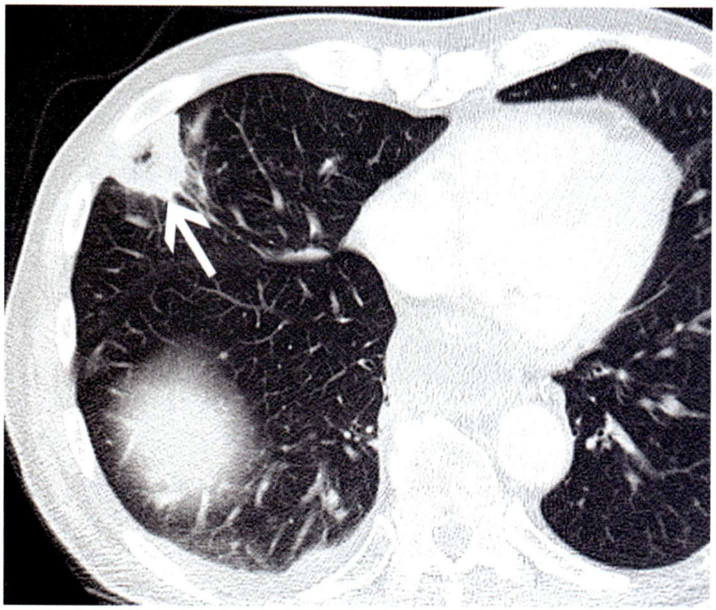

Figure 1.30a — Pulmonary Infarct Resulting From Pulmonary Embolus. CT image in lung windows shows a peripheral, wedge-shaped opacity at the base of the right middle lobe (referred to as "Hampton hump," *arrow*).

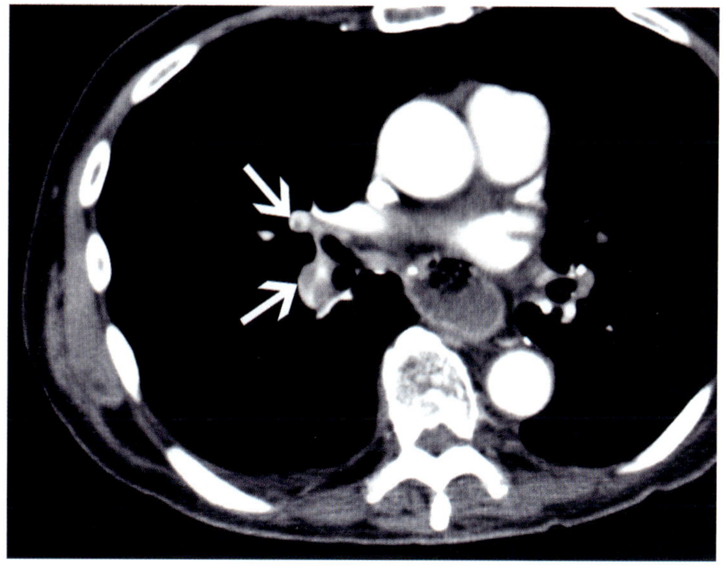

Figure 1.30b — Pulmonary Infarct Resulting From Pulmonary Embolus. Image through the more central pulmonary arteries shows filling defects in the right pulmonary arteries (*arrows*) compatible with pulmonary emboli.

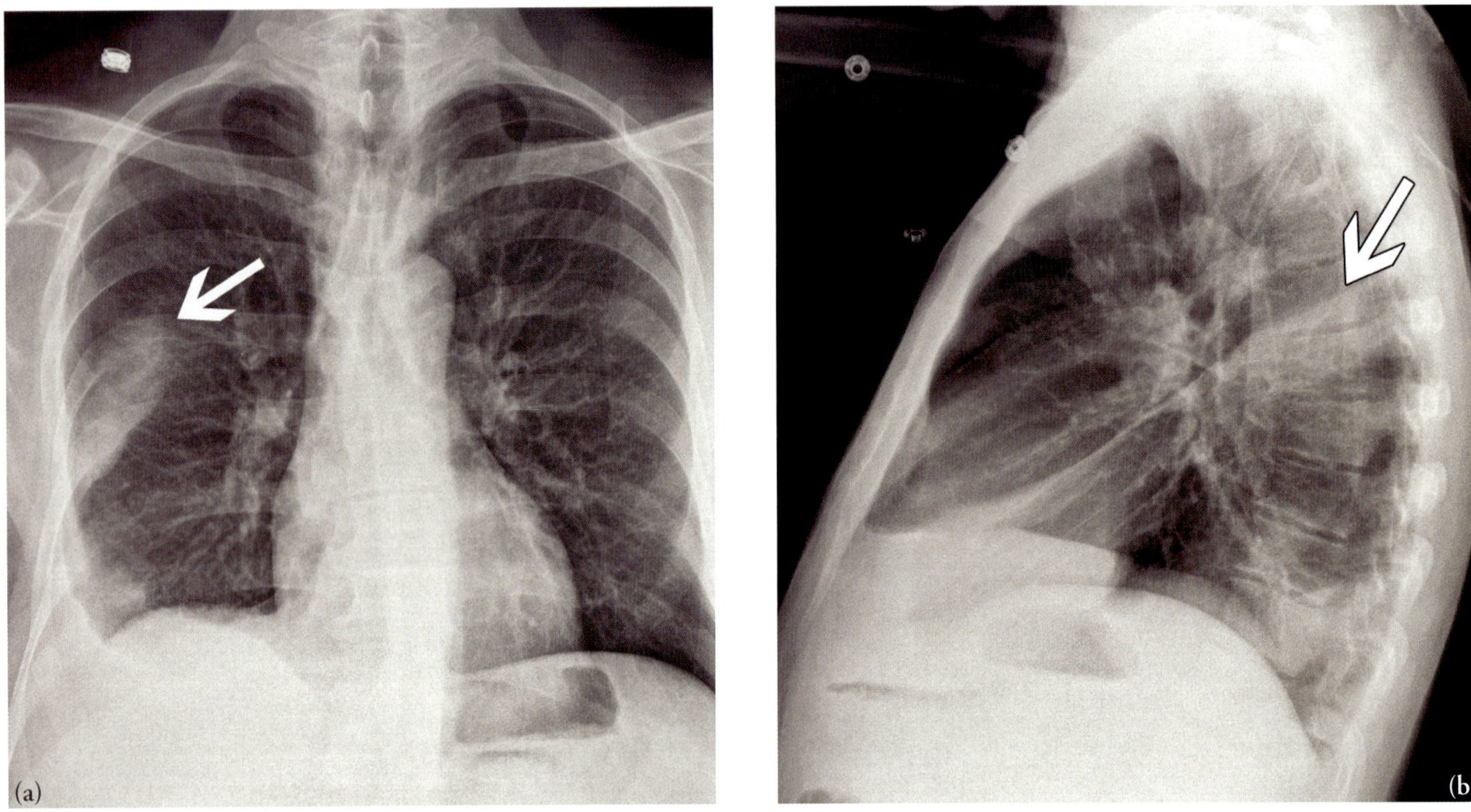

Figure 1.31(a, b) — "Pseudotumor" From pleural fluid. (a) Frontal and (b) lateral radiographs show a lenticular-shaped opacity in the right mid lung (*arrows*), which is shown on the lateral to be oriented along the major fissure.

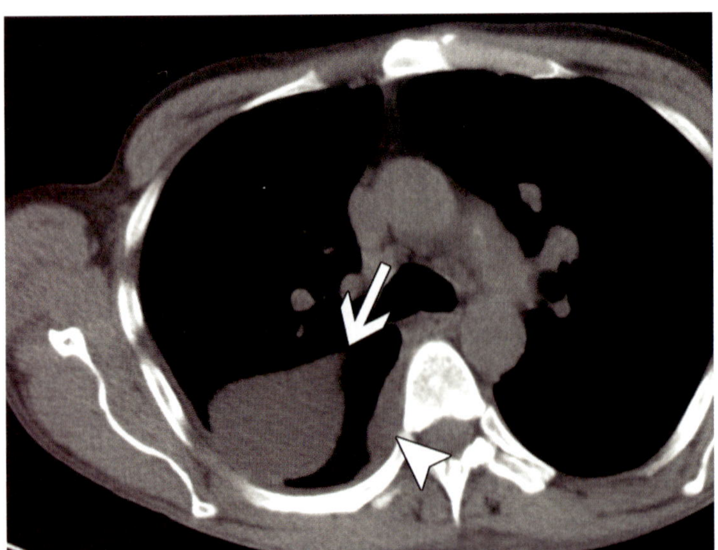

Figure 1.31c — "Pseudotumor" From pleural fluid. CT without contrast shows a homogeneous water density pleural fluid in the major fissure with tapering "beak" (*arrow*) directed along the fissure. Additional loculated fluid is also noted at the posterior medial right pleural space (*arrowhead*).

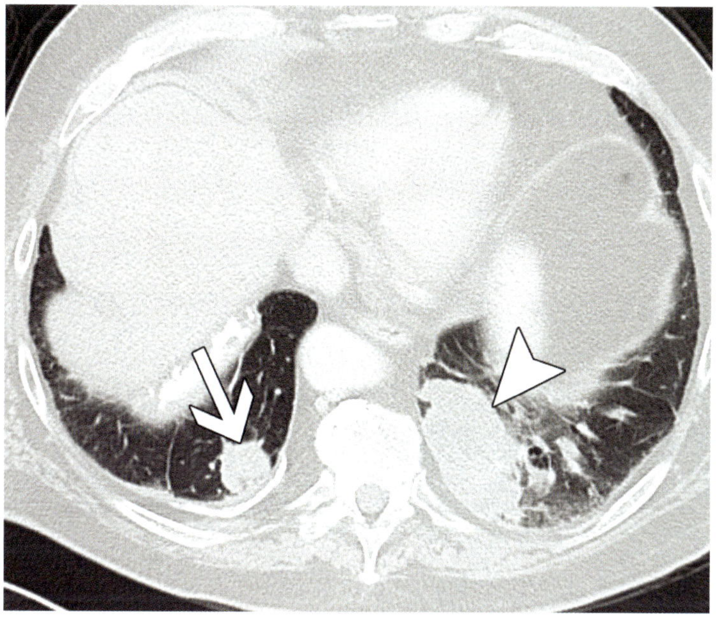

Figure 1.32a — Rounded Atelectasis. CT image shows a peripheral round nodule at the right lung base (*arrow*). Left lung base mass (*arrowhead*) represents metastatic adenocarcinoma of unknown primary.

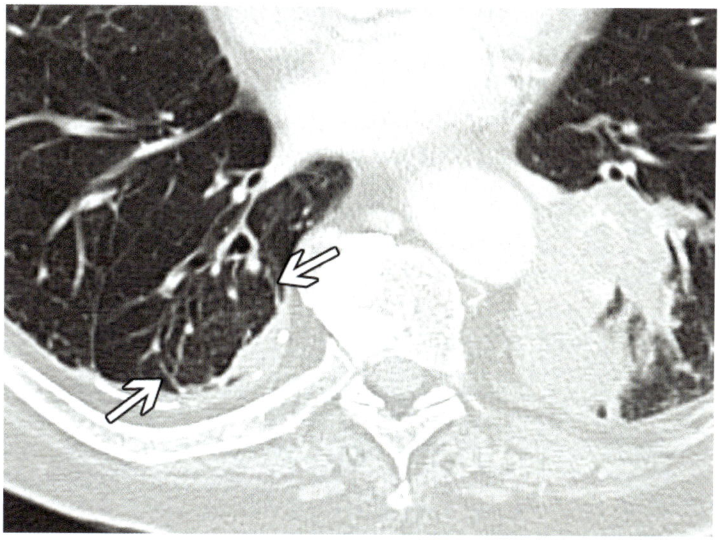

Figure 1.32b — Rounded Atelectasis. CT image slightly superior to this shows curving of pulmonary vessels into the edge of the lesion ("comet-tail" sign, *arrows*) and crowding of bronchovascular structures compatible with volume loss.

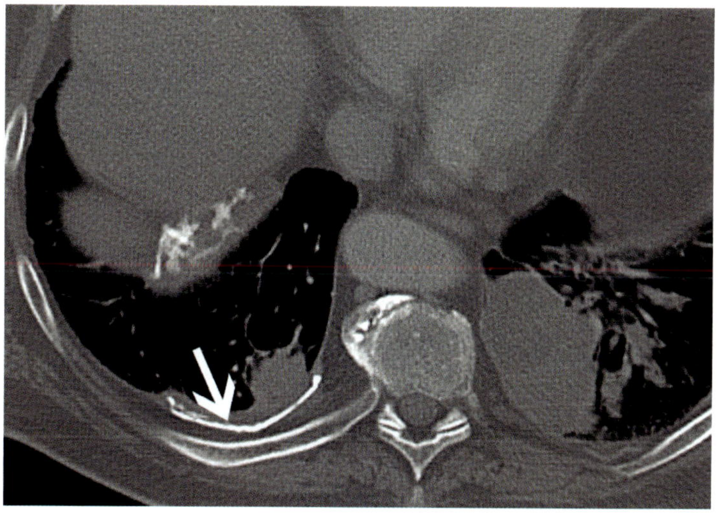

Figure 1.32c — Rounded Atelectasis. Bone windows at the level of the mass show a calcified pleural plaque (*arrow*). With this constellation of findings, the diagnosis of rounded atelectasis can be made.

RECOMMENDED READING

Collins J, Stern EJ. *Chest Radiology: The Essentials.* Philadelphia, PA: Lippincott Williams & Wilkins; 1999:284.

The International Association for the Study of Lung Cancer (IASCL) Prospective Lung Cancer Staging Project: Protocol; March 27, 2009.

Webb WR, Higgins CB. *Thoracic Imaging: Pulmonary and Cardiovascular Radiology.* Philadelphia, PA: Lippincott Williams & Wilkins; 2005:837.

Webb WR, Muller NL, Naidich DP. *High-Resolution CT of the Lung.* Philadelphia, PA: Lippincott Williams & Wilkins; 2008:617.

2

Normal Lung

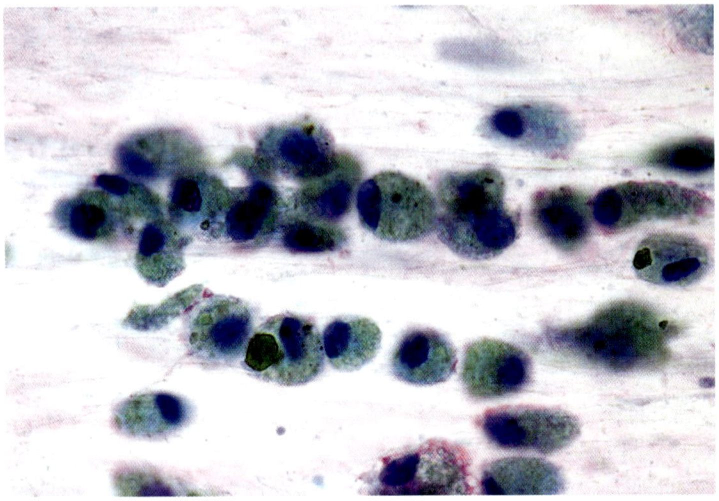

Figure 2.1a — Pigment-Laden Pulmonary Alveolar Macrophages, Bronchoalveolar Lavage [Pap Stain; High Power]. Macrophages within the alveolar spaces may contain variable amounts of pigment, which is not necessarily abnormal. Compare the macrophage at the top right-hand corner, which contains light blue cytoplasm and little pigment, to other macrophages in the field, which contain green pigment material, some of which is coarse and some of which is more granular-appearing. Most pigment is secondary to the breakdown of red blood cells and the heme moiety they contain. The presence of blood may be secondary to a previous hemorrhage. It often can be difficult to definitively characterize pigment material; if necessary, an iron stain can be performed. A patient with a history of metastatic melanoma may pose a diagnostic dilemma.

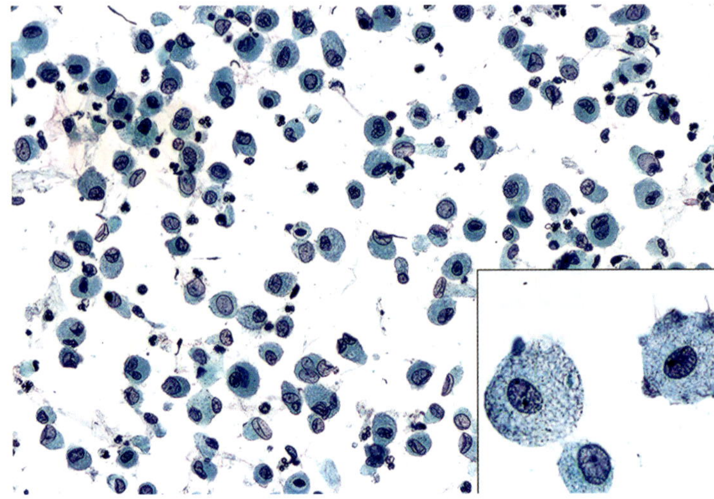

Figure 2.1b — Pulmonary Alveolar Macrophages, Bronchoalveolar Lavage [Pap Stain; Medium and High Powers]. Pulmonary alveolar macrophages reside primarily in alveolar spaces and their presence alone confirms the adequacy of a bronchoalveolar lavage procedure. The cells have foamy and abundant cytoplasm and oval- to-hyphen-shaped nuclei. The chromatin pattern is bland, with distinct yet small nucleoli. Some cells are binucleate. If macrophages are not seen in an otherwise benign bronchoalveolar lavage, the procedure should be reported as inadequate rather than negative for malignancy.

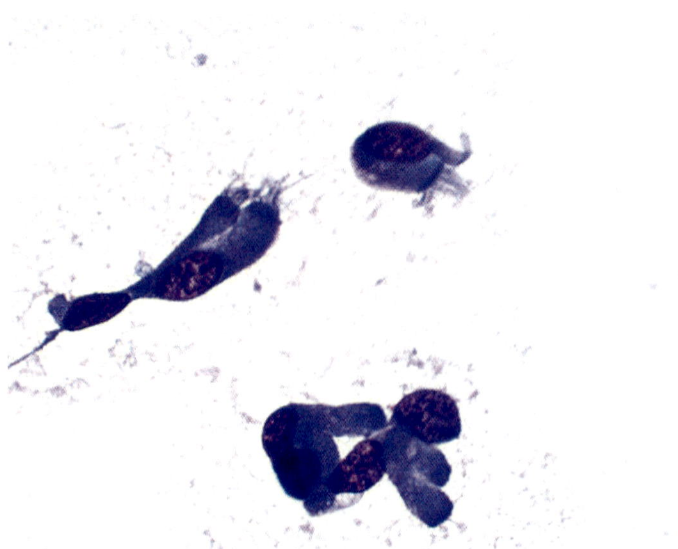

Figure 2.2a — Benign Respiratory Epithelial Cells, Fine Needle Aspiration [Diff-Quik Stain; High Power]. Benign ciliated respiratory epithelial cells are often present in the background of fine needle aspiration, bronchial brushing and washing, and bronchoalveolar lavage specimens. They have round-to-oval nuclei with regular borders. The cells most often have a columnar shape and are ciliated; the cilia attach to a terminal bar that may be seen as a dense, flat area at the apex of the cell. While cilia may not always be seen in all preparations or in every cell, the presence of cilia and/or a terminal bar is a reassuring finding. Reactive bronchial epithelial cells can have atypical morphologies that mimic adenocarcinoma, as will be demonstrated in later chapters.

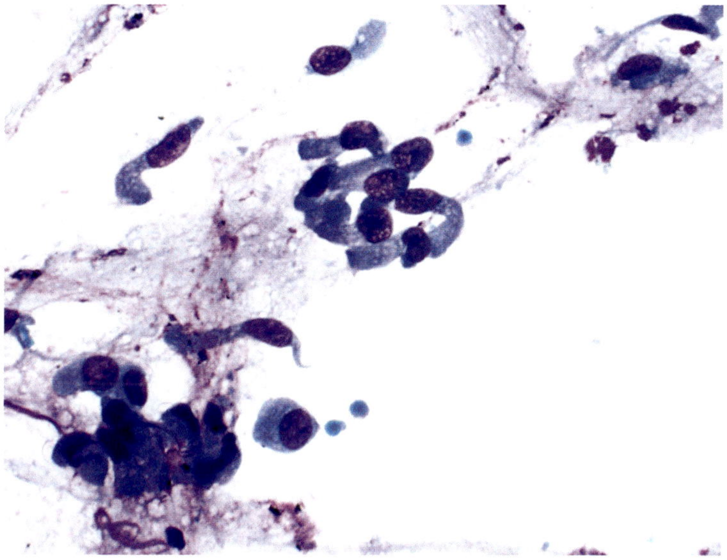

Figure 2.2b — Benign Respiratory Epithelial Cells, Fine Needle Aspiration [Diff-Quik Stain; Medium Power]. The field contains numerous benign respiratory epithelial cells, both singly and in a small fragment. This field contains cells without discernable cilia, but terminal bars can be identified. Note the blandness of the chromatin and similarity of nuclei between the cells.

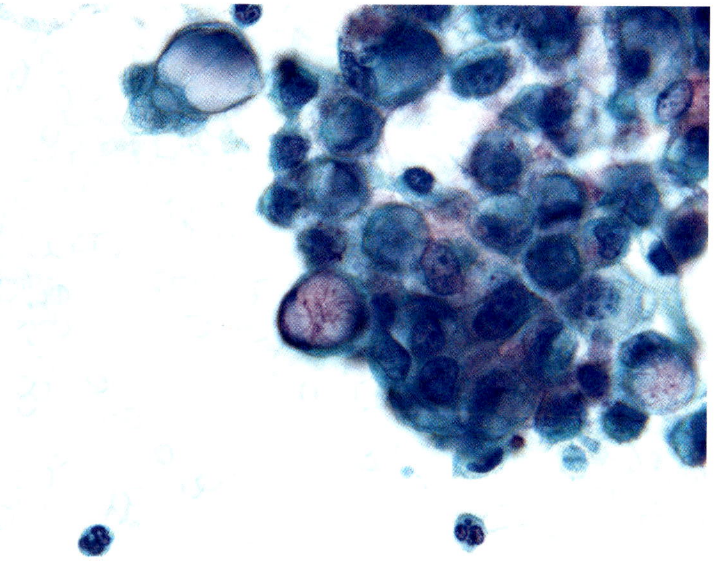

Figure 2.2c — Goblet Cells, Bronchial Brushing [Pap Stain; High Power]. Goblet cells can be found within the respiratory tract and are intermixed with ciliated bronchial respiratory cells. The mucin contained in goblet cells may appear pink-staining on the Pap stain and have overlap with pink-staining cilia attached to the end of columnar cells. Furthermore, some conditions may result in goblet cell hyperplasia in which goblet cells are more prominent. This may be initially mistaken for adenocarcinoma, but the cells are typically scant, have bland nuclear features, and are intermixed with at least a few ciliated cells.

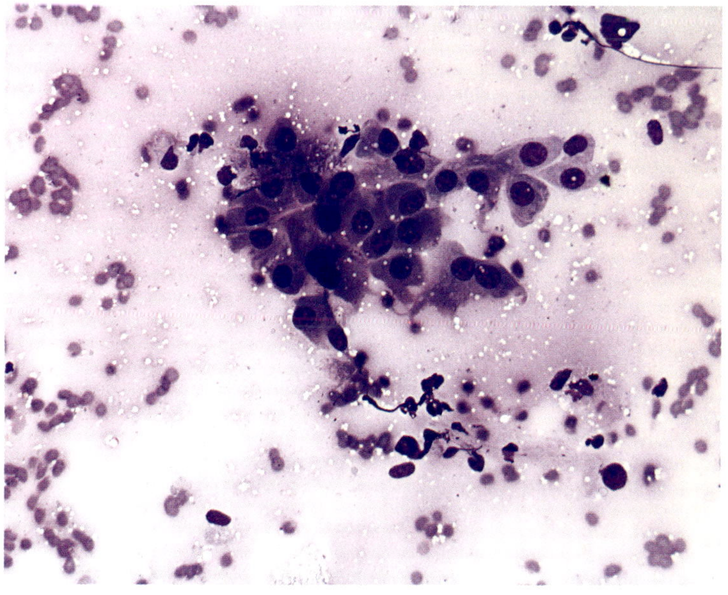

Figure 2.3a — Benign Mesothelial Cells, Fine Needle Aspiration [Diff-Quik Stain; High Power]. The cells are large, but have round nuclei with regular borders and low nuclear-to-cytoplasmic ratios. Small slits or "windows" between some cells can be seen, indicating a mesothelial origin. The Diff-Quik stain allows for better visualization of the cellular cytoplasm, which may have an amphophilic or "two-toned" appearance. The differential diagnosis would include neoplasms in which cytoplasm is often preserved with round nuclei, such as renal cell carcinoma, melanoma, thyroid carcinoma, and prostate carcinoma.

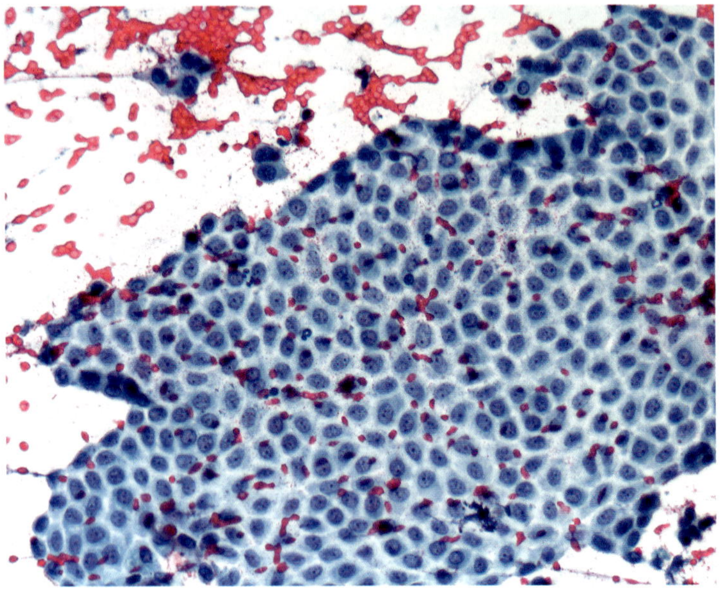

Figure 2.3b — Benign Mesothelial Sheet, Fine Needle Aspiration [Pap Stain; Medium Power]. These benign cells form a honeycomb-like pattern in a monolayer sheet; occasionally, this sheet may fold over on itself and appear more complex. By contrast, mesotheliomas tend to have more complex architecture, with three-dimensional structures and rigid projections within fragments. In this case, the cells lack atypical features; in reactive conditions, mesothelial cells can often have markedly typical appearance and have significant overlap with carcinoma or mesothelioma.

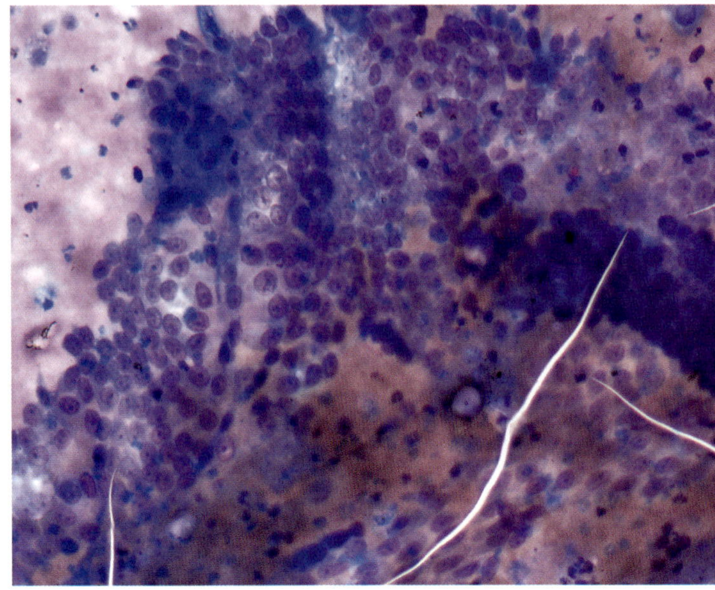

Figure 2.3c — Benign Mesothelial Sheet, Fine Needle Aspiration [Diff-Quik Stain; Medium Power]. Here the cells are slightly disorganized within the sheet and have prominent nucleoli and mild anisonucleosis. However, the nuclei are fairly monotonous appearing and the monolayer architecture of the sheet suggests a mesothelial origin. Typically only small fragments of mesothelium will be sampled on a fine needle aspiration procedure; if a large number of fragments are seen, a neoplastic process needs to be excluded.

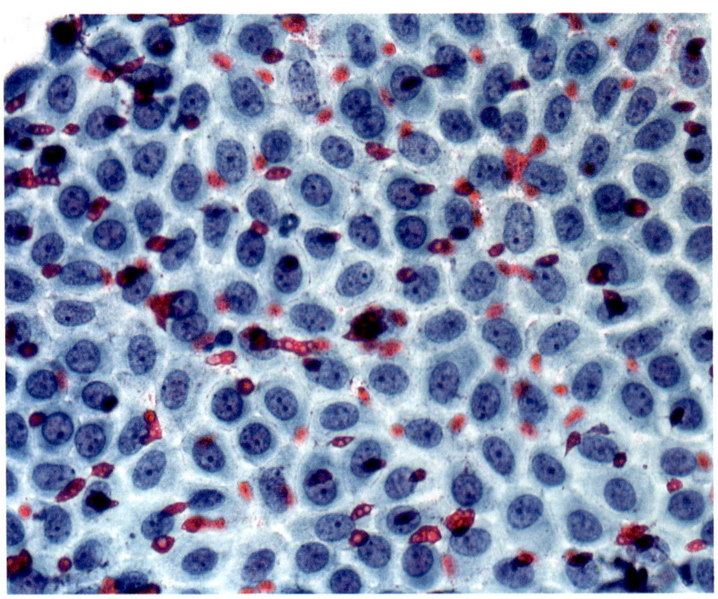

Figure 2.3d — Benign Mesothelial Sheet, Fine Needle Aspiration [Pap Stain; High Power]. Transthoracic fine needle aspiration passes through the pleural lining and thus specimens may be contaminated with benign mesothelial cells. If a lesion is particularly hard to aspirate, these mesothelial sheets may be the only epithelial cells seen and may be mistaken for sampling of the lesion in an unsatisfactory sample. Here, the cells are evenly spaced within a monolayer sheet, with regular nuclear borders and bland chromatin. Note the distinct cell borders and small "windows" between cells.

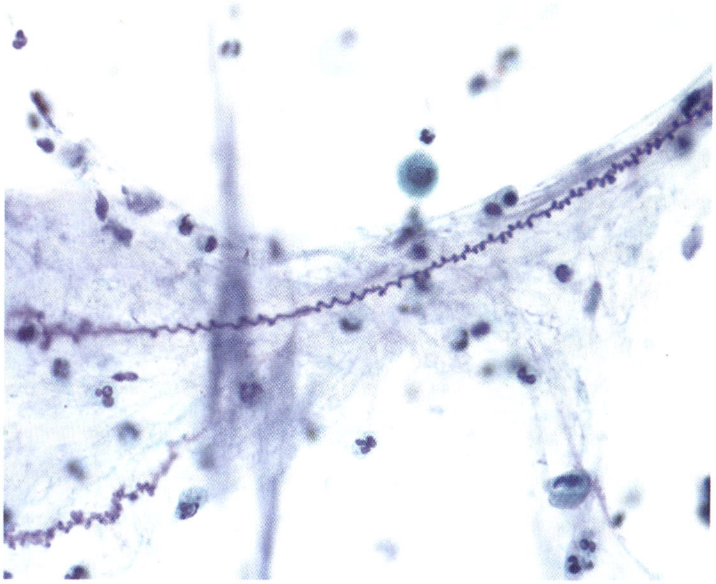

Figure 2.4a — Curschmann's Spirals, Sputum [Pap Stain; Medium Power]. Curschmann's spirals appear suspended, banner-like, in this image. The spirals are composed of dense mucinous secretions and are formed as these secretions become inspissated to form a cast of the encasing airway.

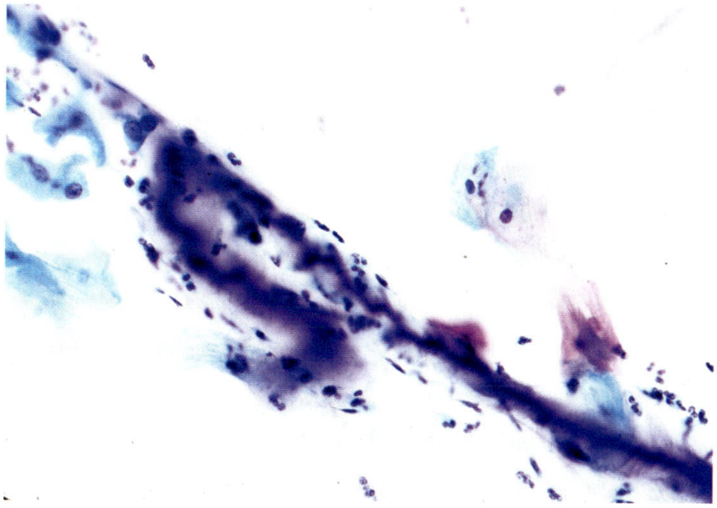

Figure 2.4b — Curschmann's Spirals [Diff-Quik Stain; High Power]. At higher magnification, the surface has a "wrapped" or banded appearance. The tight bundle of mucus is embedded within a mucoid background. Curschmann's spirals are nonspecific, and may be seen in patients with increased mucus production for any reason.

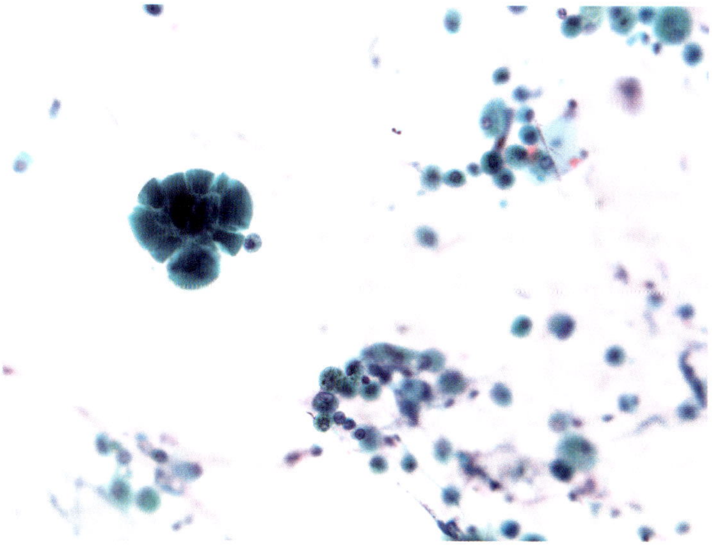

Figure 2.5a — Corpora Amylacea [Pap Stain; Medium Power]. Corpora amylacea may be found in bronchoalveolar (BAL) specimens. They appear as dense, lamellated concretions and may have cracking artifact around the edges, as seen in this image. Also seen are the pulmonary alveolar macrophages and scattered neutrophils, which give an indication of size. Corpora amylacea are incidental findings in BAL specimens and have no known significance.

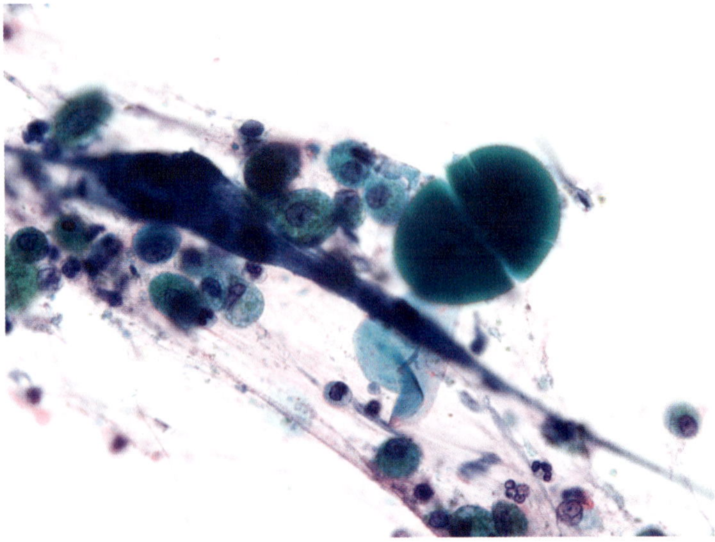

Figure 2.5b — Corpora Amylacea [Pap Stain; High Power]. In the lung, corpora amylacea are found within scattered alveoli. The primary differential diagnosis is pulmonary alveolar microlithiasis. Pulmonary alveolar microlithiasis is an autosomal recessive condition in which the alveoli become filled with calcified bodies. Corpora amylacea do not calcify, and are not seen in the quantity that the calcified secretions of pulmonary alveolar microlithiasis are seen.

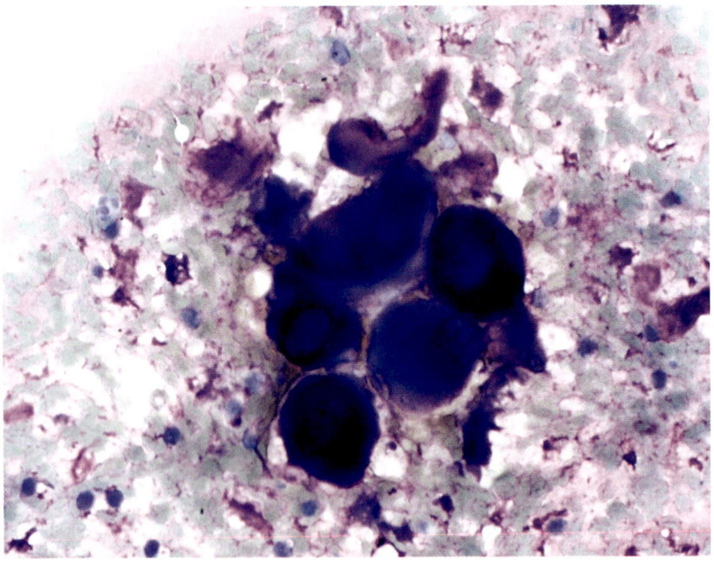

Figure 2.6a — Large Airway Cartilage, Fine Needle Aspiration [Diff-Quik Stain; High Power]. The blue-magenta colored globules are somewhat reminiscent of the globules of adenoid cystic carcinoma, but the material is not homogenous and is of low cellularity. When the needle passes through large airways, cartilage may be sampled and cause initial confusion. Generally only small amounts will be present on a fine needle aspiration specimen, though inexperienced operators may sample more connective tissue, cartilage, nerve, and/or adipose tissue than lesional tissue.

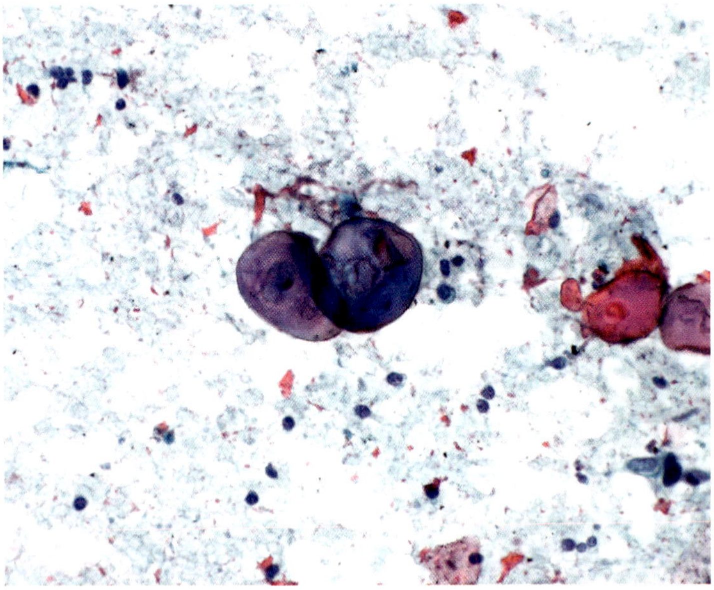

Figure 2.6b — Large Airway Cartilage, Fine Needle Aspiration [Pap Stain; High Power]. Less alarming on a Pap stain, fragments of cartilage may still provide a distraction. The balls have smooth yet irregular edges and internal spaces in which a chondrocyte typically resides, though the chondrocyte may not be readily identifiable. Note the spectrum of staining in this field—some cartilage is more blue and violet, while other cartilage appears pink (right side of the field).

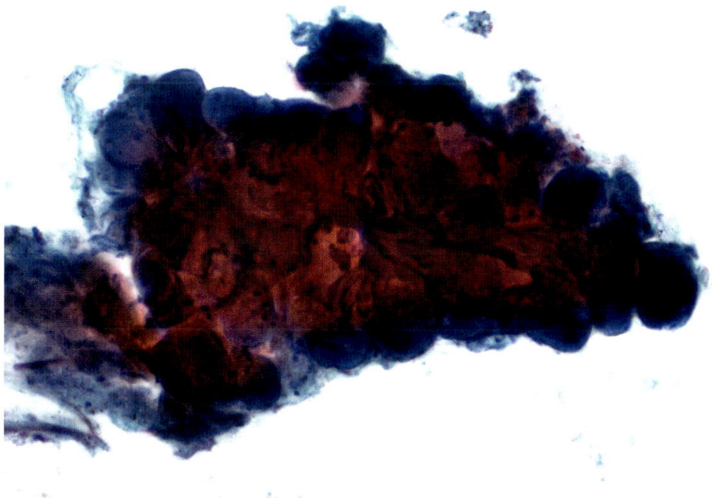

Figure 2.7 — Large Airway Salivary Tissue, Fine Needle Aspiration [Pap Stain; High Power]. The presence of benign salivary tissue on fine needle aspiration suggests sampling has taken place near a large airway space. Note the regular lobular architecture seen in this "mini-biopsy." The lobules are attached to a central duct that may be difficult to see in a three-dimensional structure. A nonneoplastic finding, only rare salivary tissue should be seen on a lung fine needle aspiration specimen. Salivary gland tissue reminds us that salivary gland neoplasms may develop within the lung.

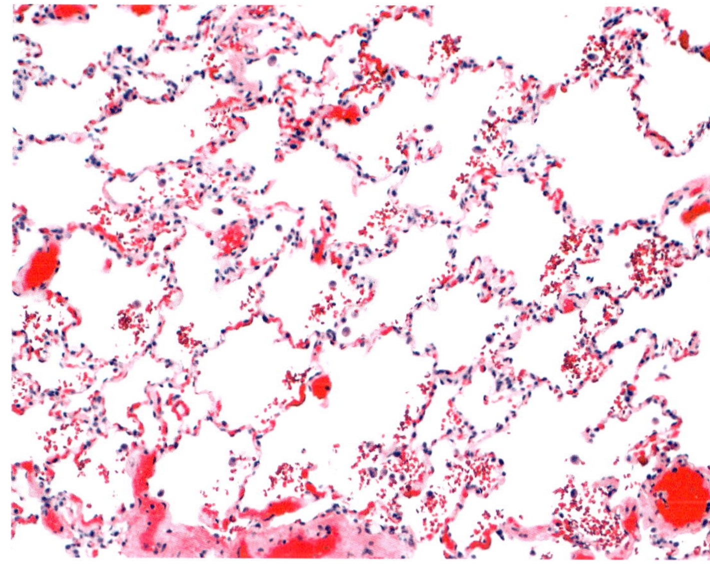

Figure 2.8 — Alveoli, Lobectomy [H&E Stain; Medium Power]. Peripherally, the lung is composed of thin-walled air sacs. These thin walls hold the capillaries and are the surfaces through which gas exchange occurs. Occasional intra-alveolar histiocytes may be present.

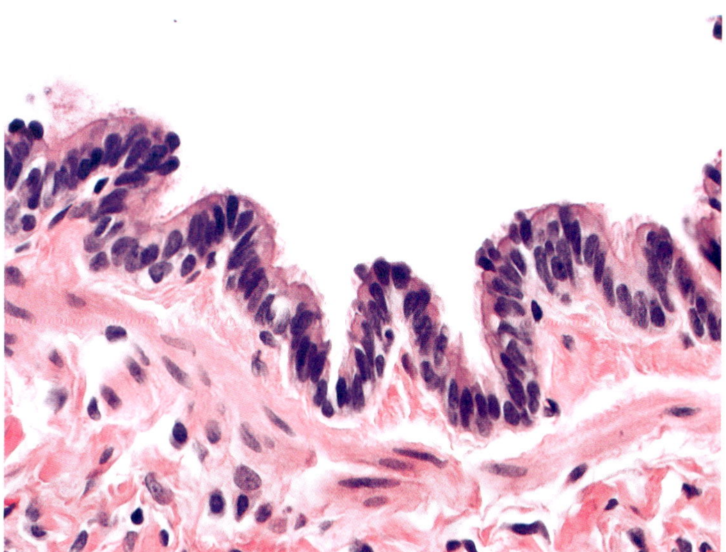

Figure 2.9 — Respiratory (Bronchiolar) Epithelium, Lobectomy [H&E Stain; High Power]. At high magnification, the bronchi and bronchioles are lined by columnar, ciliated epithelium. Long delicate cilia are easily discerned above the terminal bar in this case. A small band of smooth muscle is present beneath the epithelium with underlying occasional mast cells within fibroconnective tissue.

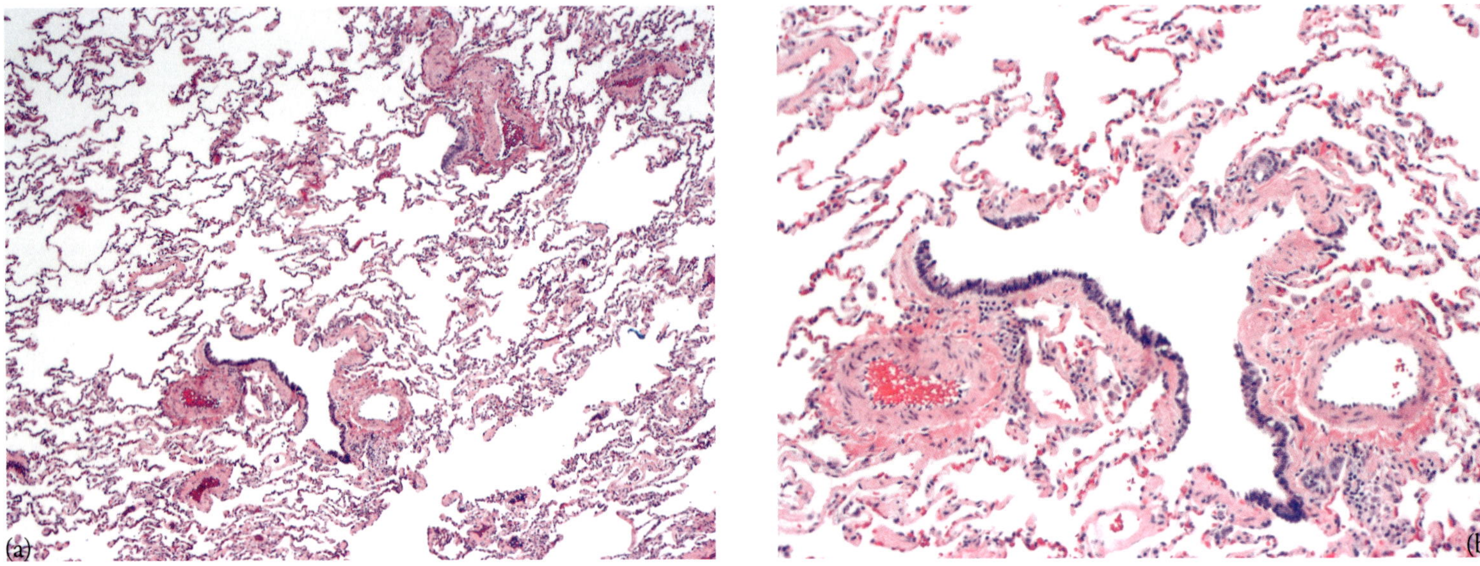

Figure 2.10(a, b) — Terminal Bronchiole, Lobectomy [H&E Stain; Low and Medium Powers]. The conducting system reaches its conclusion with the terminal bronchioles. The terminal bronchiole is the smallest airway with respiratory epithelium without alveoli in the walls. Here a terminal bronchiole, accompanied by small arteries, opens into respiratory bronchioles and the alveolar system.

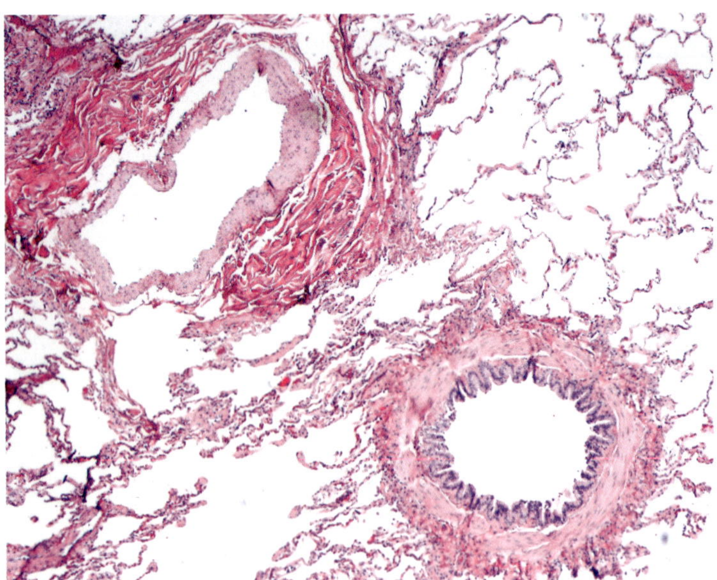

Figure 2.11 — Bronchiole and Artery, Lobectomy [H&E Stain; Low Power]. The conducting airways of the lung are accompanied by arteries along their path. The arteries are similar in caliber to the airway. These two course together all the way from the hilum to the terminal bronchioles.

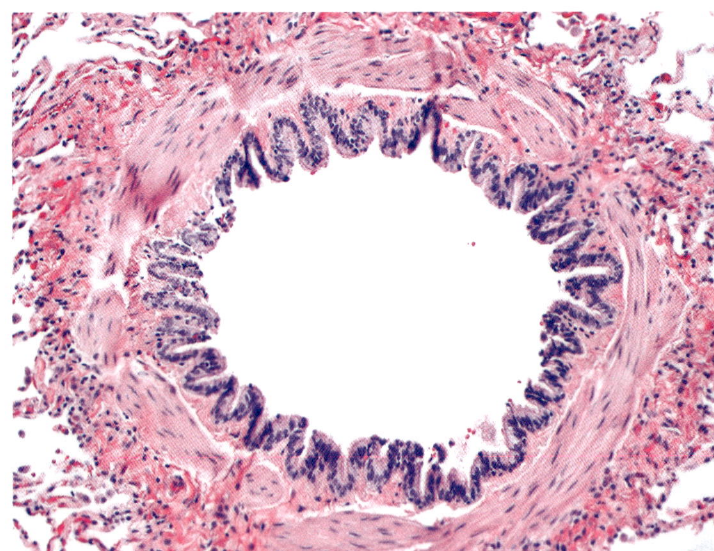

Figure 2.12 — Bronchiole, Lobectomy [H&E Stain; Medium Power]. Bronchioles are part of the conducting system of the lung and are lined by the same pseudostratified ciliated epithelium of the bronchi with smooth muscle walls, but lack cartilage by definition. The infolded epithelium has a loose supporting tissue and elastic tissue to allow it to expand with dilation of the airway.

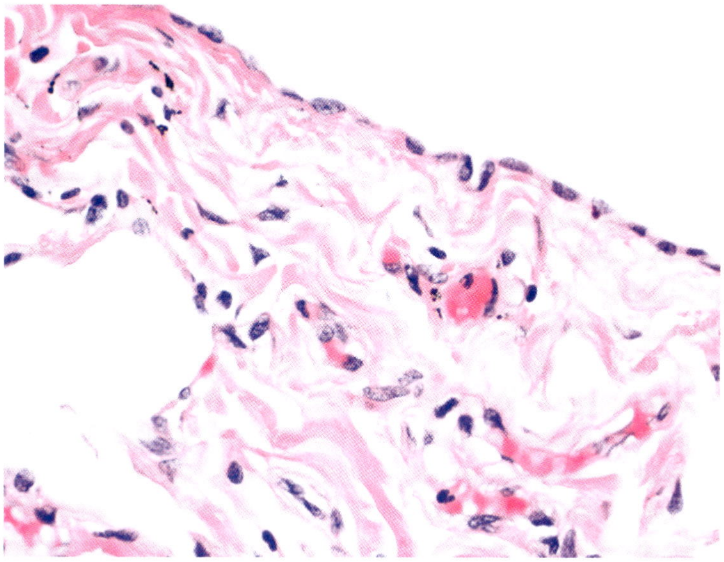

Figure 2.13 — Normal Pleura, Wedge Resection [H&E Stain; High Power]. Under normal conditions, a single layer of flattened mesothelial cells line the pleural surfaces of both the lung (visceral pleura) and the inner thoracic cavity (parietal pleura). Beneath this layer is a thin area of fibrovascular connective tissue with scattered fibroblasts and thin vessels, as well as the elastic layer. This elastic layer is not well-visualized by H&E, and special elastic stains may be needed to see it. Breach of this elastic layer by tumor cells is considered visceral pleura invasion and is now reported in lung carcinoma staging.

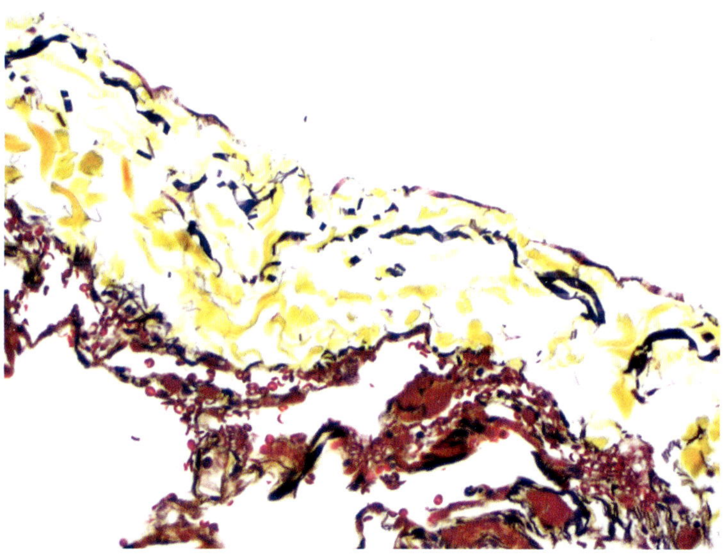

Figure 2.14 — Normal Pleura, Wedge Resection [Movat Pentachrome Special Stain; High Power]. When pleural sections are stained with special stains that highlight elastic fibers, such as the Movat Pentachrome as seen here, the submesothelial elastic layer is readily visible as thick black fibers that run parallel to the surface. In this stain, the mature collagenous tissue of the pleura stains yellow, and the mesothelium and blood in the scant lung tissue below the pleura stain a dusky red. Elastic tissue is also appreciated in the lung septae.

3

Reactive Changes and Benign Lung Lesions

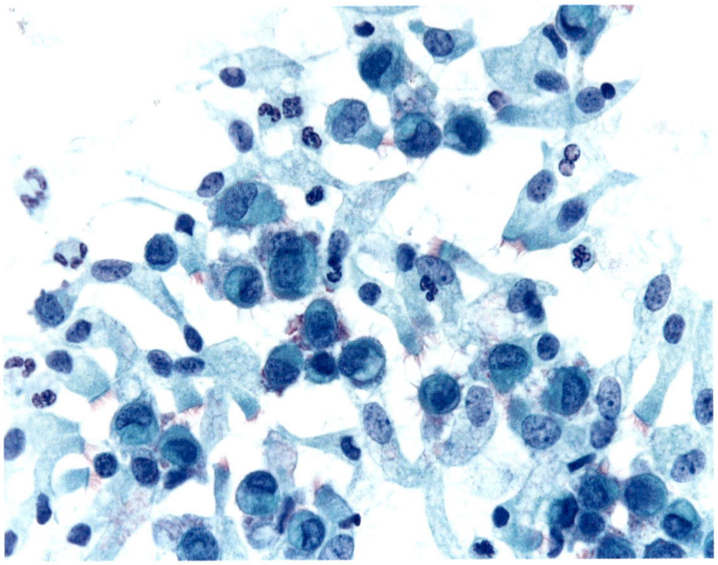

Figure 3.1a — Reactive Epithelial Cells, Bronchial Brushing [Pap Stain; High Power]. The majority of cells shown are bronchial respiratory epithelial cells, though they demonstrate various morphologies with various shapes and sizes. Some cells are round while other cells have a columnar or flask-like appearance. The nuclear-to-cytoplasmic ratios vary tremendously, with some cells appearing to have very little cytoplasm. The presence of pink cilia is evidence that these cells are benign, and is an important finding in the rounder cells that lack a distinct terminal bar.

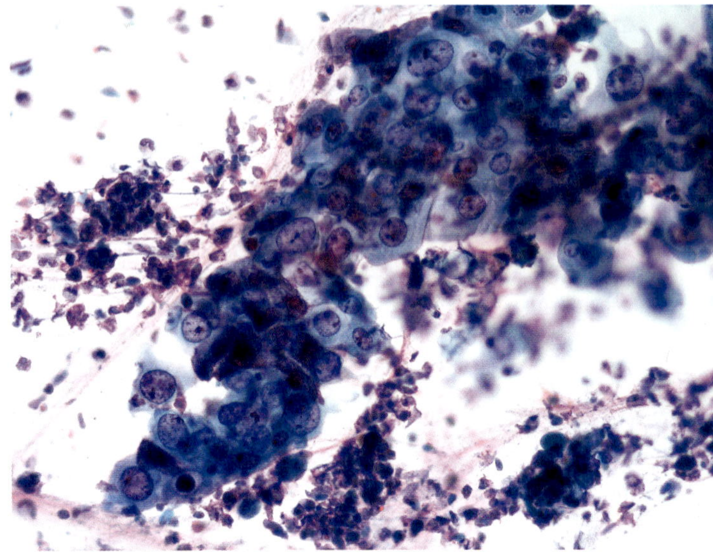

Figure 3.1b — Reactive Epithelial Cells, Bronchial Brushing [Pap Stain; High Power]. The fragment of cells in this field appears markedly atypical. Some cells have extremely large nuclei with high-to-cytoplasmic ratios and cause concern for malignancy. However, the nuclear borders are round and regular and the chromatin pattern is bland. The most reassuring finding is the presence of pink cilia at the edge of some cells, as well as a distinct terminal bar at the bottom of the field. The presence of wispy, pink mucin in the background, which can coat cells and mimic cilia, is a confounding factor. Once some cells in the fragment are determined to be benign, the remainder of the cells can be dismissed as benign as well.

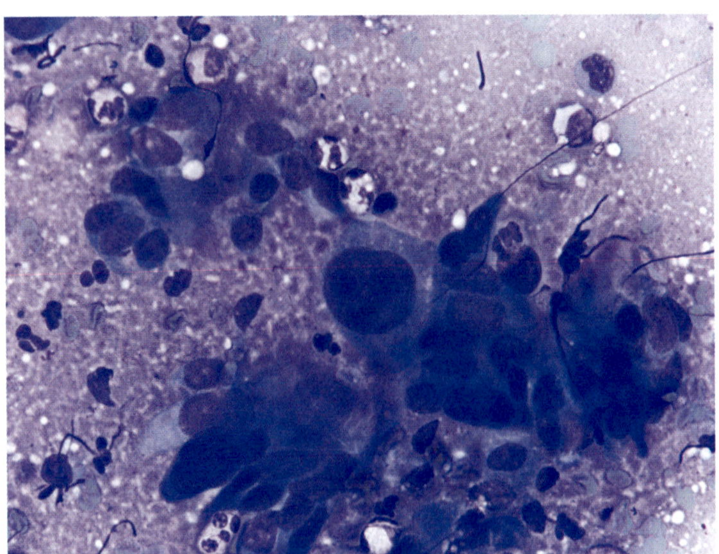

Figure 3.1c — Reactive Atypia, Bronchial Brushing [Diff-Quik Stain; High Power]. The center cell in this brushing demonstrates the dramatic reactive atypia occasionally encountered in pulmonary specimens. The adjacent glandular cells show focal nuclear overlap and enlargement with mild pleomorphism, but careful examination reveals preservation of apical cilia, suggesting benignity. Other findings in favor of a reactive atypia include the many background and epithelial-associated neutrophils and the smooth nuclear borders and even chromatin, even in the very large center cell. Dramatic atypia may be encountered after radiation and/or chemotherapy.

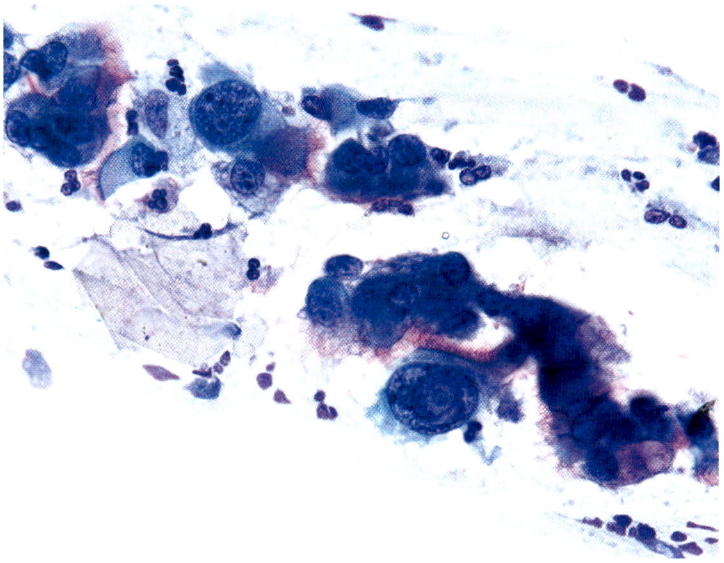

Figure 3.1d — Reactive Atypia, Bronchial Brushing [Pap Stain; High Power]. Scattered cells stand out among the more reassuringly reactive ciliated glandular background in this brush specimen. These large cells are alarming, but have a chromatin pattern identical to their reactive neighbors as well as smooth nuclear borders and both appear to have a terminal bar with cilia, providing additional reassurance. Reactive bronchial cells may also have nuclear grooves, which are visible in some cells in this image. Bronchial irritation may result in cells with nuclei 10-20x larger than seen in normal bronchial cells.

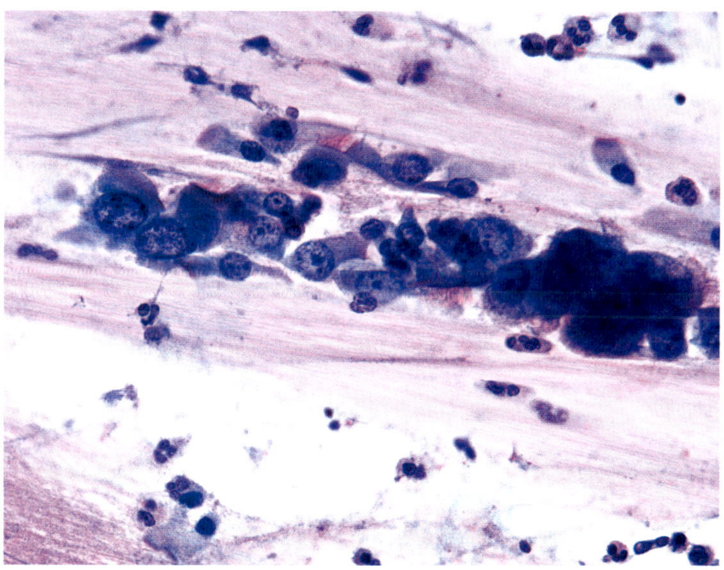

Figure 3.2a — Reactive Atypia, Bronchial Brushing [Pap Stain; High Power]. This image shows the typical features of reactive bronchial respiratory cells, chiefly nuclear enlargement, pleomorphism, coarse chromatin with prominent nucleoli, and a "jumbled" arrangement. It is important to note the presence of a terminal bar and cilia on the atypical cells, which strongly favors reactive atypia. Scattered normal bronchial cells are present in the background for comparison. Reactive atypia may be seen in any condition that causes airway irritation, including infections, prior procedures, and chronic illness.

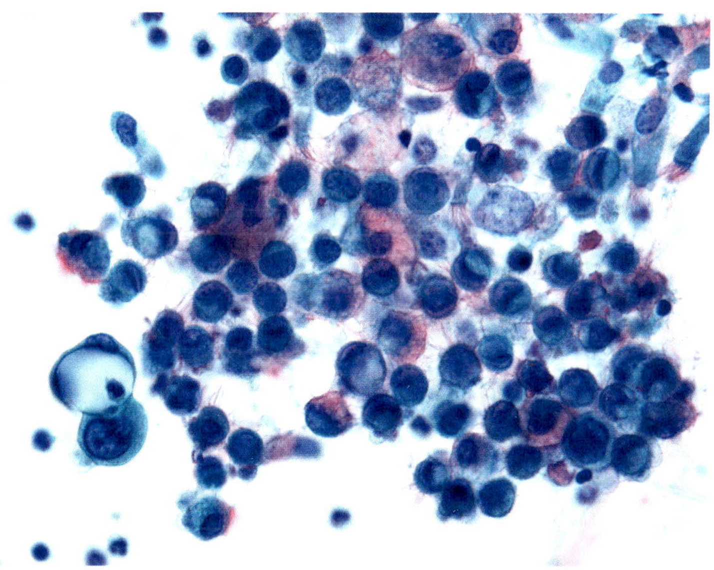

Figure 3.2b — Reactive Atypia, Bronchial Brushing [Pap Stain; High Power]. Numerous cells with swollen cytoplasm with a single vacuole are most striking in this image. While this may raise concern for adenocarcinoma, the background of reactive respiratory epithelium favors goblet cell metaplasia, a feature of chronic airway irritation. Goblet cell metaplasia may be particularly prominent in patients with cystic fibrosis.

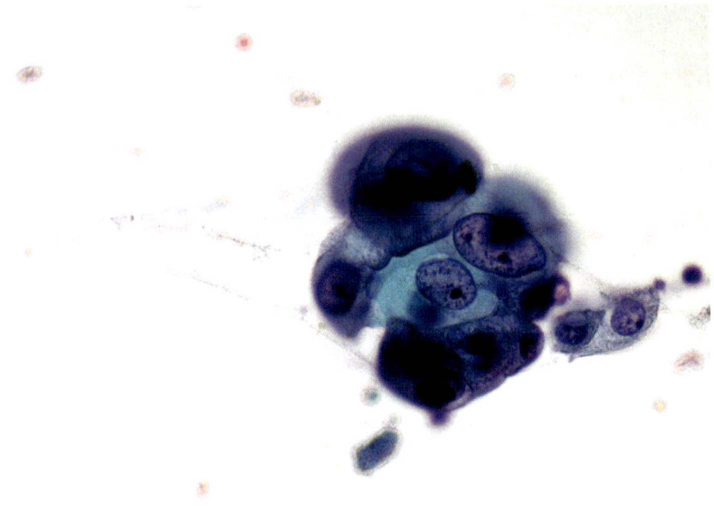

Figure 3.2c — Reactive Atypia, Bronchial Brushing [Pap Stain; High Power]. The dramatic nuclear enlargement of reactive bronchial epithelium is easily appreciated in this photograph. The nuclei in the center are several times larger than those at the periphery, and all display an open, coarsened chromatin with conspicuous nucleoli. There is a suggestion of a terminal bar in the center cells, but cilia are not easily appreciated. Immunohistochemistry cannot readily distinguish reactive from malignant cells, and careful attention to cellular details and context is crucial to avoid overdiagnosis of reactive changes as malignant.

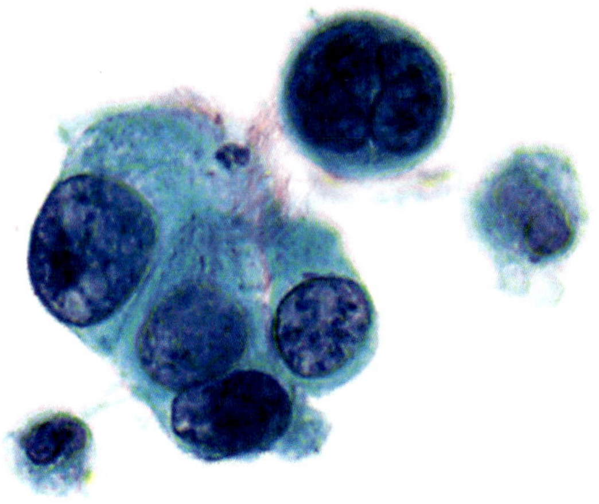

Figure 3.3a — Reactive Atypia, Bronchoalveolar Lavage [Pap Stain; High Power]. Benign bronchial cells undergo morphologic alterations to a variety of injurious stimuli including inflammatory disease, various organisms, chemoradiation, inhaled irritants, asthma, toxic fumes (including oxygen toxicity), and pharmaceutical agents. These alterations typically include a variety of nuclear changes that mimic non–small cell carcinoma including enlargement, hyperchromasia, irregular and coarse chromatin distribution, and nucleolomegaly. Bronchial cilia may become either inconspicuous or lost altogether. In this image, marked nuclear enlargement along with the appearance of a distinct nucleolus (cell at the far left) is seen. Reddish cilia are barely perceptible. These changes may occur in single cells, and also in bronchial cell clusters.

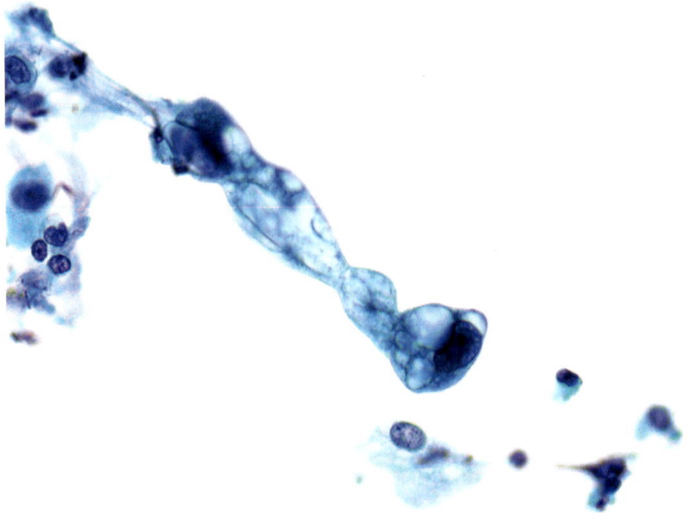

Figure 3.3b — Reactive Atypia, Bronchoalveolar Lavage [Pap Stain; High Power]. In this example of reactive atypia, two cells exhibit marked nuclear enlargement, as well as coarse cytoplasmic vacuolization reminiscent of adenocarcinoma. Clinical history and radiologic findings are critical pieces of information needed to avoid a misdiagnosis of malignancy. In a patient such as this individual with acute and diffuse lung injury and the absence of a discrete lung mass, such cells should be interpreted with caution. Sequential bronchoalveolar lavage specimens may be necessary from such patients to assure a correct diagnosis.

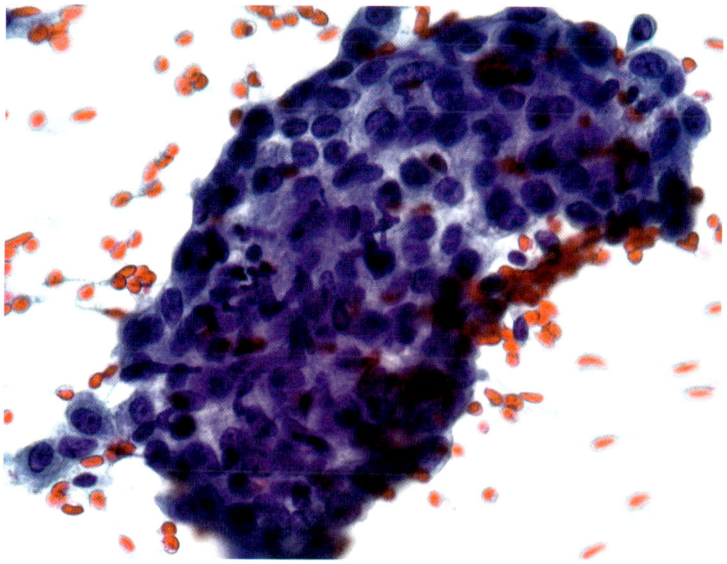

Figure 3.4a — Reactive Atypia, Fine Needle Aspiration [Pap Stain; High Power]. A cluster of reactive bronchial epithelial cells illustrates again the nuclear pleomorphism that typifies reactive atypia, but with the retention of smooth nuclear contours and a more open chromatin. The latter two features help to distinguish reactive cellular changes from malignant ones. Additionally, in reactive processes the cell-cell borders are maintained and the nuclei do not generally overlap. Architecturally, the streaming pattern and associated inflammatory cells also suggest a reactive rather than neoplastic process. Benign reactive atypia typically shows a spectrum of changes, rather than an abrupt transition.

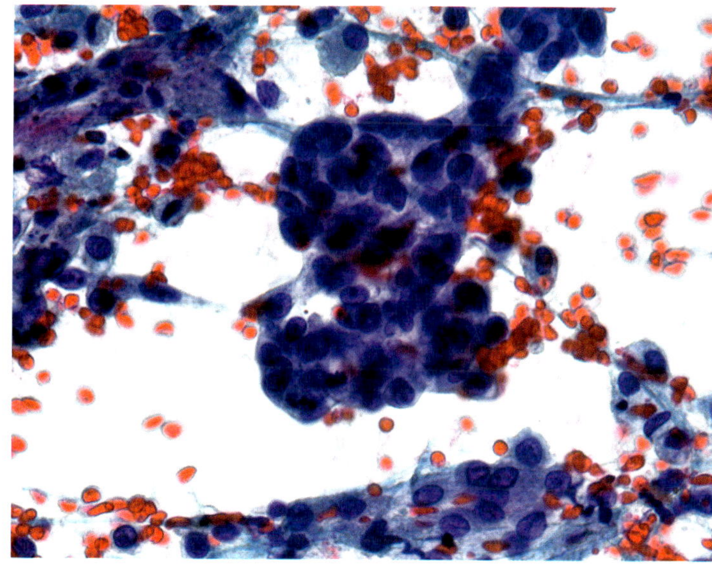

Figure 3.4b — Reactive Atypia, Fine Needle Aspiration [Pap Stain; High Power]. At first glance, the central cluster of cells is concerning for adenocarcinoma, given the prominent nuclear atypia with conspicuous nucleoli and multiple mitotic figures (lower left of the central cluster). However, the overall architecture still displays the "streaming" quality that points to reactive, rather than malignant, changes. Additionally, the nuclear changes in the center cluster are similar to those in the bottom half of the image, where the benign nature of the cells is less in question. Chronic obstructive pulmonary disease can be a cause for airway irritation and reactive cellular changes.

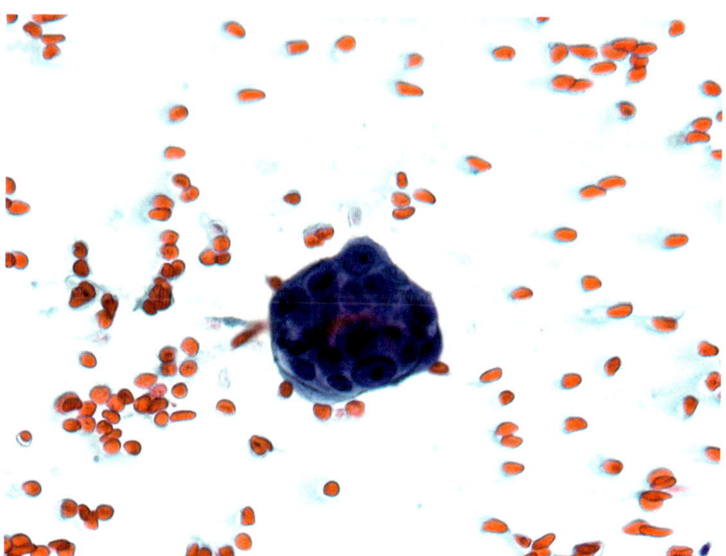

Figure 3.4c — Reactive Atypia, Fine Needle Aspiration [Pap Stain; High Power]. The cells in this small cluster from a fine needle aspiration have a wide range of reactive nuclear changes, including variable size, shape, and presence/prominence of nucleoli. The cluster is small and isolated with a clean background. The smooth nuclear contours and even, open chromatin are also well displayed. Reactive changes may also be associated with systemic chemotherapy or radiation therapy for other malignancies.

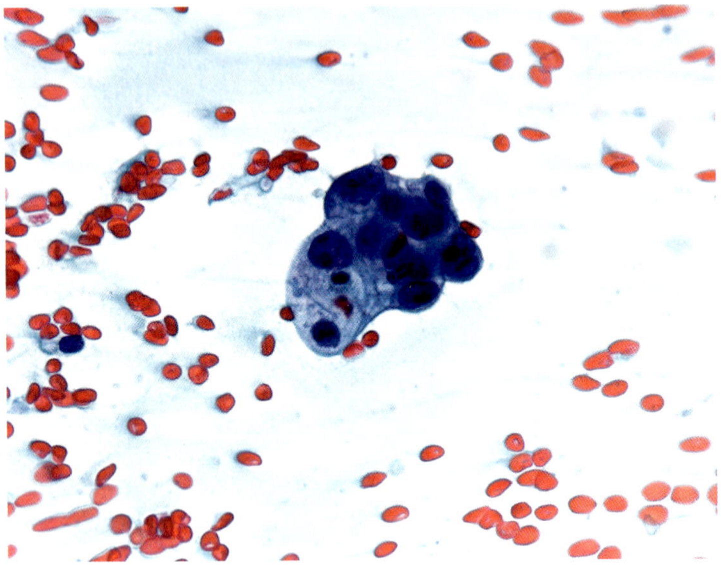

Figure 3.4d — Reactive Atypia, Fine Needle Aspiration [Pap Stain; High Power]. This image again illustrates the spectrum of changes seen in reactive cells, with enlarged nuclei with multiple nucleoli co-existing with smaller nuclei. Additional significant findings are that of an intra-epithelial neutrophil and other inflammatory cells within the cluster. The presence of inflammatory cells is reassuring of the reactive nature of the atypia, particularly if there are no other features of malignancy anywhere else in the specimen.

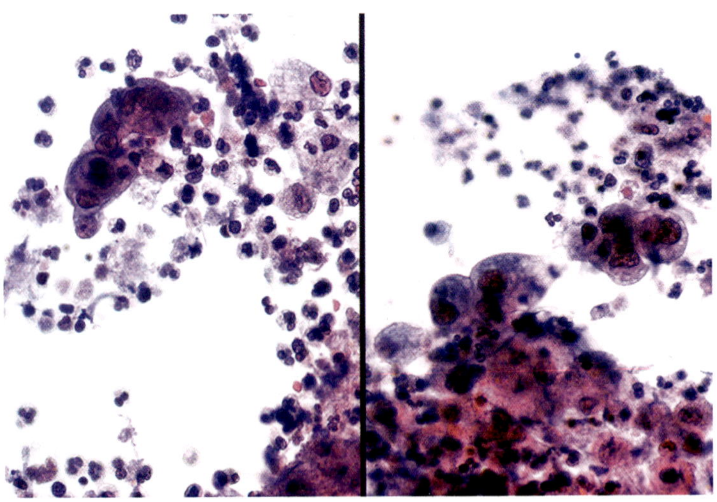

Figure 3.5a — Acute Pneumonia, Bronchoalveolar Lavage [Pap Stain; High Power]. Bronchoalveolar lavage fluid from a patient with acute pneumonia demonstrates abundant neutrophils, foamy pulmonary alveolar macrophages, and a few reactive pneumocytes. Exudative pneumonia, as seen here, is often a result of pyogenic bacteria, such as Streptococcus pneumonia.

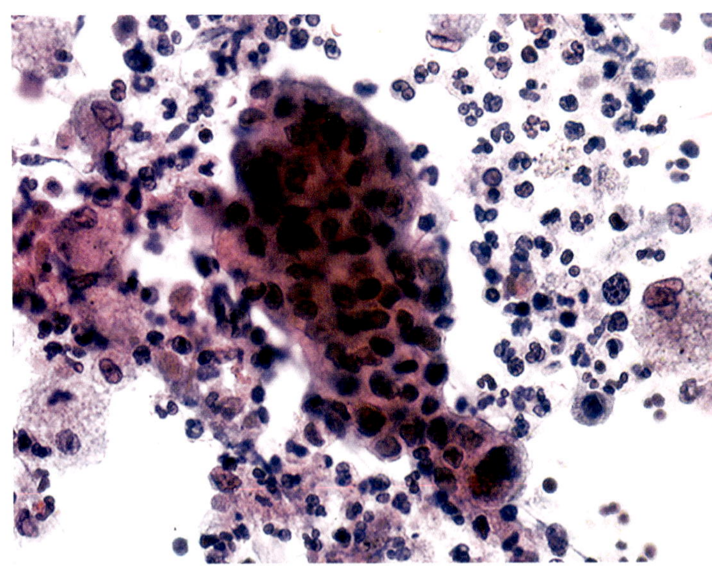

Figure 3.5b — Acute Pneumonia, Bronchoalveolar Lavage [Pap Stain; High Power]. Acute exudative pneumonia, characterized by abundant neutrophils and scattered foamy histiocytes, as well as a cohesive cluster of atypical epithelial cells. These cells likely represent reactive pneumocytes that have sloughed off, but the degree of atypia could cause concern for carcinoma. Careful attention to the background and radiographic correlation are needed.

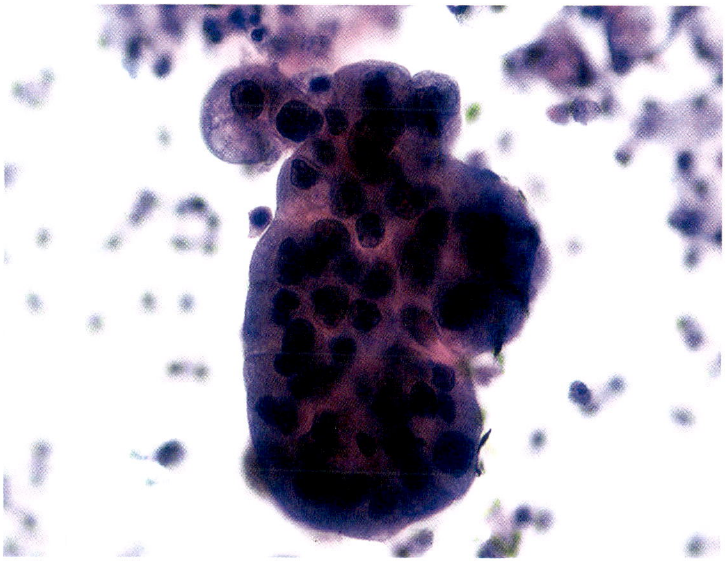

Figure 3.5c — Acute Pneumonia, Bronchoalveolar Lavage [Pap Stain; High Power]. One cluster of reactive pneumocytes demonstrates variably enlarged nuclei with occasional nucleoli. The cells maintain a relatively low nuclear-to-cytoplasmic ratio with ample vacuolated cytoplasm. At times, it may not be possible to tell whether the changes represent pneumonia superimposed on a neoplasm, or dramatic reactive changes. In such cases, repeat sampling after resolution of the acute infection may be warranted.

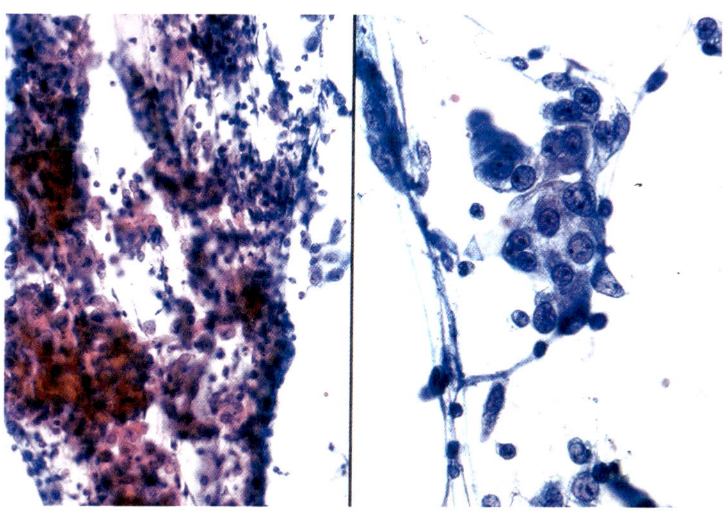

Figure 3.6a — Acute Pneumonia, Bronchial Brushing [Pap Stain; High Power]. Brushings from a patient with acute pneumonia contain clusters and aggregates of surface epithelium with admixed acute inflammation [left panel]. The striking reactive changes in the epithelial cells are evident on the right. Despite the nuclear variability and prominent nucleoli, the nuclear borders remain smooth and the nuclear-to-cytoplasmic ratio is minimally increased.

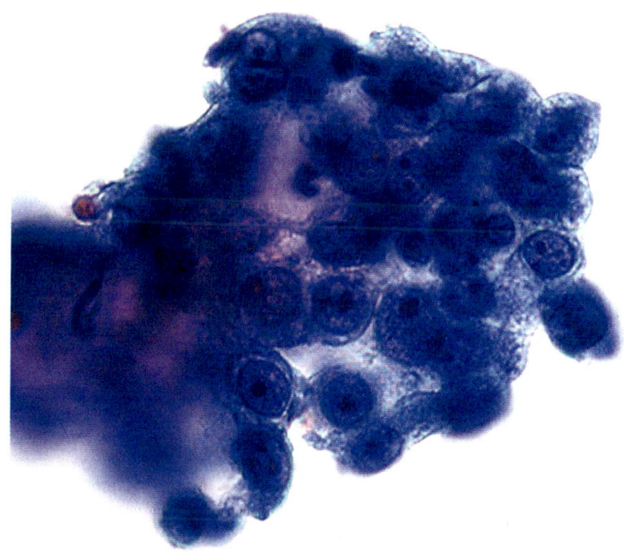

Figure 3.6b — Acute Pneumonia, Bronchial Brushing [Pap Stain; High Power]. This image gives another view of the reactive changes that can be seen in a patient with pneumonia, particularly the increased nuclear size, open chromatin, and prominent nucleoli. Features that point to a reactive process include the smooth nuclear borders and the preserved cell-cell borders.

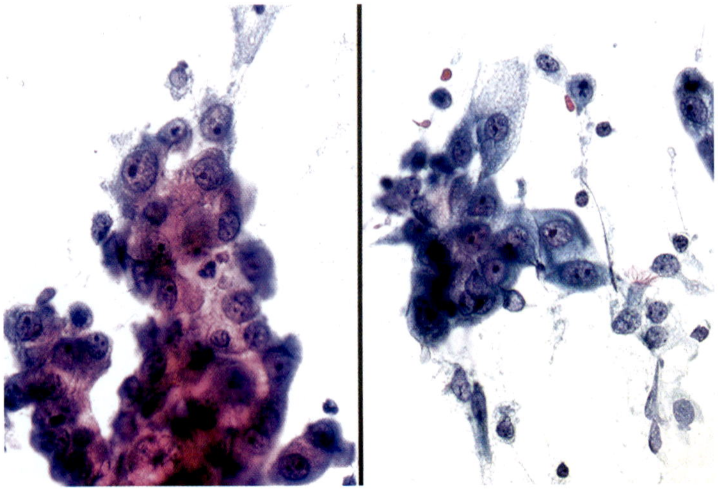

Figure 3.6c — Acute Pneumonia, Bronchial Brushing [Pap Stain; High Power]. The striking atypia that can accompany an infectious pneumonia is again visible. The panel on the left contains a cohesive cluster of reactive bronchial epithelium, with vacuolated cytoplasm, enlarged nuclei, and nucleoli. The right hand panel has at the center-right a ciliated benign bronchial epithelial cell for comparison. This internal control shows how enlarged the reactive cells may be.

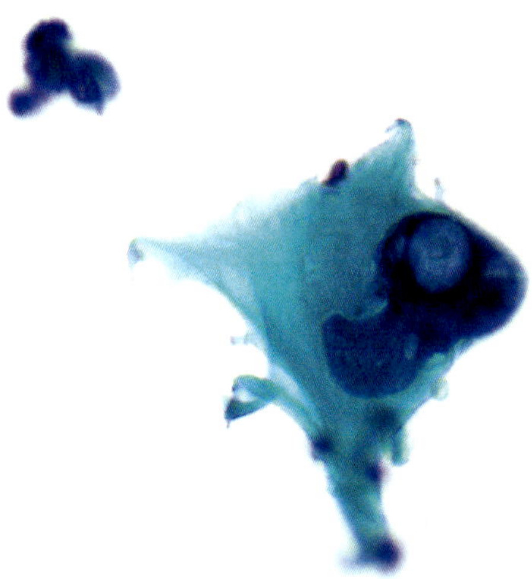

Figure 3.7 — Radiation-Induced Atypia, Bronchoalveolar Lavage [Pap Stain; High Power]. Radiation to the lung occurs as treatment for a variety of malignancies, for preconditioning prior to bone marrow transplantation, or less often from environmental exposure. Injury may be acute or chronic. Its effects on the cytomorphology of bronchial cells and pneumocytes are similar. These effects typically affect individual single cells, and include marked nuclear enlargement, often bizarre nuclear pleomorphism, intracytoplasmic and even intranuclear vacuolization (as seen in this cell), and multinucleation. Because cytoplasmic enlargement also occurs, the nuclear-cytoplasmic ratio is often preserved. Though not present in this image, cytoplasmic polychromasia is another manifestation of radiation-induced cellular atypia.

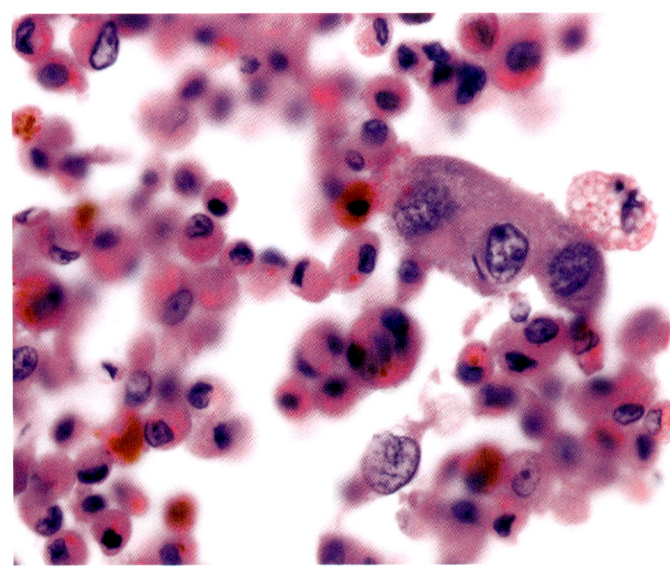

Figure 3.8a — Busulfan Treatment Effect, Bronchoalveolar Lavage [H&E Stain; High Power]. Busulfan is an alkyl sulfonate chemotherapeutic agent used to treat some hematopoietic malignancies and as a conditioning agent prior to bone marrow transplant. Interstitial pulmonary fibrosis ("busulfan lung") is one toxic side effect seen in patients treated with busulfan. Busulfan can also cause atypical cytologic changes throughout the body, including nuclear enlargement, irregular nuclear borders, coarsely granular chromatin, macronucleoli, and cytoplasmic vacuolization. Seen here on a cell block preparation, atypical epithelioid cells with enlarged nuclei and an irregular chromatin pattern stand out in a background of macrophages and inflammatory cells.

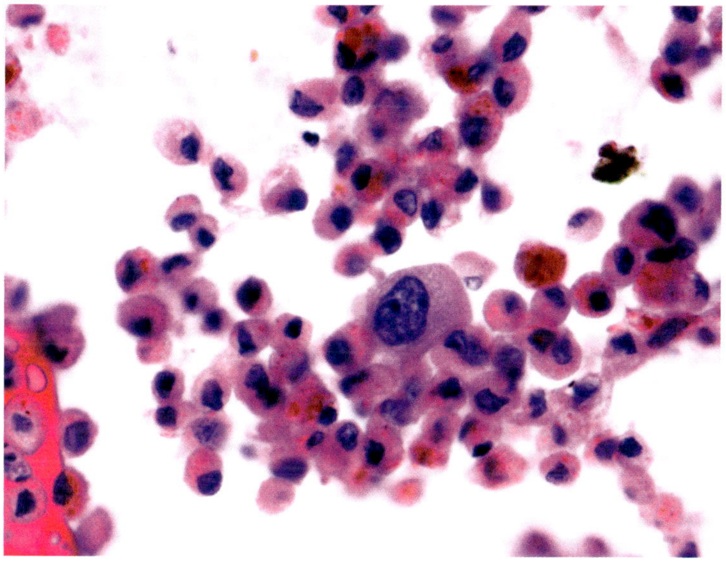

Figure 3.8b — Busulfan Treatment Effect, Bronchoalveolar Lavage [H&E Stain; High Power]. Cancer patients may be immunosuppressed and susceptible to lung infections. Bronchoalveolar lavages may be taken for the purposes of culture, with radiation and/or chemotherapy-induced changes seen in the specimen. If the history is unknown, these cells may be suspicious for dysplasia and/or malignancy. In this case, the atypical cell has a large amount of cytoplasm in spite of its enlarged nucleus with irregular borders and coarse chromatin.

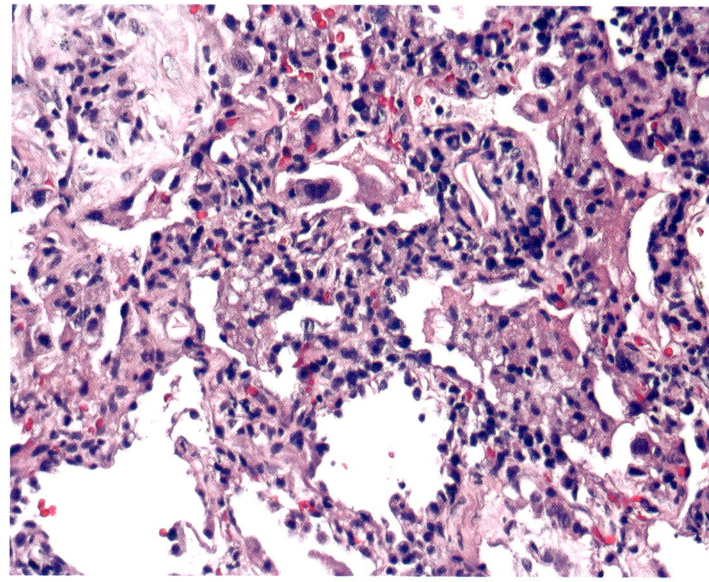

Figure 3.8c — Chemotherapy-Induced Atypia, Biopsy [H&E Stain; High Power]. Reparative changes in the setting of chemotherapy may be associated with mass-like consolidation, and may have overlapping cytologic features with malignancy, as in this lung section. Epithelial cells are enlarged, with maintenance of the nuclear-to-cytoplasmic ratio (cytomegaly). There is nuclear pleomorphism and variable hyperchromasia; nucleoli are frequent. In some instances, mitoses may be readily identified. The interstitium contains a lymphoplasmacytic infiltrate with foamy histiocytes, and organizing pneumonia is present at the upper left. In contrast, the component cells of a malignant process manifest coarser chromatin and significant nuclear membrane irregularities; inflammation may be present, but the neoplastic cells predominate. An additional consideration is viral infection, from which chemotherapy effect cannot be confidently distinguished without viral diagnostic studies.

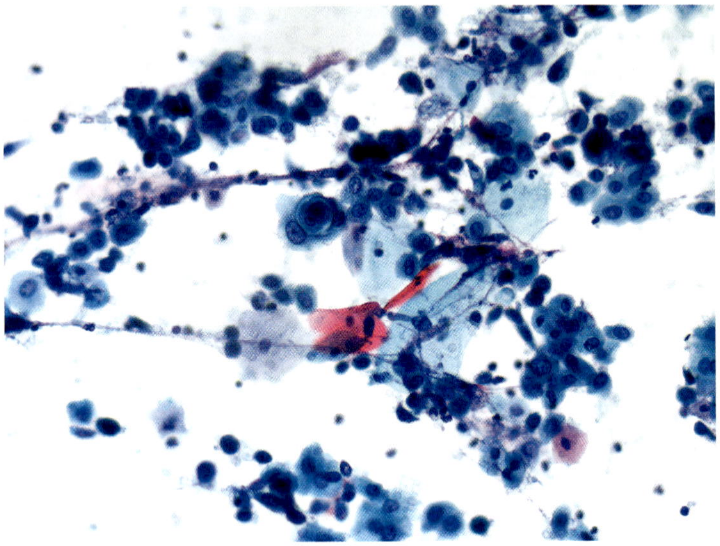

Figure 3.9a — Squamous Metaplasia, Sputum [Pap Stain; High Power]. The tracheobronchial mucosa may undergo squamous metaplasia in response to a variety of insults. The unexpected presence of cells with dense, squamoid cytoplasm and orangeophilic keratinization may cause the consideration of a dysplastic squamous lesion or even squamous cell carcinoma. Here, the formation of a squamous pearl can be seen in the center of the field. Metaplastic squamous cells can be seen in the background; they are slightly hyperchromatic, but have regular nuclear borders and low nuclear-to-cytoplasmic ratios. Irregular cytoplasmic extensions, often seen in squamous cell carcinoma, are absent, and there is minimal size variation among the nuclei. Squamous metaplasia may be seen in bronchial brushings and washings, sputum specimens, and bronchoalveolar lavages.

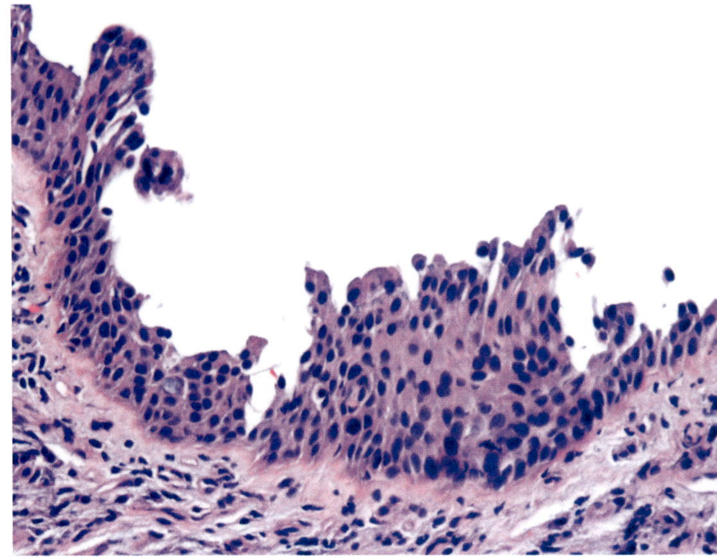

Figure 3.9b — Squamous Metaplasia of Bronchus, Endobronchial Biopsy [H&E Stain; Low Power]. This mucosal surface shows incomplete immature squamous metaplastic replacement of the respiratory epithelium in this endobronchial biopsy. The surface cells retain a columnar cytology, and there is a residual mucin vacuole at the lower left. Squamous metaplasia develops in the bronchial mucosa of smokers; while it may be an early preneoplastic change, it may persist for years without progression, and can regress with smoking cessation.

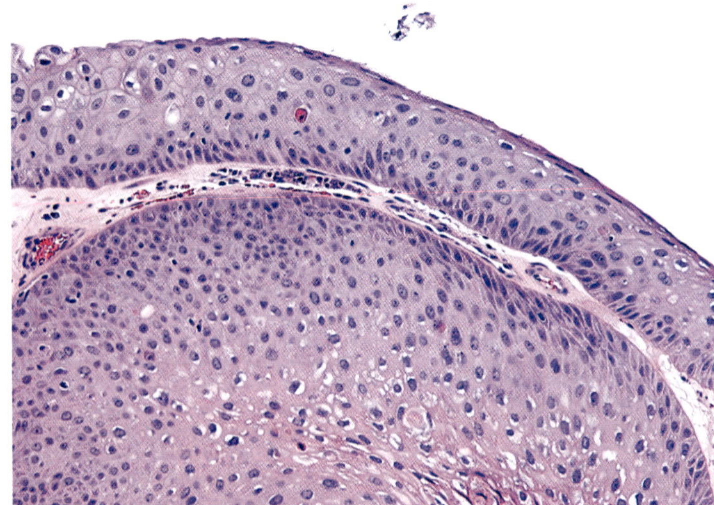

Figure 3.9c — Mild Squamous Dysplasia, Endobronchial Biopsy [H&E Stain; Low Power]. This squamous metaplastic process has completely replaced the respiratory epithelium, and extends into the subepithelial duct below. Mild dysplasia is defined by acanthosis, mild anisocytosis and pleomorphism, and expansion of the basilar zone to fill the bottom one third of the epithelium, with surface maturation and a virtual absence of mitoses above the basal layer.

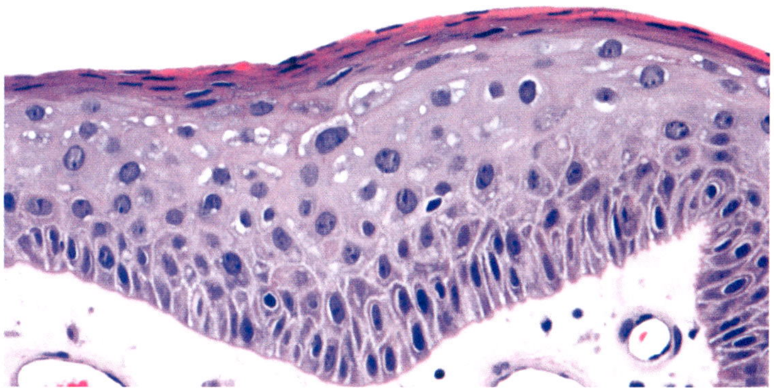

Figure 3.9d — Mild Squamous Dysplasia, Endobronchial Biopsy [H&E Stain; High Power]. Higher magnification shows vertical orientation of the cells in the lower one third of the epithelium, a well-defined intermediate/"prickly" zone, and surface maturation with slight parakeratosis. Such changes are not uncommon in the bronchi of smokers, and may give rise to false-positive lymph node transbronchial needle aspiration specimens if traversed to access the node.

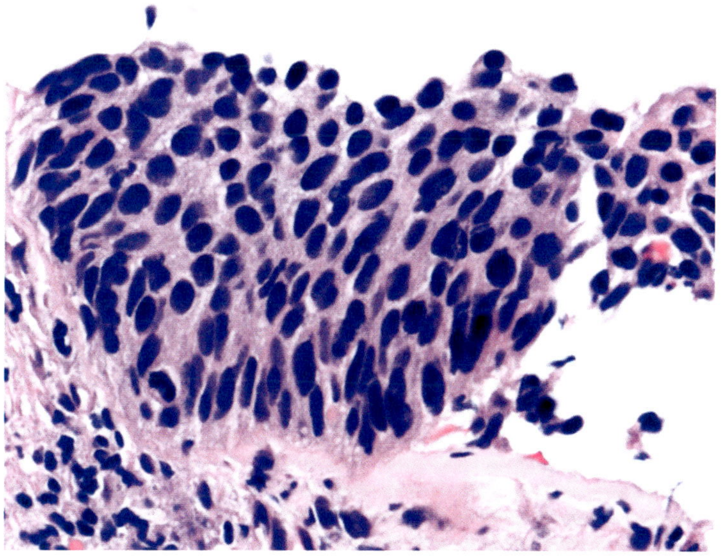

Figure 3.9e — Squamous Cell Carcinoma in Situ, Endobronchial Biopsy [H&E Stain; High Power]. There is full-thickness replacement of the epithelium by immature squamous cells, with vertical orientation of densely hyperchromatic nuclei throughout the lesion. Similar mucosal changes may be present in patients with bronchogenic carcinomas of all histologic subtypes; inadvertent sampling of such a mucosal lesion (brushing, transbronchial needle aspiration, fragmented biopsy) may contribute to confusion about the histologic subtype of an adjacent adenocarcinoma or small cell carcinoma.

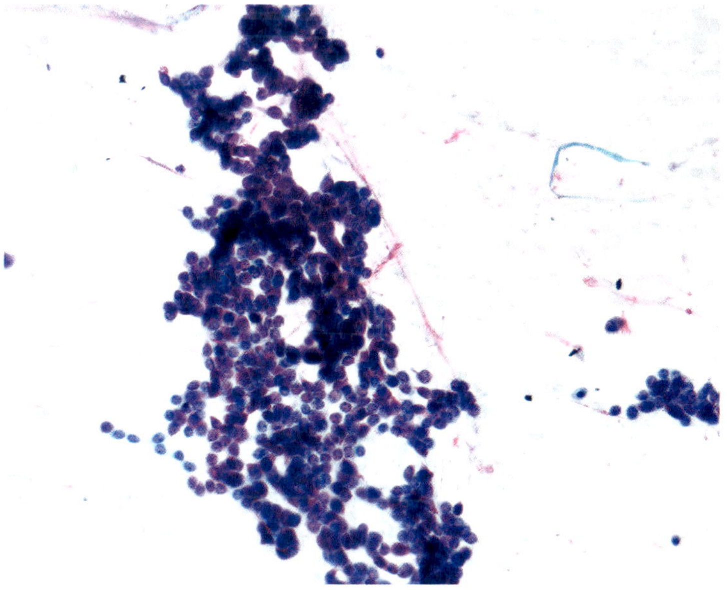

Figure 3.10a — Reserve Cell Hyperplasia, Bronchial Brushing [Pap Stain; Medium Power]. Bronchial reserve cells proliferate as a reaction to injury to the surface epithelium. In some instances, the proliferation can be quite exhuberant and mimic a neoplastic process. Reserve cells are typically small and have high nuclear-to-cytoplasmic ratios. This can result in an impression of small cell carcinoma.

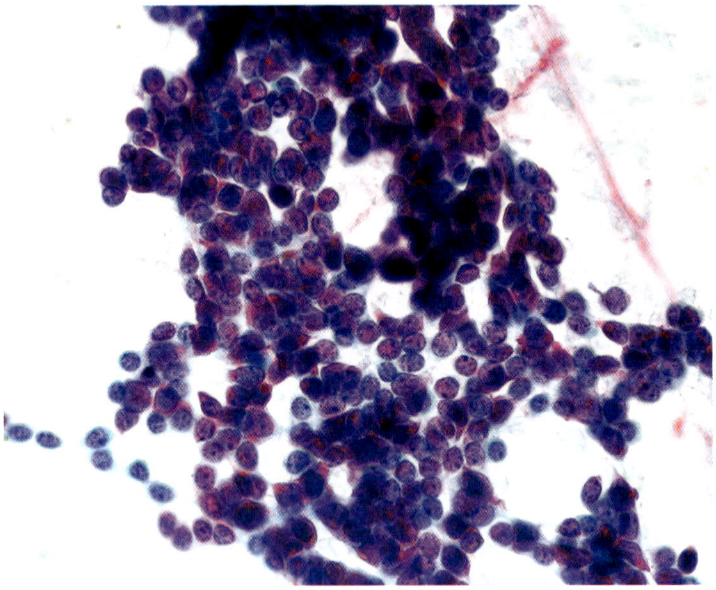

Figure 3.10b — Reserve Cell Hyperplasia, Bronchial Brushing [Pap Stain; Medium Power]. On closer examination, reserve cells have a bland chromatin pattern and may possess small chromocenters. While nuclei may appear to mold against each other, a feature of small cell carcinoma, there is little nuclear size variation, an absence of karyorrhexis and mitotic figures, and lack of the "smearing artifact" often seen in small cell carcinomas.

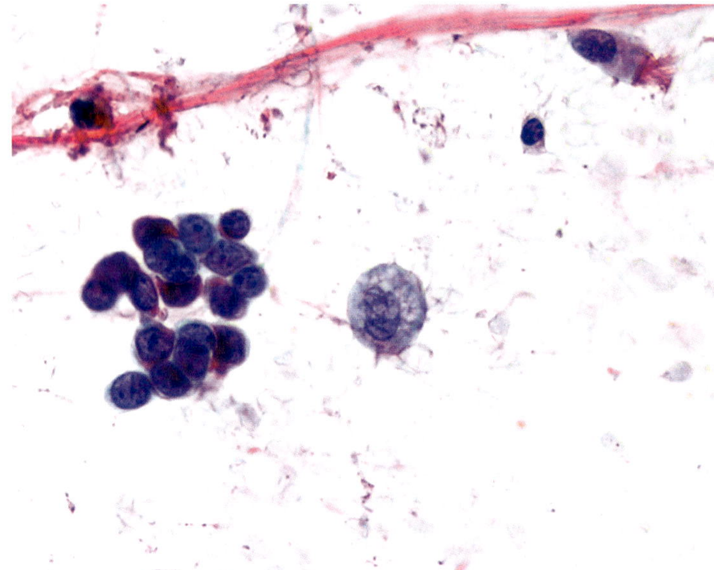

Figure 3.10c — Reserve Cell Hyperplasia, Bronchial Brushing [Pap Stain; Medium Power]. The small size of the cells can be compared to the ciliated bronchial respiratory epithelial cell and pulmonary alveolar macrophage also seen in the field. In many instances, reserve cell hyperplasia is a focal finding, and recognizing these cells allows one to dismiss them as likely benign rather than representing the focal sampling of a small cell carcinoma.

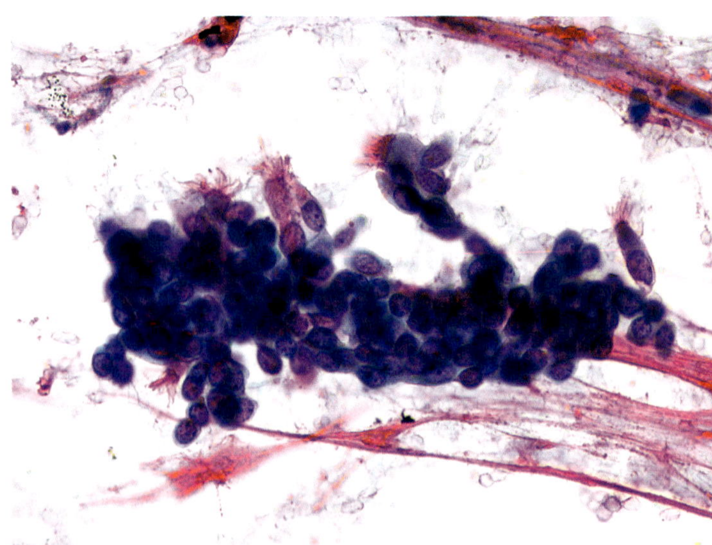

Figure 3.10d — Reserve Cell Hyperplasia, Bronchial Brushing [Pap Stain; Medium Power]. If more fields are examined, reserve cells in association with overlying ciliated respiratory epithelial cells may be observed. This confirms that the small cells are benign. Note the similarity in chromatin quality and nuclear size between the ciliated cells and the reserve cells. The reserve cells simply do not have cilia and contain much less cytoplasm than the overlying epithelial cells.

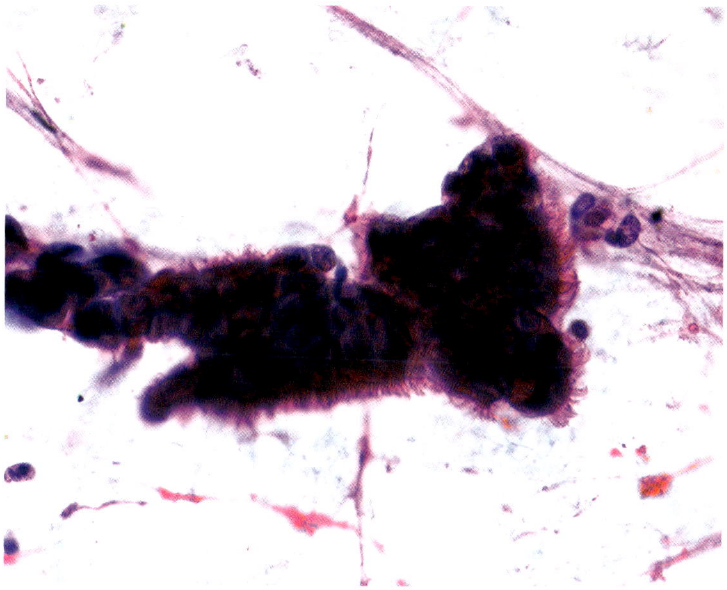

Figure 3.11a — Reserve Cell Hyperplasia, Bronchial Brushing [Pap Stain; Medium Power]. There is no question that this fragment is benign, as the edges clearly contain abundant cilia. However, note the crowded and hyperchromatic nature of the cells in the middle of the fragment, in this case representing reserve cell hyperplasia. If the cilia is not clearly identified, the flat terminal bars may suggest these are benign cells. Otherwise, they would be suspicious for a carcinoma.

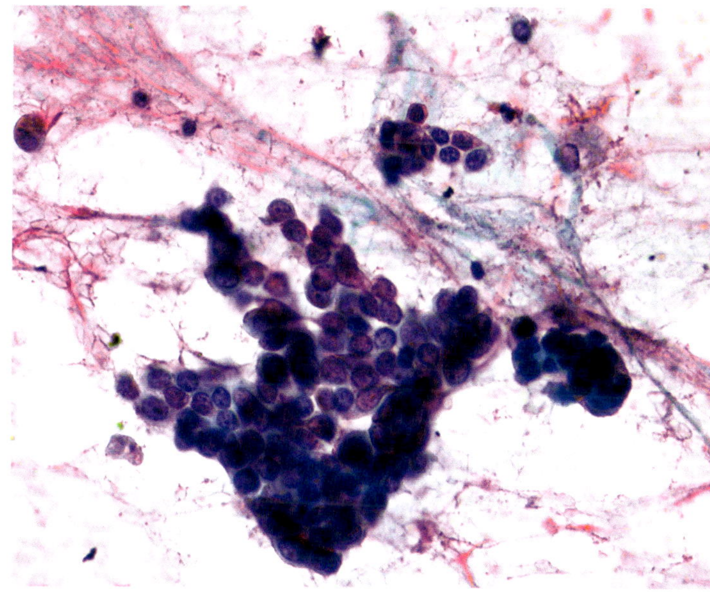

Figure 3.11b — Reserve Cell Hyperplasia, Bronchial Brushing [Pap Stain; Medium Power]. Here cilia is not clearly identified on cells that are likely benign bronchial respiratory epithelial cells, given the flat edge seen at the bottom of the field. The multi-layered nature of the fragment suggests that there is also a proliferation of reserve cells, though here the nuclei do not overlap as much and the differential diagnosis may include an adenocarcinoma rather than a small cell carcinoma. Note the bland nature of the chromatin, which suggests these are not malignant cells.

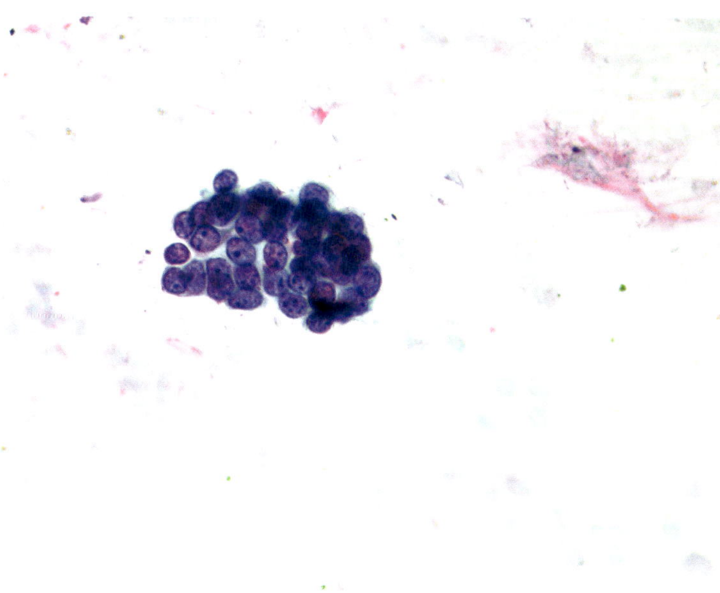

Figure 3.11c — Reserve Cell Hyperplasia, Bronchial Brushing [Pap Stain; Medium Power]. These reserve cells have very little cytoplasm but the chromatin makes a misdiagnosis of small cell carcinoma unlikely. The differential diagnosis should include a well-differentiated adenocarcinoma resulting in a careful review of the entire specimen and clinicoradiologic impression.

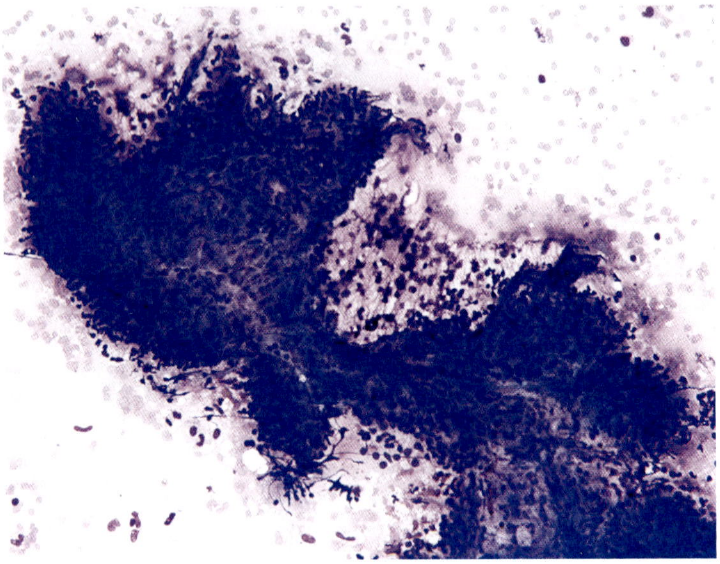

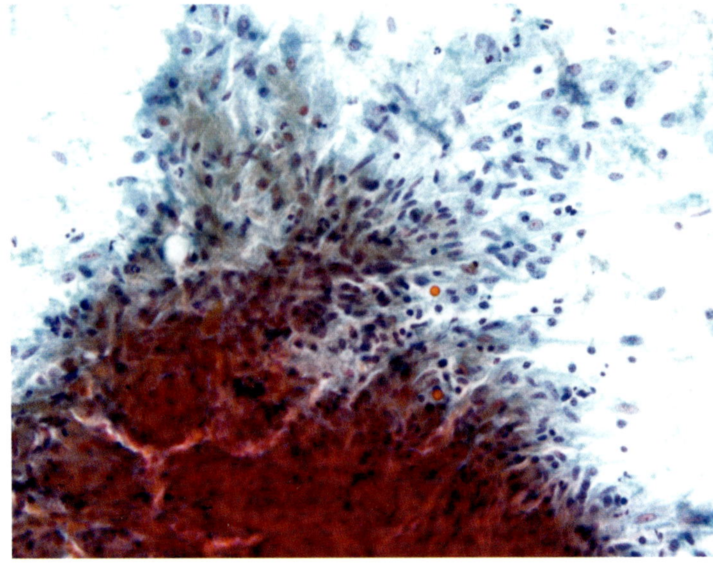

Figure 3.12a — Nonnecrotizing Granuloma [Diff-Quik Stain; Low Power]. Granulomatous inflammation in the lung occurs as a response to infectious disease, the presence of foreign material, and idiopathic causes. Of the latter, pulmonary sarcoidosis is one of the more commonly encountered in cytopathology with more than 90% of sarcoidosis patients having some form of pulmonary involvement. Patients with parenchymal disease may or may not have hilar adenopathy. Nonnecrotizing granulomas in fine needle aspiration smears from endobronchial ultrasound-guided procedures or transbronchial needle aspirates are scattered as individual fragments of variable size and shape. As in this image, these are tightly clustered, often in 3-dimensional microfragments due to their high cellularity of epithelioid histiocytes. Lymphocytes commonly accompany these clusters, and on occasion multinucleated giant cells are seen. By definition, other causes of granulomatous inflammation such as fungi, acid-fast bacilli, and parasitic infection must be excluded.

Figure 3.12b — Nonnecrotizing Granuloma [Pap Stain; Medium Power]. Sarcoidosis is a worldwide disease affecting all races and nearly all ages. At the edge of this nonnecrotizing granuloma, a syncytial cluster of epithelioid histiocytes displays nuclear features of hypo-or euchromasia, oval and elliptical/spindled nuclei, and evenly dispersed chromatin. The moderately abundant interdigitating cytoplasm creates a syncytial cell cluster. Although a few small lymphocytes are present near the top of this image, a necrotizing acute inflammatory infiltrate and cellular necrosis are absent.

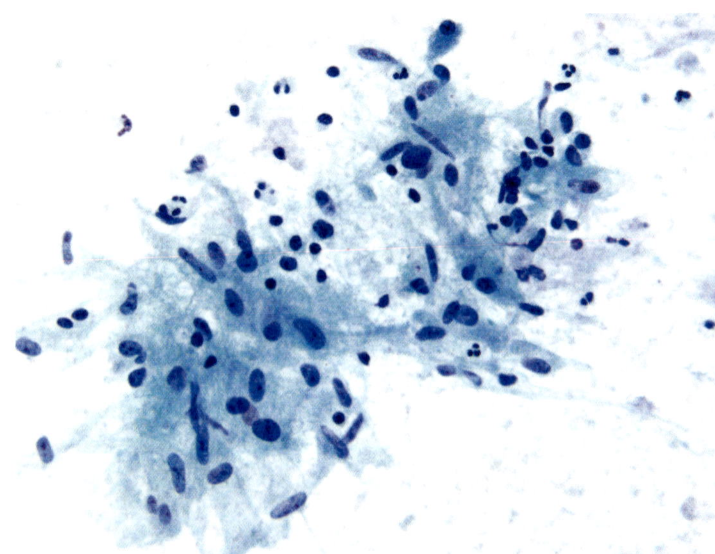

Figure 3.12c — Nonnecrotizing Granuloma [Pap Stain; High Power]. High power of a much more loosely clustered collection of epithelioid histiocytes emphasizes the large size of these cells, as well as their characteristic elongated/elliptical nuclear contour. A number of fanciful adjectives have been ascribed to the nuclei of these cells including "boomerang," "banana," and "footprint in the sand" shape because a percentage of them have a slight indentation on one side of the nucleus producing this contour. Notice the variation in size of these nonnecrotizing granulomas when comparing this image with Figure 3.12a. A major differential diagnostic consideration of nonnecrotizing granulomas when they are this small and one is sampling mediastinal lymph nodes is to distinguish them from dendritic-lymphocytic aggregates. Dendritic cells have long cytoplasmic processes as seen here, but lack the elongated, often indented nuclei of epithelioid histiocytes.

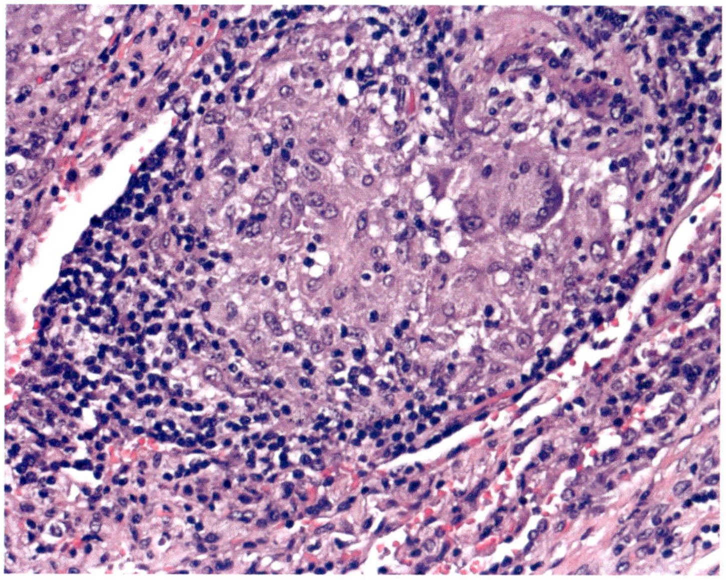

Figure 3.12d — Granuloma, Biopsy [H&E Stain; High Power]. This well-formed granuloma consists of an aggregate of macrophages with abundant vacuolated eosinophilic cytoplasm ("epithelioid" change), bean-shaped nuclei with open chromatin, and crisp dot-like nucleoli; a nuclear fold may be present. A multinucleated macrophage (giant cell) is near the right edge of the granuloma. There is a peripheral rim of lymphocytes with admixed plasma cells. Organism stains may reveal an etiology. In small biopsies and cytologic specimens, differential considerations include neuroendocrine tumorlet (higher nuclear-to-cytoplasmic ratio, less open chromatin, synaptophysin- and chromogranin-positive), primary and metastatic epithelioid neoplasms (keratins, others), and meningothelial nodule (whorled; epithelial membrane antigen- and progesterone receptor-positive, synaptophysin-negative).

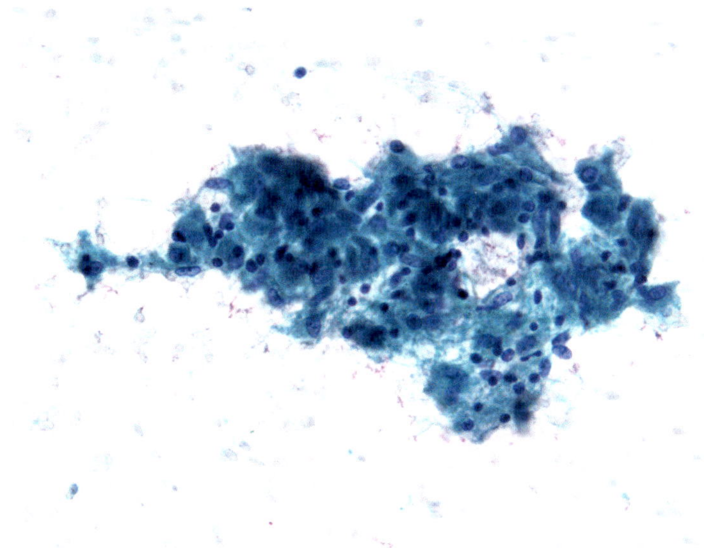

Figure 3.13a — Sarcoidosis, Fine Needle Aspiration [Pap Stain; Medium Power]. The granulomatous inflammation pictured consists of epithelioid histiocytes with an even admixture of small lymphocytes. The histiocytes are arranged in tight aggregates with grungy-appearing cytoplasm but no background necrotic debris. The differential diagnosis includes infection, inhalation of other foreign materials, and interstitial lung diseases. The diagnosis of sarcoidosis is based on both clinical and pathologic findings, and infection must be excluded before the diagnosis can be made.

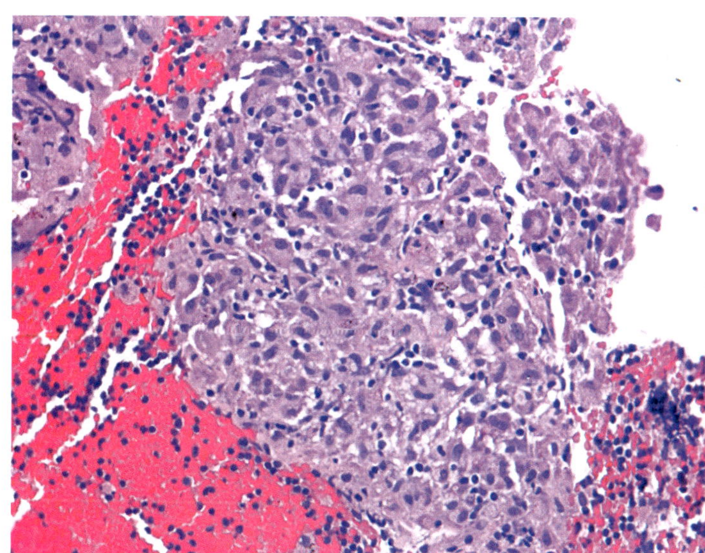

Figure 3.13b — Sarcoidosis, Fine Needle Aspiration [H&E Stain; Medium Power]. This cell block image shows the typical histologic features of sarcoid-type granulomas: epithelioid histiocytes admixed with lymphocytes in small, nonnecrotizing aggregates. The histocytes have abundant pink cytoplasm with some pigment inclusions seen in this image. Sarcoidosis typically affects young females, with a predilection for African-Americans.

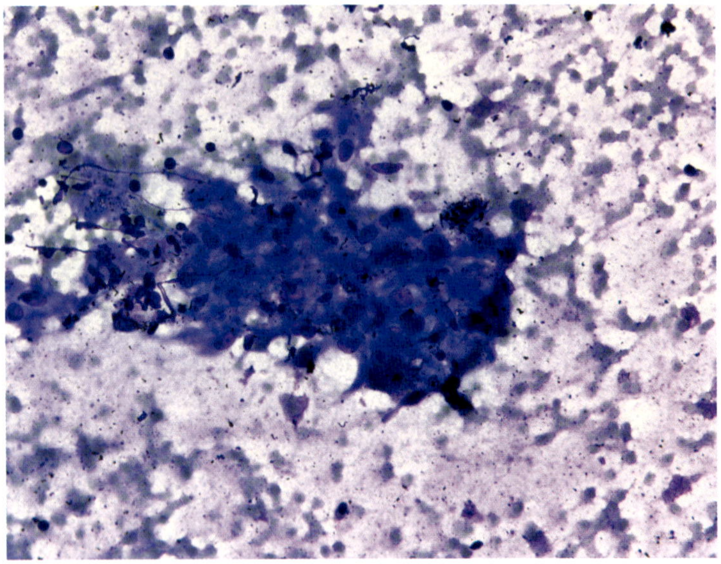

Figure 3.13c — Sarcoidosis, Fine Needle Aspiration [Diff-Quik Stain; High Power]. This Diff-Quik stained smear shows a single epithelioid granuloma from a patient with sarcoidosis. Numerous crushed lymphocytes can be appreciated as fine dark blue streaks among the histocyte nuclei. The background is remarkable for the absence of necrosis and presence of only scattered small lymphocytes. In the lung, sarcoidosis may present with hilar adenopathy, with or without small pulmonary nodules, but over time may progress to pulmonary fibrosis.

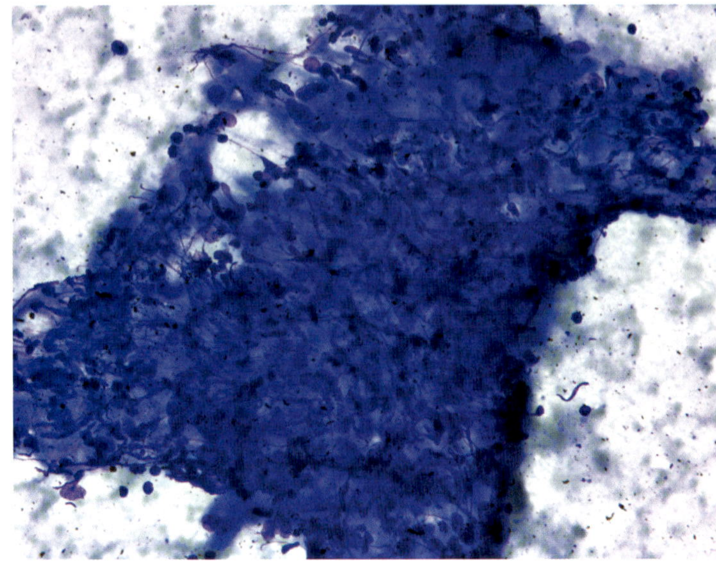

Figure 3.13d — Sarcoidosis, Fine Needle Aspiration [Diff-Quik Stain; High Power]. This high power view shows the oval histiocyte nuclei interspersed among "crushed" lymphocytes. These nuclei are most readily appreciated along the perimeter of this aggregate, and are recognizable by their round to oval shape, open chromatin, and single nucleolus. Giant cells may be a feature seen in sarcoid-associated granulomas, although not appreciated in this image. Sarcoidosis is often a systemic disease, and can affect liver, lung, spleen, bone, and skin, among others.

Figure 3.14a — Sarcoidosis, Fine Needle Aspiration [H&E Stain; Medium Power]. This cell block image shows again the histologic features of sarcoidosis-associated granulomas: tight, epithelioid histiocytes with pink cytoplasm, associated lymphocytic infiltrate composed primarily of T cells, and no evidence of necrosis. Asteroid bodies, the poetic term for stellate inclusions within giant cells, may be seen in cases of sarcoidosis, but are not specific to the diagnosis. Anthracotic pigment may also be seen within the histiocytes of sarcoidosis. The etiology of sarcoidosis remains unknown at present, but sarcoidosis may arise due to an altered immune response to an environmental exposure.

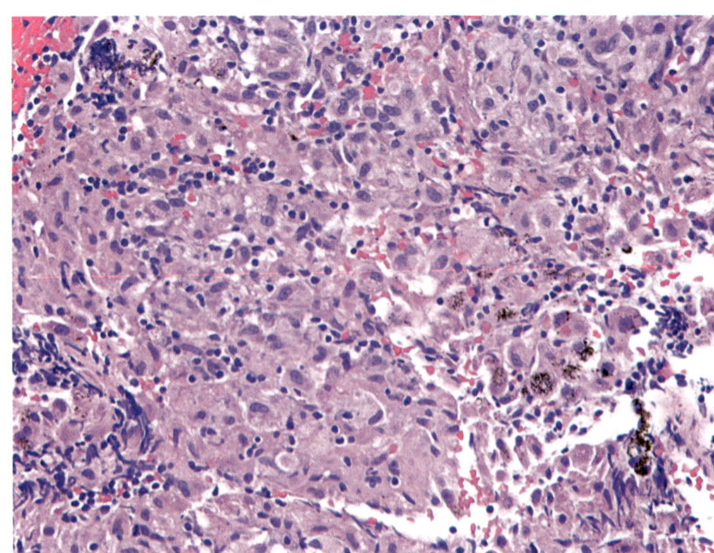

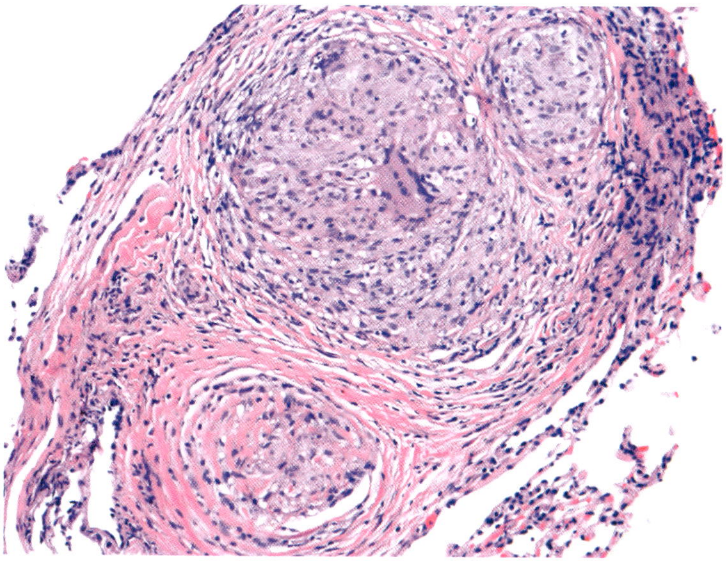

Figure 3.14b — Sarcoidosis, Transbronchial Biopsy [H&E Stain; Low Power]. A peribronchilar cluster of three nonnecrotizing epithelioid granulomas shows the typical features of sarcoidosis in a transbronchial biopsy. Two multinucleated cells are present in the largest granuloma. A rim of scar tissue is present around the granuloma at the bottom. As granulomas coalesce and scar, nodules of a centimeter or more may result, occasionally mimicking mass lesions. Granulomatous infections should always be excluded with stains and cultures.

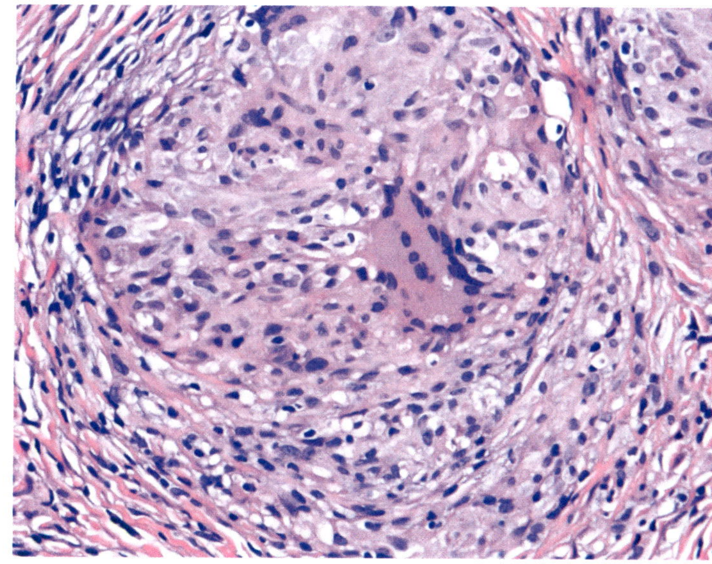

Figure 3.14c — Sarcoidosis, Transbronchial Biopsy [H&E Stain; High Power]. The component histiocytes of sarcoid granulomas have abundant eosinophilic cytoplasm and plump, open nuclei (hence the term "epithelioid"). In fine needle aspirations or exfoliative samples, they may mimic epithelial processes, including carcinoma. Epithelioid histiocytes have elongated or bean-shaped nuclei, often grooved, and abundant vacuolated cytoplasm; mitoses are rare. Immunohistochemical stains (CD68+, keratin-) can be helpful in equivocal cases.

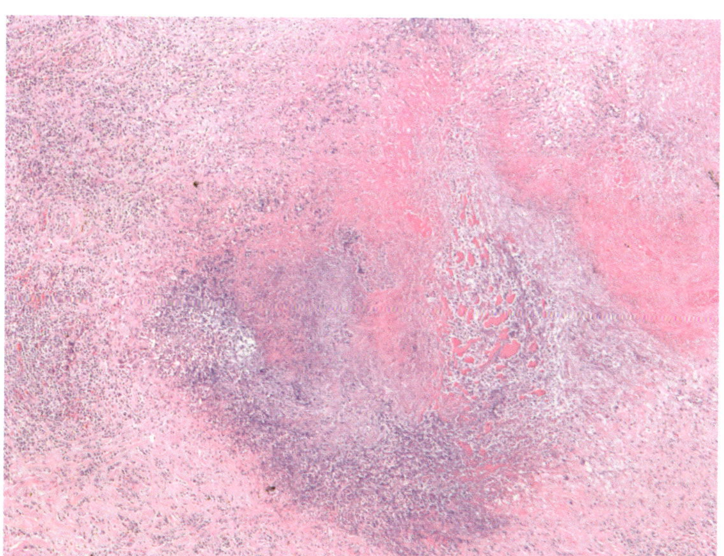

Figure 3.15a — Rheumatoid Nodule, Transbronchial Biopsy [H&E Stain; Low Power]. This rheumatoid nodule has a geographic, necrobiotic center and an incomplete rim of palisading histiocytes. An outer rim of mixed lymphocytes is present at left. Adjacent lymphocytic angiitis may occasionally be demonstrable. Rheumatoid nodules are almost always subpleural. Granulomatous infection must be assiduously excluded; a mycobacterial polymerase chain reaction may be required in some cases.

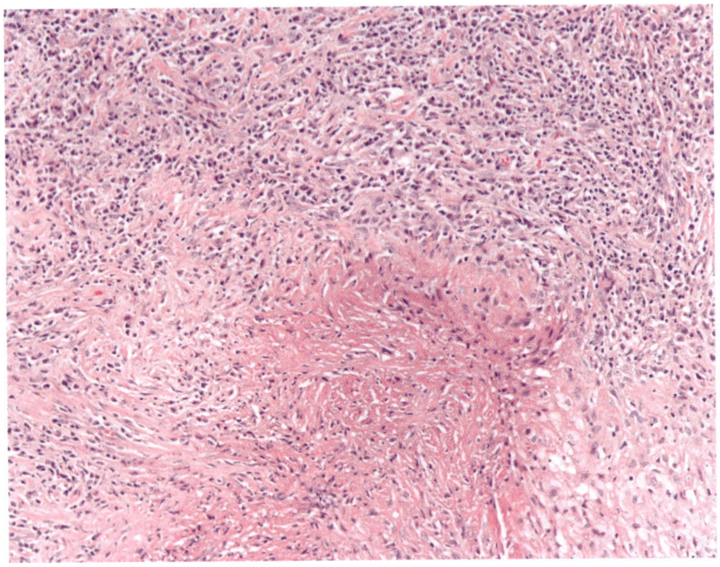

Figure 3.15b — Rheumatoid Nodule, Wedge Biopsy [H&E Stain; High Power]. An area of impending necrobiosis is hypereosinophilic. A focus of palisading histiocytes is present, just left of the center. A multinucleated histiocyte is present at right of the center. The outer rim of lymphocytes is at the top.

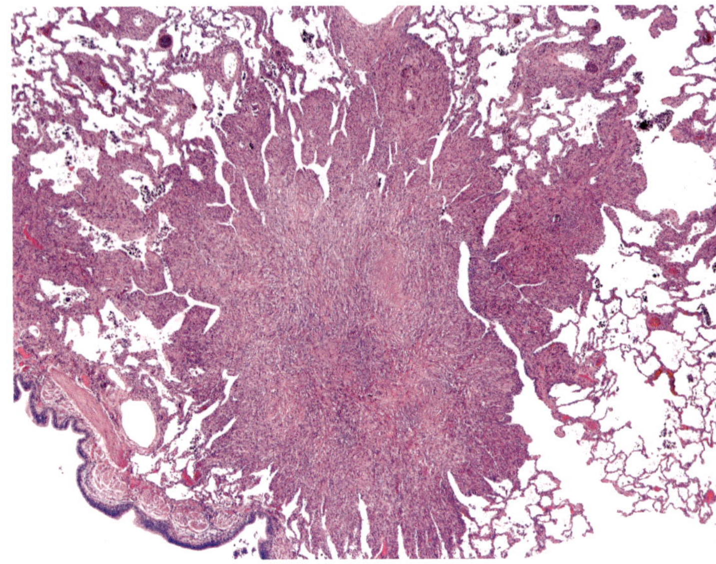

Figure 3.16a — Dust Macule, Biopsy [H&E Stain; Low Power]. In advanced pneumoconiosis, fibrotic nodules may reach a centimeter or more in diameter and create a mass lesion. This macule from a coal worker is a parabronchiolar stellate aggregate of histiocytes with a small central scar. At low power the stellate arrangement may suggest Langerhans Cell Histiocytosis (Langerin, S100, and CD1a positive).

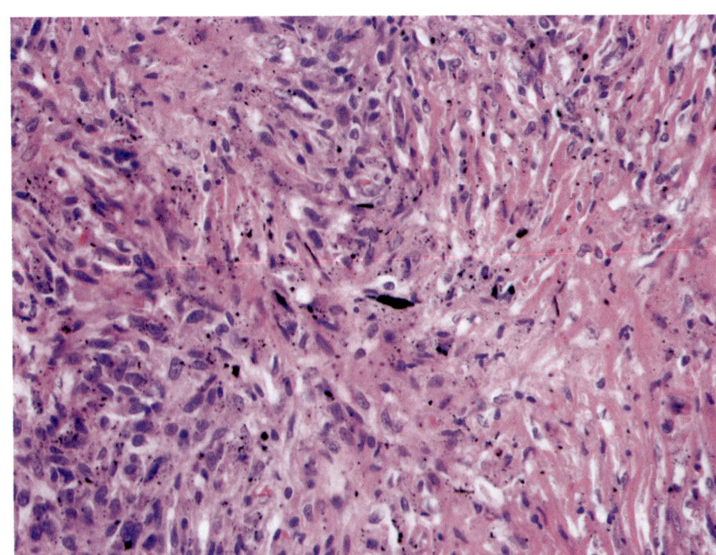

Figure 3.16b — Dust Macule, Biopsy [H&E Stain; High Power]. On higher power, the macule is composed of both spindled and epithelioid histiocytes, with abundant background collagen. Chunky and granular anthracotic material is present. These patients have impaired macrophage function and an increased risk for mycobacterial infection; an acid fast bacilli (AFB) stain is therefore indicated.

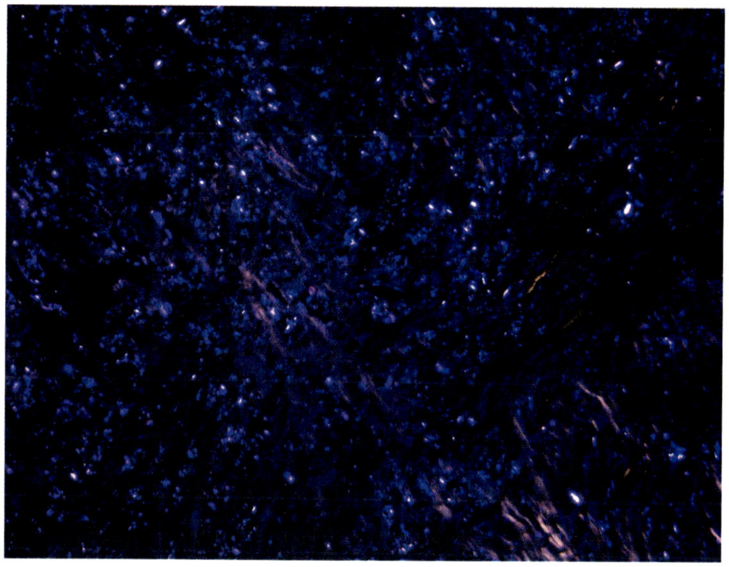

Figure 3.16c — Dust Macule, Biopsy [Polarized H&E Stain; Low Power]. Polarization of macules typically shows numerous polarizable particles, which cannot be further identified without specialized referral techniques. Most dust exposures are mixed; silica is a common component.

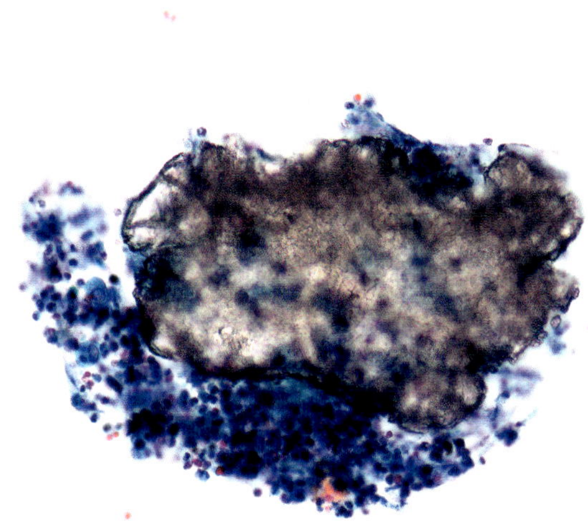

Figure 3.17 — Aspirated Peanut, Bronchial Washing [Pap Stain; Medium Power]. There is a fragment of tan-brown, refractile, amorphous material surrounded by histiocytes, lymphocytes, neutrophils, and scattered red blood cells in this bronchial wash. The material appears foreign. Aspirated foreign material may not be readily identifiable, but correlation with clinical history and ingestions may be helpful. In this case, the material was subsequently identified as peanut (*Arachis hypogaea*).

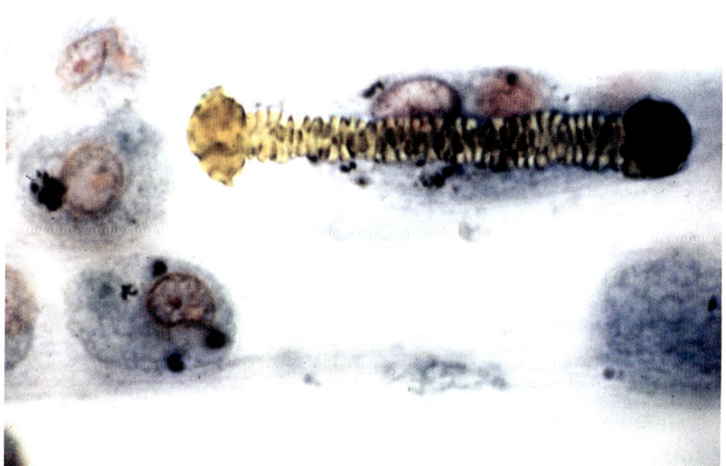

Figure 3.18a — Asbestos Body, Bronchoalveolar Lavage [Pap Stain; High Power]. The asbestos body is dumbbell-shaped and golden-brown in color. Asbestos bodies are formed from asbestos fibers and coated with an iron-rich protein matrix. The iron gives the golden-brown color and iron stains can be used to highlight the bodies if any doubt exists. In tissues, asbestos bodies are associated with fibrosis of peribronchial, lung, and pleural tissues.

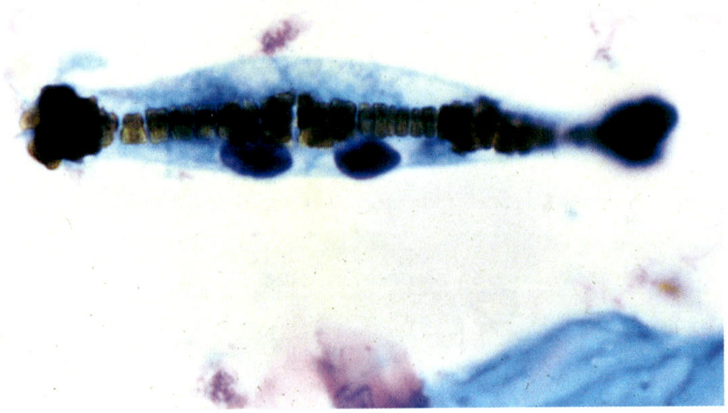

Figure 3.18b — Asbestos Body, Bronchoalveolar Lavage [Diff-Quik Stain; High Power]. In this image, the asbestos body has a thin, beaded appearance with two larger swellings on the end. The body appears to be within a histiocyte. Asbestos bodies may be found in peripheral lung tissue with associated fibrosis but in patients with more exposure will appear in sputum and have been reported in lymph nodes as well. Patients with asbestos exposure may be asymptomatic, or may present with severe dyspnea and restrictive lung disease.

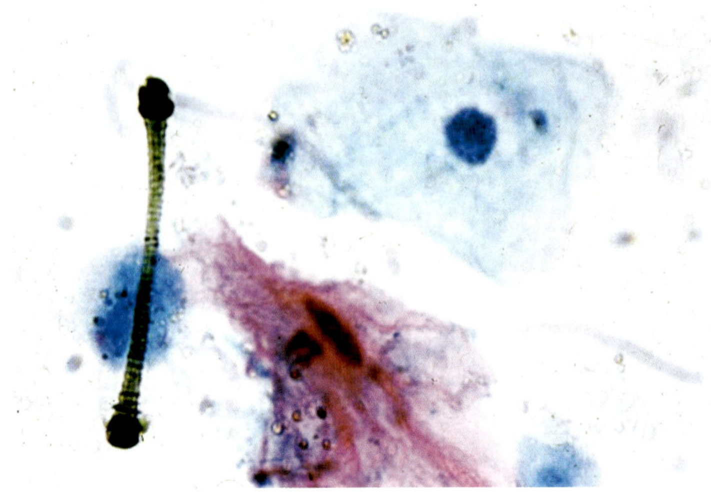

Figure 3.18c — Asbestos Body, Bronchoalveolar Lavage [Pap Stain; High Power]. The beaded and dumbbell-shaped asbestos body rests with exfoliated superficial squamous cells in this image. The true asbestos body has a fine, thin, and delicate core with the beaded deposition along the length, and accentuation at the ends to give the characteristic appearance. The differential diagnosis includes ferruginous bodies from other exposures, such as coal dust. These other bodies lack the delicate core of the true asbestos body.

Figure 3.19a — Amyloid, Fine Needle Aspiration [Diff-Quik Stain; Medium Power]. Pulmonary amyloidosis is divided into systemic and localized types. In the lung, it is further subdivided into tracheobronchial, nodular, diffuse alveolar septal, and pleural subtypes. The nodular form mimics neoplastic or granulomatous disease, and is usually solitary. These nodular deposits average 3 cm in diameter, but some over 10 cm have been described. Smears are extremely hypocellular, perhaps acellular, and contain smudged, somewhat "glassy or waxy" acellular material dispersed in irregularly shaped thin and thick fragments. In Romanowsky-stained smears, amyloid is densely basophilic. Globule formation as seen in alveolar proteinosis is usually absent.

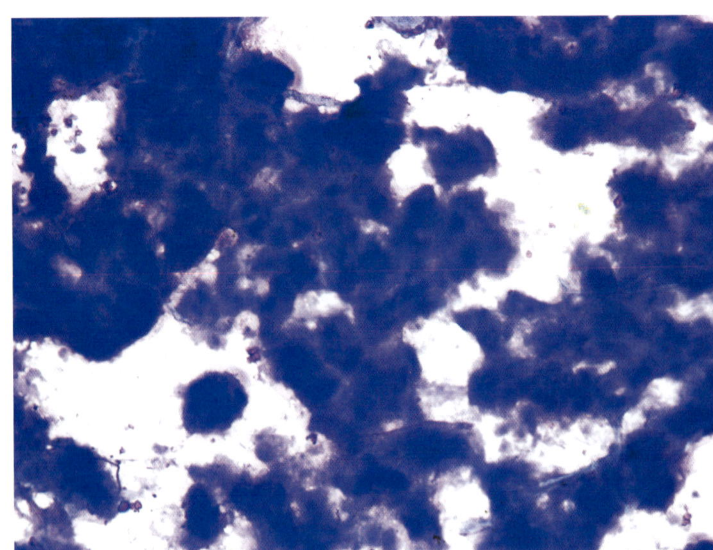

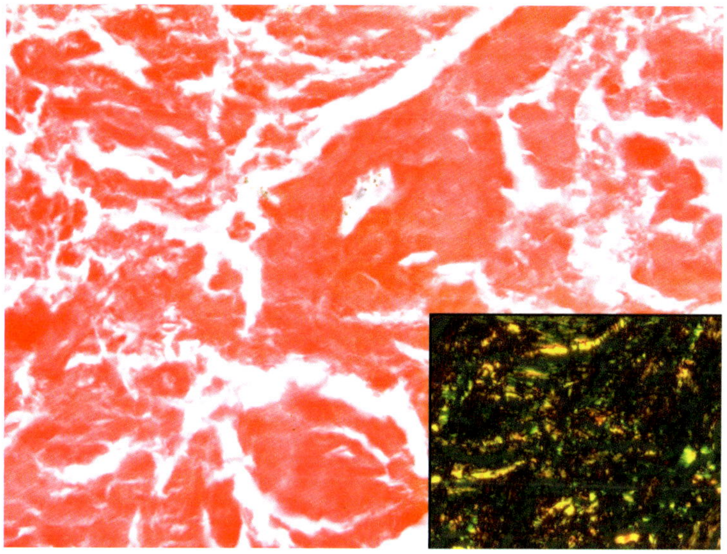

Figure 3.19b — Amyloid, Fine Needle Aspiration [Congo Red Special Stain; Medium Power]. Nodular pulmonary amyloid may be associated with pulmonary lymphoma and lymphoid interstitial pneumonia. In this Congo red-stained slide, amyloid exhibits an intense reddish-orange coloration. Polarization shows the expected yellow-green birefringence [inset]. Amyloid nodules (amyloidoma) may undergo calcification, ossification, and a multinucleated giant cell reaction–all of which may be captured with fine needle aspirates of this lesion.

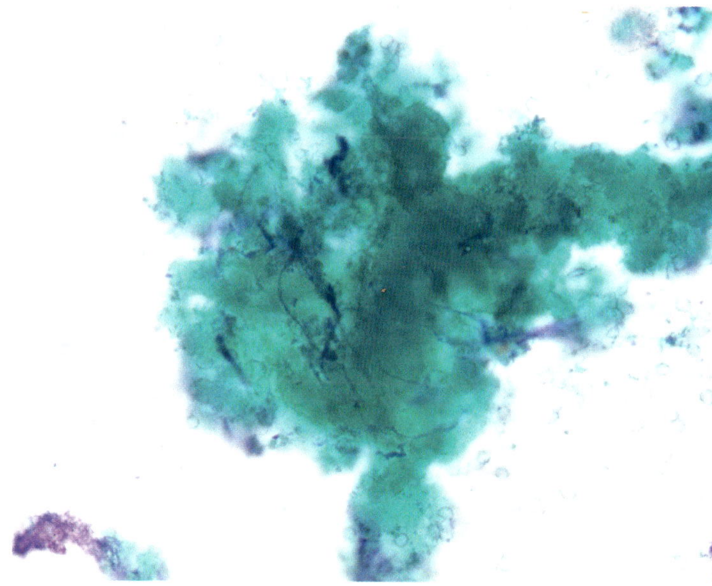

Figure 3.19c — Amyloid, Fine Needle Aspiration [Pap Stain; Medium Power]. A fragment of opaque cyanophilic amyloid contains a few deeply embedded spindle-shaped fibroblast nuclei. These fragments have irregularly contoured edges that are somewhat ragged in appearance. Amyloid lacks the "spongy/foamy" character of *Pneumocystis jirovecii* infection. Note the absence of inflammatory cells including plasma cells.

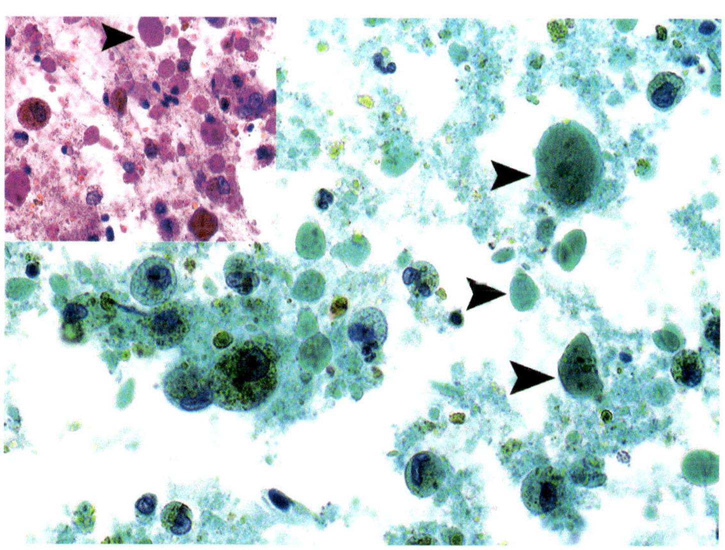

Figure 3.20a — Alveolar Proteinosis, Bronchoalveolar Lavage [Pap Stain; Medium Power]. Surfactant globules of dense cyanophilic proteinaceous material [arrowheads] are scattered among acellular debris and macrophages. These dense globules are absent in exogenous lipid pneumonia, which is in the differential diagnosis of pulmonary alveolar proteinosis. PAS-stain [inset] highlights the intense PAS-positivity of these globules, which is resistant to diastase predigestion. This globular material is negative with mucicarmine and Congo red, but may show lipid (Oil Red O) staining. A more specific test includes immunohistochemical staining of these globules for surfactant apoprotein, such as surfactant protein A. Though not seen in this field, flat plate-like cholesterol crystals are occasionally seen.

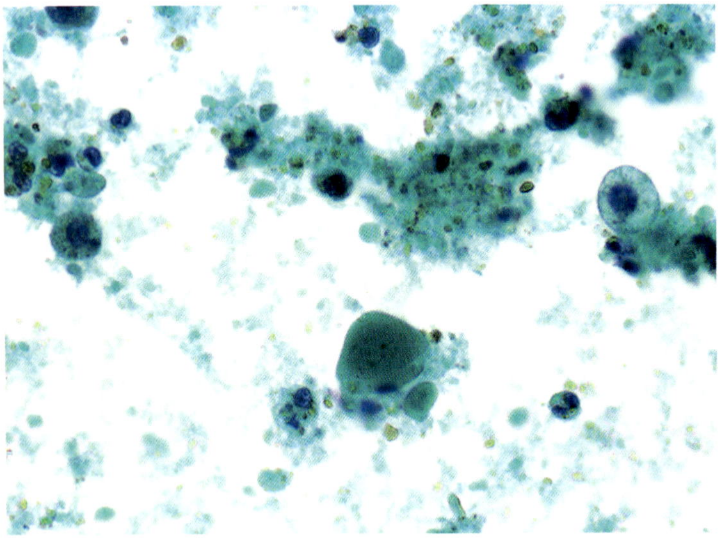

Figure 3.20b — Alveolar Proteinosis, Bronchoalveolar Lavage [Pap Stain; High Power]. Pulmonary alveolar proteinosis, a rare disease, is divided into idiopathic primary (90% of cases), secondary, and congenital forms. It is helpful to correlate the cytopathology with radiographic imaging that classically displays a "butterfly" pattern of severe pulmonary edema, which results from a massive accumulation of surfactant. This image shows an abundance of amorphous granular debris, occasional pigmented macrophages, and a few globules. Gross examination of this fluid appears cloudy, milky, or even purulent, often with visible flocculent material.

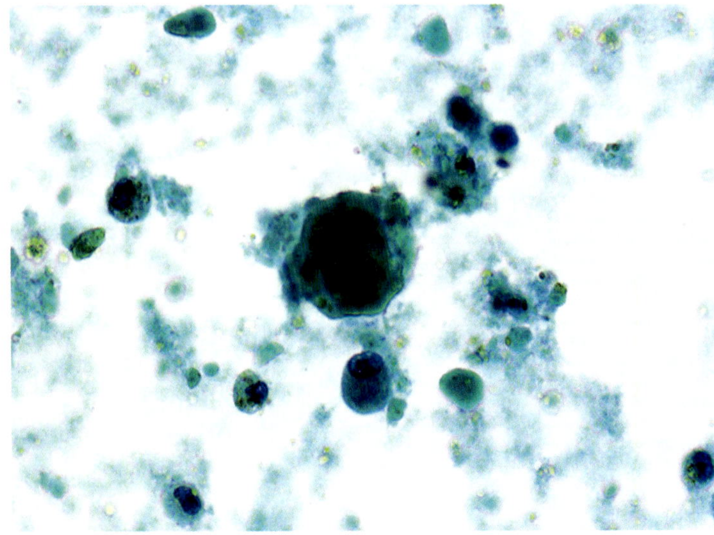

Figure 3.20c — Alveolar Proteinosis, Bronchoalveolar Lavage [Pap Stain; High Power]. Bronchoalveolar lavage specimens of pulmonary alveolar proteinosis are typically devoid of bronchial cells and consist primarily of macrophages seen here that are variably pigmented with granular material distributed both intra- and extracellularly. This fluid is coarser and lacks the foamy "soap-bubble" character of alveolar exudate seen in *Pneumocystis jirovecii* infection. Gomori methenamine silver (GMS) staining for organisms is negative in pulmonary alveolar proteinosis. Note the absence of other inflammatory cells such as lymphocytes and neutrophils, helping to exclude a pneumonitic process. Eosinophils have been described in an occasional patient.

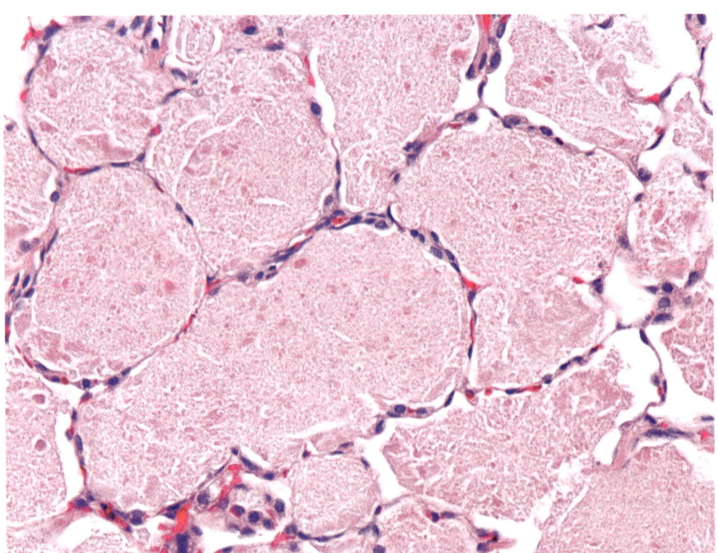

Figure 3.20d — Alveolar Proteinosis, Biopsy [H&E Stain; High Power]. Alveolar spaces are filled and distended by coarsely granular, paucicellular, brightly eosinophilic material with occasional clefts, comprised of surfactant and degenerating macrophages. There is minimal or no inflammation. The material is brightly Periodic acid-Schiff (PAS)- and PAS-diastase-positive. Alveolar proteinosis should be distinguished from transudative edema (paler, not granular, PAS-negative), early diffuse alveolar damage (brightly eosinophilic, PAS-negative), and the foamy exudates associated with Pneumocystis infection (PAS-negative, Gomori methenamine silver-positive).

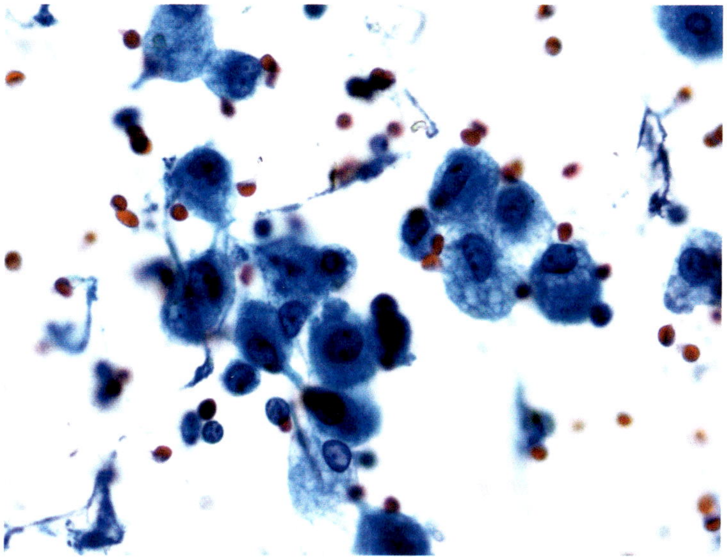

Figure 3.21a — Lipoid Pneumonia, Bronchoalveolar Lavage [Pap Stain; High Power]. Numerous foamy macrophages are present in loose clusters. The slightly curved, hyphen-shaped nuclei possessed by some cells reveals their histiocytic origin. The cytoplasm is packed with small vacuoles containing an unknown substance. Special stains for iron, mucin, and lipid can help identify substances contained in macrophages that are not easily identified on routine stains.

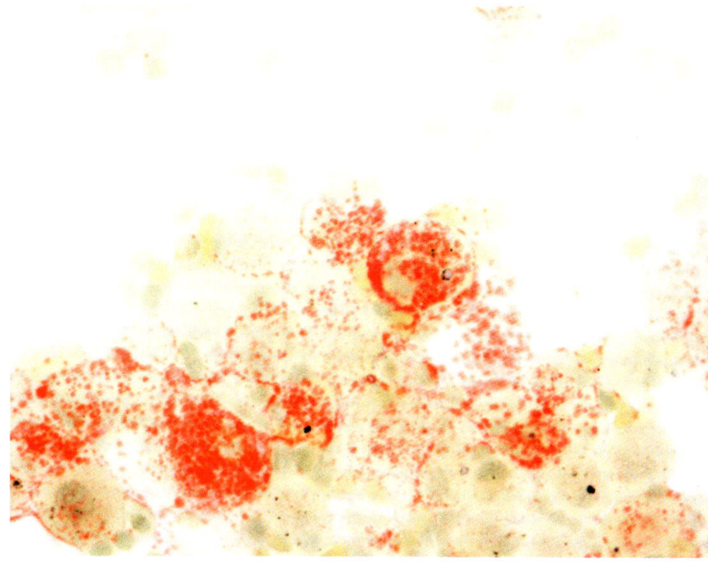

Figure 3.21b — Lipoid Pneumonia, Bronchoalveolar Lavage [Oil Red O; High Power]. This smear was air-dried and then stained with Oil Red O so that any lipid material in the preparation is preserved, then highlighted by Oil Red O. The lipid vacuoles contained in the macrophages now appear red, proving that these alveolar macrophages have been exposed to lipids, which is not a normal happening in the airways. In this case, the patient was a chronic user of a medical product containing petroleum jelly, which over time entered her airway.

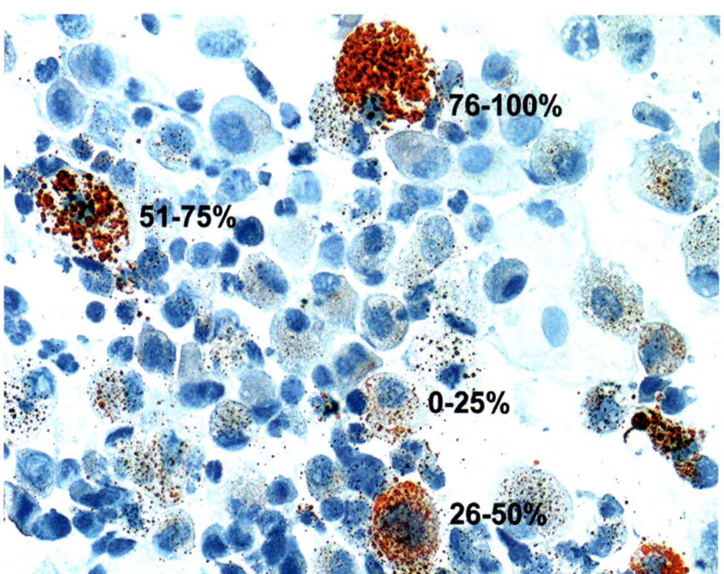

Figure 3.21c — Lipid-Laden Pulmonary Alveolar Macrophages, Bronchoalveolar Lavage [Oil Red O Special Stain; High Power]. The presence of lipid in pulmonary alveolar macrophages is abnormal and may be caused by a tracheoesophageal fistula or aspiration. Because lipid is removed on routine cytologic preparations, special preparation with Oil Red O allows the detection of lipid material, which stains red. This field demonstrates pulmonary alveolar macrophages that are positive for Oil Red O to varying degrees.

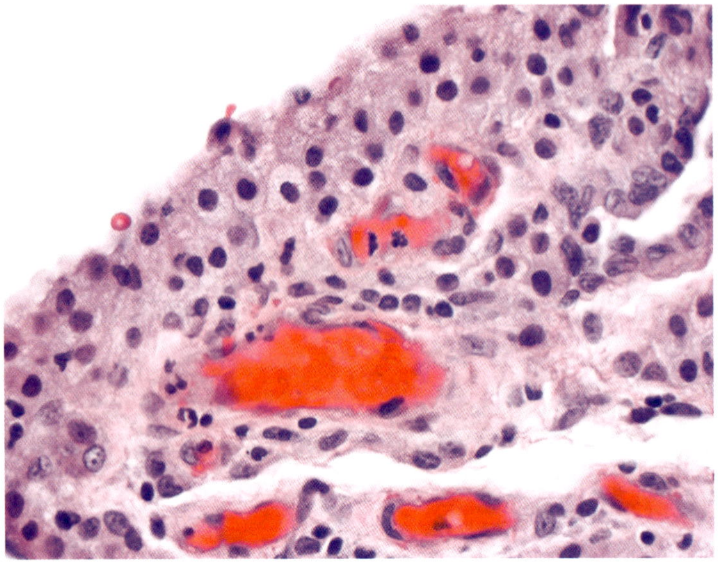

Figure 3.22a — Reactive Mesothelial Cells, Wedge Resection [H&E Stain; High Power]. Fibrinous pleural adhesions may occur after any injury to the pleura. In this image, reactive mesothelial cells proliferate with surrounding vessels and chronic inflammation. The reactive cells are larger and atypical and form complex epithelial structures, but never invade deep into fatty tissues of the chest wall or into lung parenchyma. Normal pleura and a scant amount of peripheral lung are present at the bottom of the image.

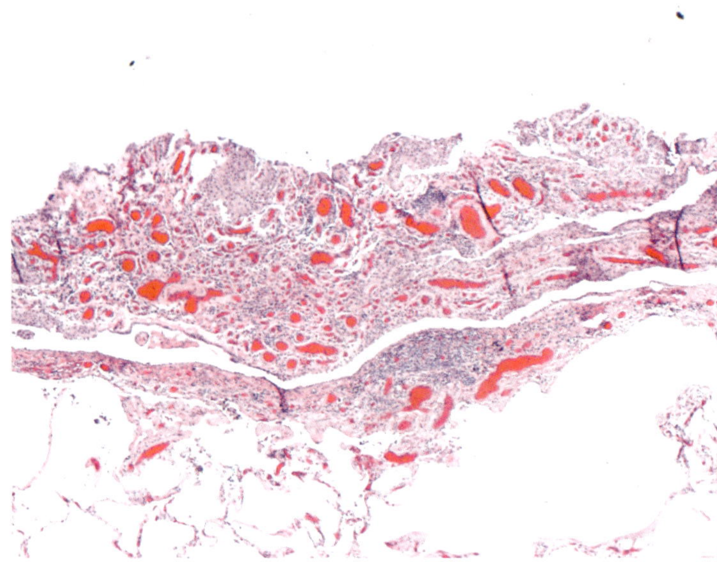

Figure 3.22b — Reactive Mesothelial Cells, Wedge Resection [H&E Stain; Low Power]. Reactive mesothelial cells (top) are much larger than the normal attenuated pleural lining (bottom). The reactive mesothelial cells have moderate pink cytoplasm and enlarged, round to oval nuclei with open chromatin and visible nucleoli. Some have mild nuclear membrane irregularities (folds, grooves), the surface is thickened, and the cells appear somewhat disordered. Notice the admixed inflammatory cells, both acute and chronic. The reactive mesothelial cells have occasional intercellular "windows," or spaces between the cells.

4

Infectious Lung Lesions

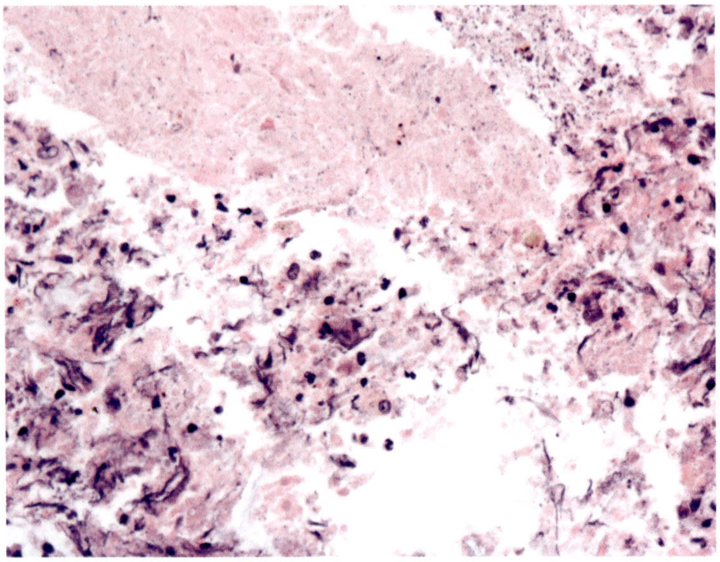

Figure 4.1a — Tuberculosis, Fine Needle Aspiration [H&E Stain; High Power]. This fine needle aspiration came from a right apical cavitary mass in a woman with a positive PPD and exposure to tuberculosis through family members. The field contains necrosis and macrophages. The presence of necrosis with granulomatous inflammation should raise concern for infectious organisms, in particular mycobacteria and yeast, and staining for these organisms should be performed.

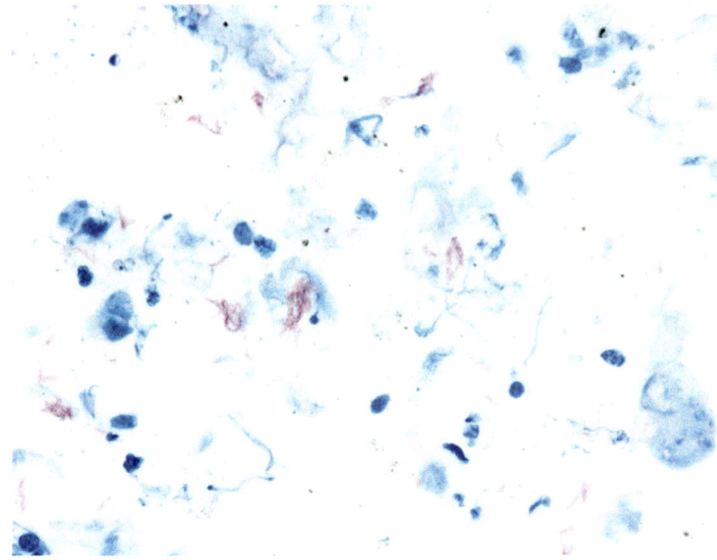

Figure 4.1b — Tuberculosis, Fine Needle Aspiration [Ziehl–Neelsen Special Stain; High Power]. The Ziehl–Neelsen stain is an acid-fast stain useful for the detection of mycobacteria and other acid-fast organisms. Because the sensitivity for detection on tissue sections is low, cultures should also be taken at the time of biopsy and patients with suspected tuberculosis infection should not be dismissed due to negative staining. In this case, the stain highlights the organism in a hot pink color. The organisms "cord" together, forming small rope-like structures.

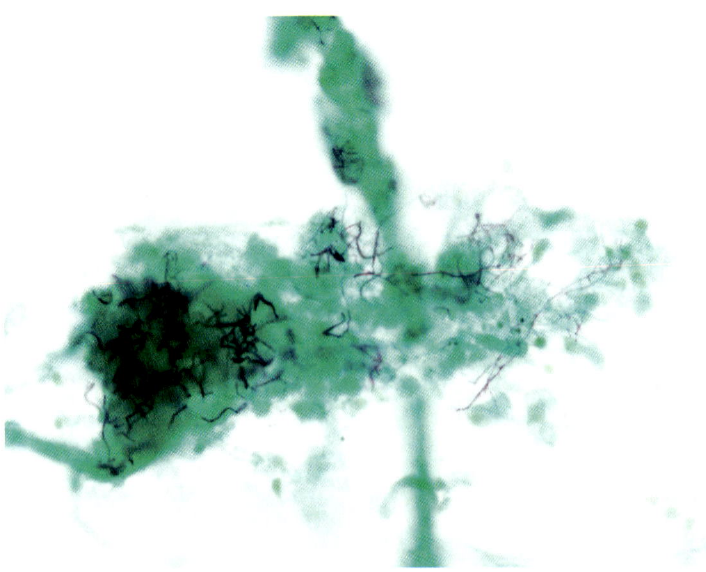

Figure 4.2 — *Nocardia*, Bronchoalveolar Lavage [Gomori Methenamine Silver Special Stain; High Power]. Pulmonary nocardiosis is caused by infection with *Nocardia asteroids* or *Nocardia brasiliensis* and is most common in patients with weakened immune systems. The organism is typically found in soil and may be inhaled with dust in the air. Nocardia are gram positive and weakly acid-fast bacteria with a branching, rod-shaped growth. Here, the organisms are demonstrated on a Gomori methenamine silver stain.

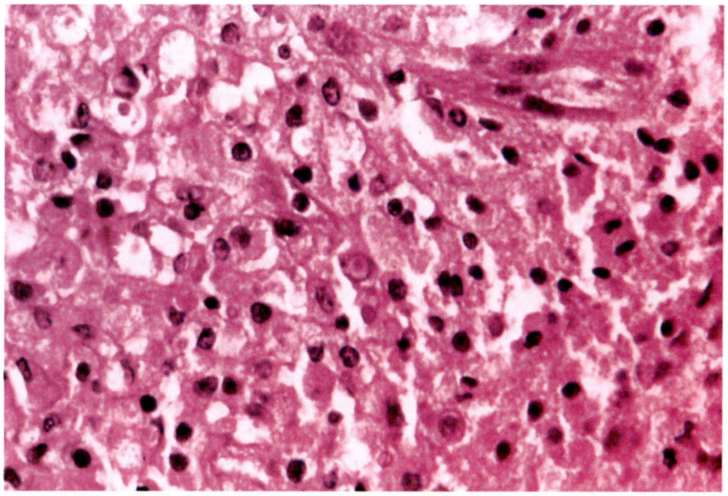

Figure 4.3a — *Rhodococcus equi*, Bronchoalveolar Lavage [H&E Stain; High Power]. *Rhodococcus equi* infection may cause malakoplakia, as demonstrated in this image. There is a diffuse dispersion of histiocytes with abundant pink granular-appearing cytoplasm and Michaelis-Gutmann bodies (round, lamellated intracytoplasmic inclusions) seen most prominently in the center of the field. Other bacterial infections (*Escherichia coli*, Proteus) may also cause malakoplakia.

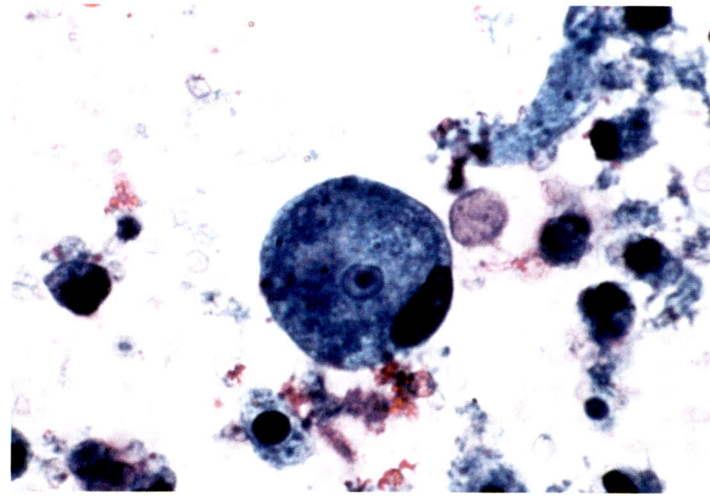

Figure 4.3b — *Rhodococcus equi*, Bronchoalveolar Lavage [Pap Stain; High Power]. On Pap-stained aspirates, Michaelis-Gutmann bodies are more readily appreciated as a lamellar intracytoplasmic inclusion in the center of the large, granular histiocyte. The Michaelis-Gutmann bodies are composed of intracellular accumulations of calcium and iron, and are thought to be a response to organisms.

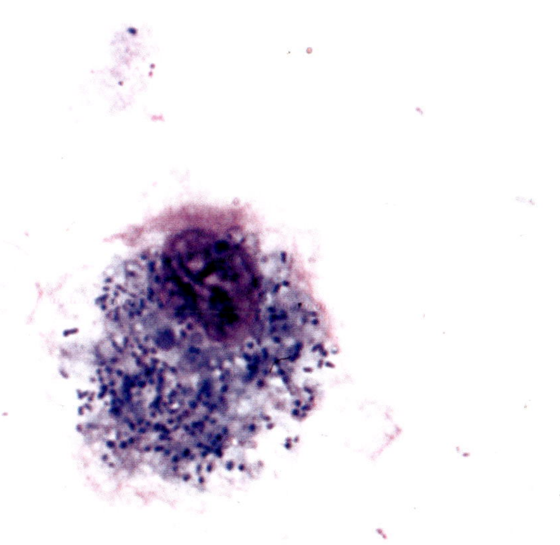

Figure 4.3c — *Rhodococcus equi*, Bronchoalveolar Lavage [Diff-Quik Stain; High Power]. *Rhodocococcus equi* is a gram-positive, partially acid-fast bacterium that can be found within histiocyte cytoplasm and may mimic true acid-fast bacilli. The infection was first described in livestock and particularly foals, but the bacterium can also be a human pathogen, particularly in immunocompromised individuals. The name *Rhodococcus* derives from the red pigment produced in cultures.

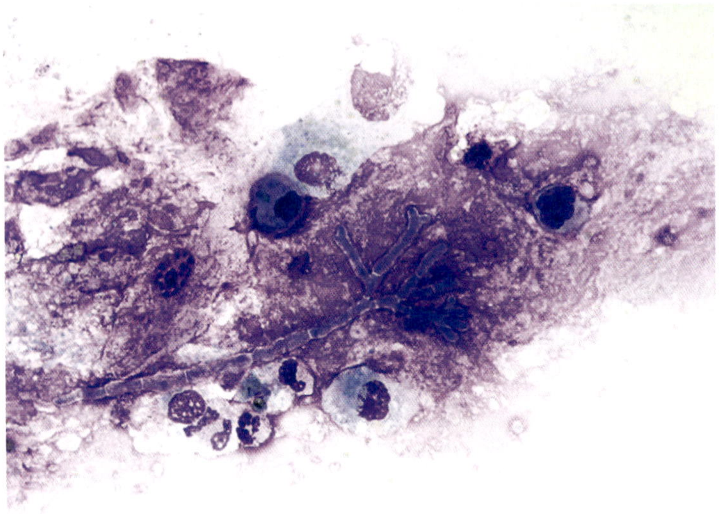

Figure 4.4a — *Aspergillus*, Bronchial Washing [Diff-Quik Stain; High Power]. This high power image from a bronchial wash shows the classic form of *Aspergillus* spp. mold—thin, septate hyphae with acute angle branching, and a background of inflammatory cells. Pulmonary aspergillosis takes many forms; ranging from a colonizer of a preexisting cavitary lesion ("fungus ball") or airway ("bronchocentric granulomatosis") to allergic disease to the potentially fatal angioinvasive disease.

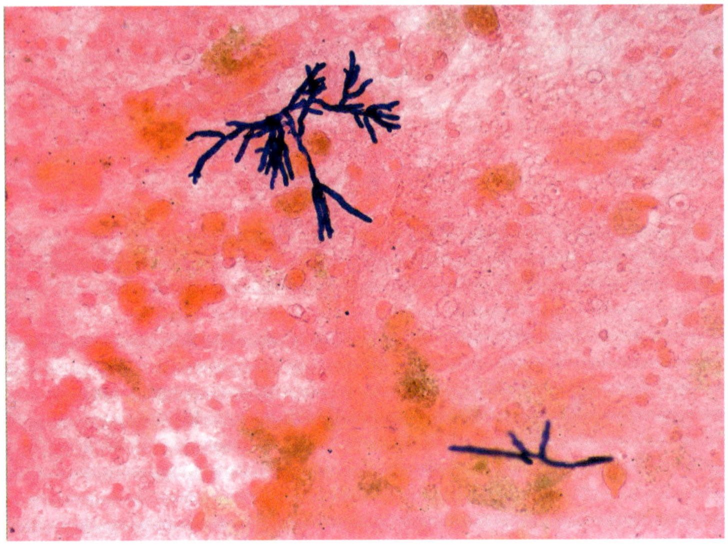

Figure 4.4b — *Aspergillus*, Bronchial Washing [Gram-Weigert Stain; High Power]. This image from another bronchial wash shows again the morphology associated with *Aspergillus*: acute angle branching and thin, septate hyphae. The diagnosis of *Aspergillus* species can be suggested by morphology, but definitive diagnosis should be made based on microbiologic studies, as other fungal species may have similar morphology.

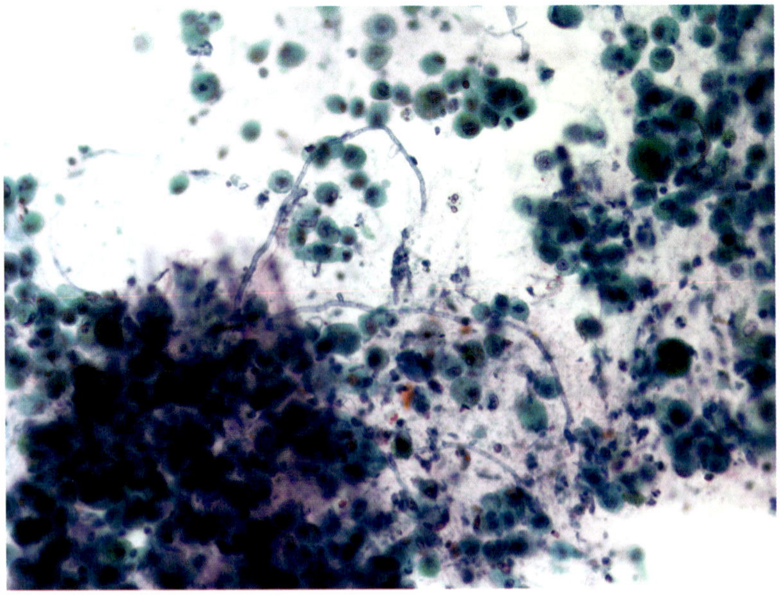

Figure 4.4c — *Aspergillus*, Bronchoalveolar Lavage [Pap Stain; High Power]. This bronchoalveolar lavage specimen is remarkable for the thin, arching fungal hyphae seen surrounded by necrotic debris, neutrophils, and abundant intra-alveolar macrophages. A possible fruiting body, resembling a broom-head, with spore formation is present at the center of the field. *Aspergillus* may be an airway contaminant, but the presence of hyphae with associated inflammatory reaction and necrosis supports the diagnosis of infection.

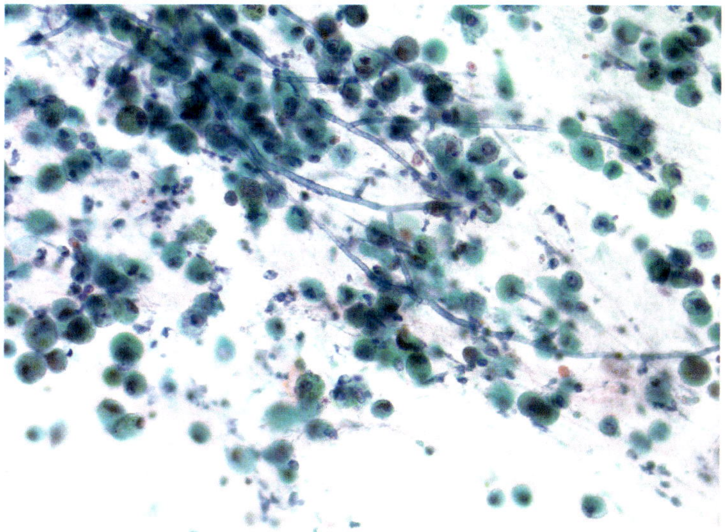

Figure 4.4d — *Aspergillus*, Bronchoalveolar Lavage [Pap Stain; High Power]. This image highlights the delicate, septate, 45-degree angle branching hyphae of *Aspergillus*, intimately associated with neutrophils and pulmonary alveolar macrophages. Invasive aspergillus is most commonly associated with decreased T cell immunity, particularly vulnerable are organ transplant recipients and leukemia patients receiving chemotherapy.

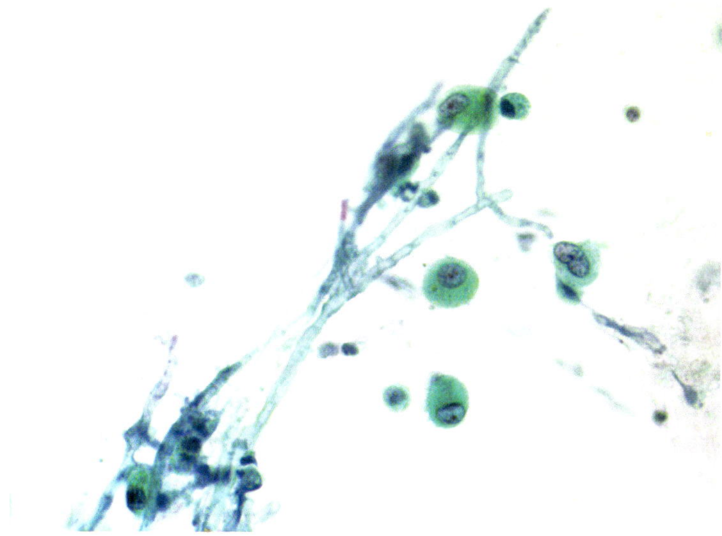

Figure 4.5a — *Aspergillus*, Bronchoalveolar Lavage [Pap Stain; High Power]. The hyphae of *Aspergillus* on high power examination reveal the thin septations and clear acute angle branching of the growing hyphae. This image also has associated pulmonary alveolar macrophages and chronic inflammatory cells. Invasive aspergillosis is usually angiocentric and the classic findings in histologic sections include thrombosed vessels with walls invaded by hyphae.

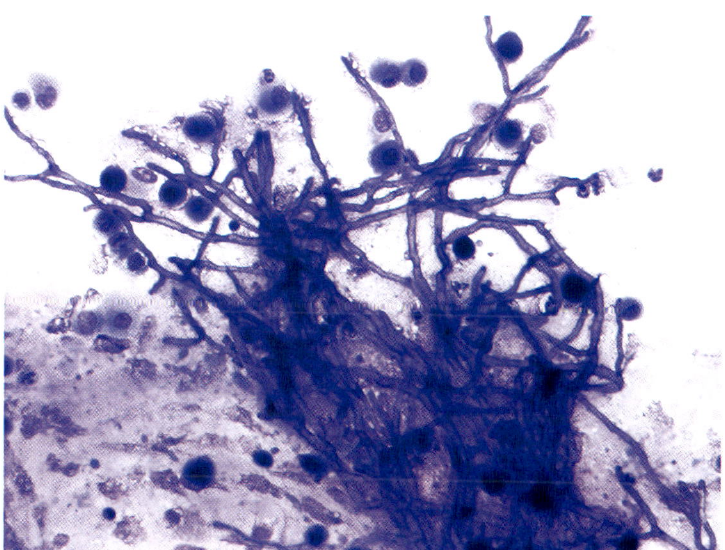

Figure 4.5b — *Aspergillus*, Bronchoalveolar Lavage [Diff-Quik Stain; High Power]. A tangled assortment of fungal hyphae dominate in this high power image of a Diff-Quik stained bronchoalveolar lavage fluid. The hyphae are thin and septate, with acute angle branching evident, best appreciated at the top of the image. The background cells are primarily pulmonary alveolar macrophages with associated inflammatory cells and proteinaceous fluid. This constellation of findings is most suggestive of pathologic involvement by *Aspergillus* spp. Allergic bronchopulmonary aspergillosis can be seen in patients with underlying asthma and an IgE-mediated reaction to the fungus, and may or may not evolve to chronic inflammation with granuloma formation.

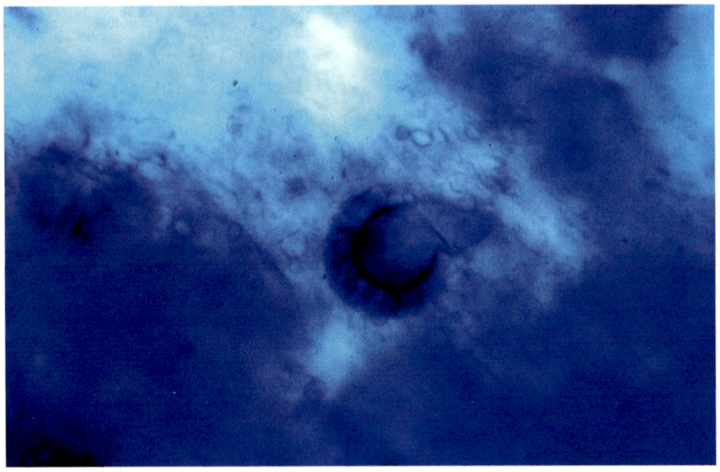

Figure 4.5c — *Aspergillus* Fruiting Body, Bronchial Washing Pap Stain; High Power]. While in most cytologic preparations *Aspergillus* spp. are seen as hyphal forms, fruiting bodies can occasionally be seen in specimens taken from cavities or airways. In this case, the conidiophore ends in a flask-shaped vesicle around which phialids and conidia are arranged. While the subspeciation of Aspergillus on cytologic preparations is usually unnecessary and challenging, the morphology seen here strongly suggests *Aspergillus* spp.; in the absence of a vesicle, the 45-degree angles formed by branching, septate hyphae are nonspecific for *Aspergillus* spp. and may be seen in other fungi, even if *Aspergillus* spp. is the usual culprit in immunocompromised patients.

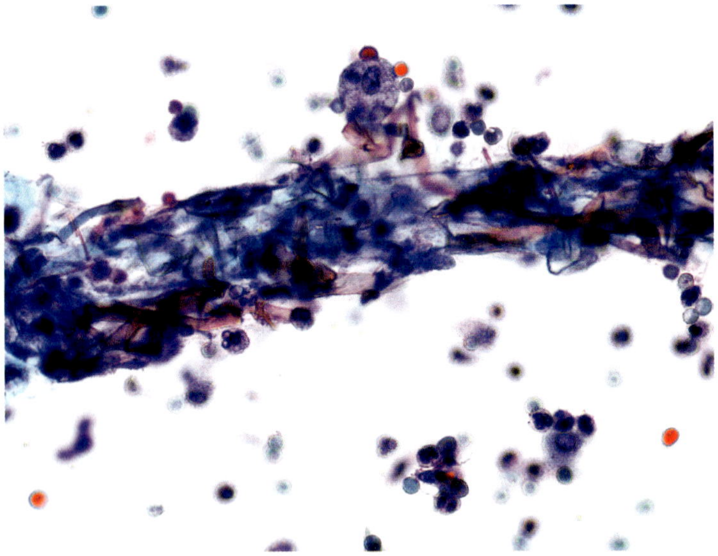

Figure 4.6a — *Mucor*, Bronchoalveolar Lavage [Pap Stain; High Power]. An aggregate of rust-colored, aseptate, "ribbon-like" hyphae stream across the center of this field of view from a bronchoalveolar lavage specimen. These hyphae also exhibit 90-degree angle branching. In the background there are scattered alveolar macrophages, neutrophils, and red blood cells. These observations all point to a diagnosis of infection by fungi of class Zygomycetes, a type of angioinvasive fungal disease usually targeting patients with decreased cellular immunity or diabetes and which may be rapidly fatal. Pulmonary infections are acquired through inhalation of environmental spores, and present as a hemorrhagic pneumonia.

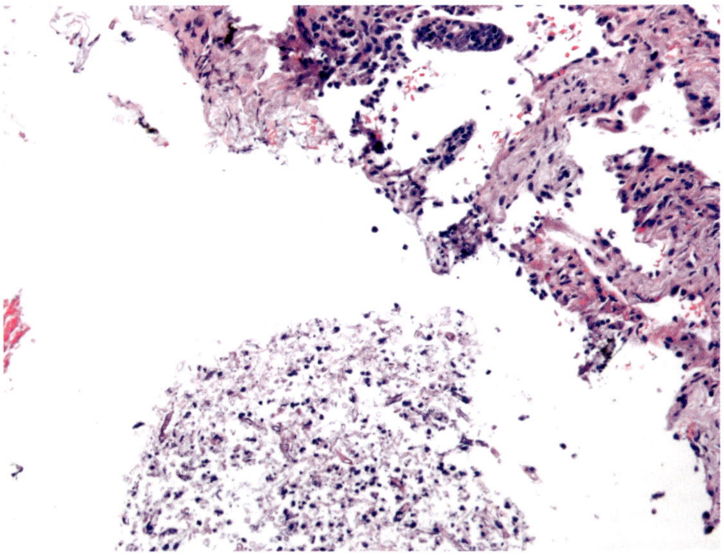

Figure 4.6b — *Mucor*, Transbronchial Biopsy [H&E Stain; Low Power]. This core biopsy was obtained from a 3.6-cm spiculated PET-avid mass in an elderly patient with recent weight loss. At upper right is inflamed parenchyma with reactive changes. At bottom center is a separate aggregate of hyphae and inflammatory cells. Chronic indolent infections are often associated with irregular peripheral fibrosis and may appear "spiculated" on imaging studies.

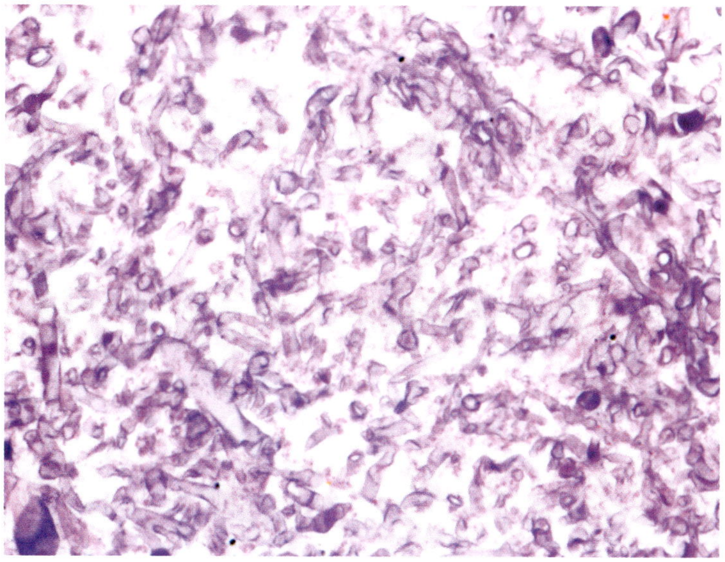

Figure 4.6c — *Mucor*, Transbronchial Biopsy [Periodic acid-Schiff (PAS)-Diastase Special Stain; High Power]. The hyphae are broad and pauciseptate, with irregular nonparallel walls and 80° to 90° angle branching. The features resemble flattened aggregates of ribbon, and are most suggestive of a zygomycete. No cultures were obtained from the small cores, as malignancy was strongly favored, pre-biopsy. In that clinical context, reactive/reparative epithelial cells may give rise to consideration of lepidic malignancy, unless the detached aggregates of hyphae with embedded inflammatory cells are carefully evaluated.

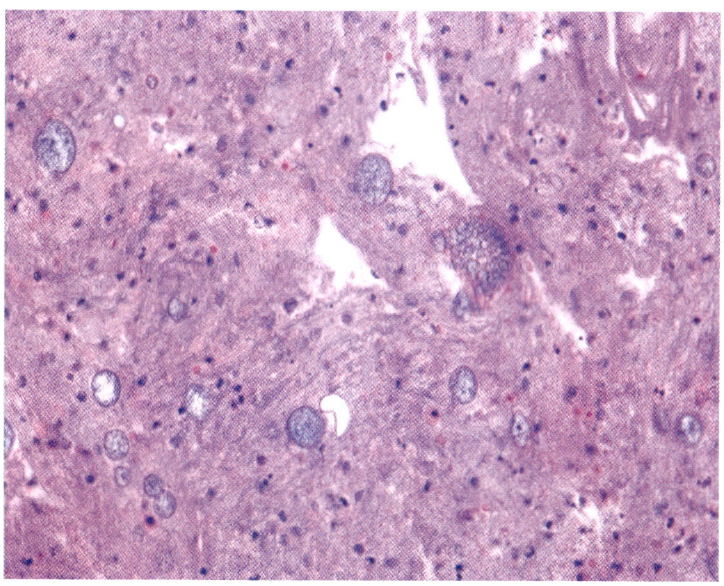

Figure 4.7a — *Coccidioides immitis*, Fine Needle Aspiration [H&E Stain; High Power]. This cell block preparation shows necrotic tissue surrounding variably sized fungal spherules and a single mature reproductive spherule with numerous small daughter cysts (center right). The reproductive spherule with the daughter cysts is a hallmark feature of *Coccidioides* infection. *Coccidioides* is endemic in the Southwestern portion of the United States as well as Mexico and Central America.

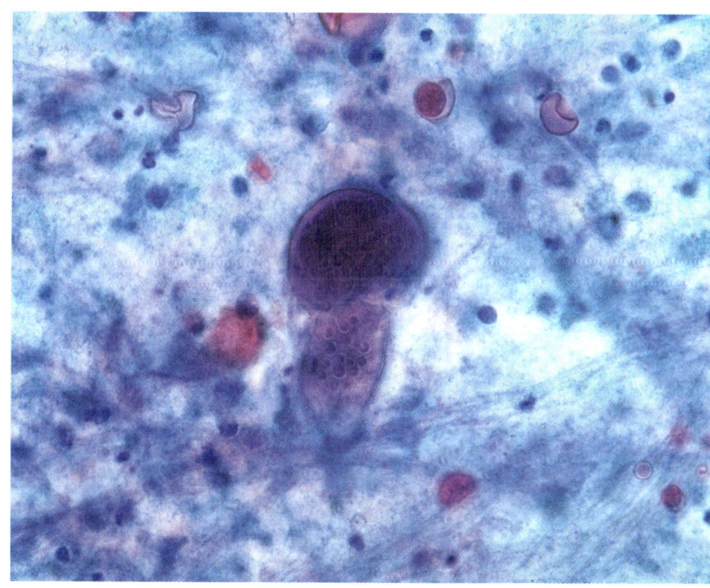

Figure 4.7b — *Coccidioides immitis*, Fine Needle Aspiration [Pap Stain; High Power]. On the Pap stain, the daughter cysts within the spherule of *Coccidioides* species are apparent. The central, mushroom-shaped reproductive spherule abounds with smaller daughter cysts. With scattered surrounding spherules and inflammatory cells, chronic infection can lead to a lung mass, which may mimic tuberculosis or malignancy clinically.

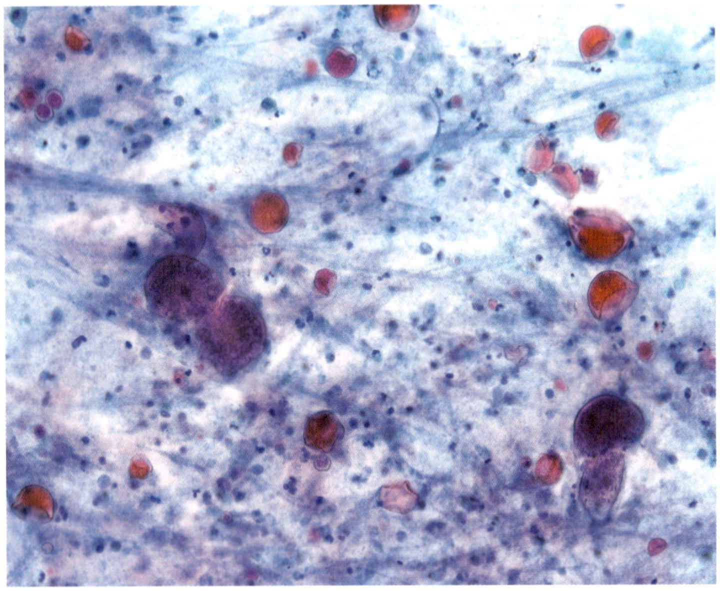

Figure 4.7c — *Coccidioides immitis*, Fine Needle Aspiration [Pap Stain; High Power]. Variably sized and indented fungal forms associate with the diagnostic reproductive spherules filled with the infectious daughter cysts. The background is typical of infection, with active inflammation and necrotic debris. *Coccidioides* infections often induce a necrotizing granulomatous inflammatory response in the lung.

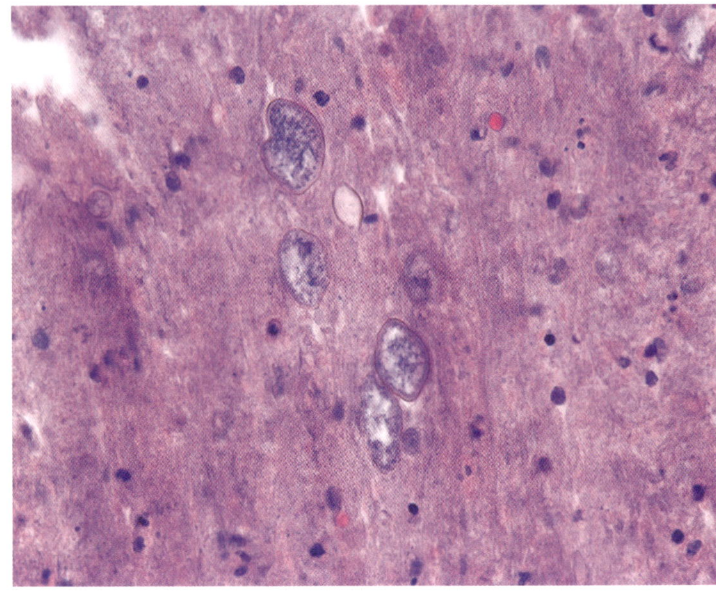

Figure 4.7d — *Coccidioides immitis*, Fine Needle Aspiration [H&E Stain; High Power]. The center of this image displays several fungal forms of *Coccidioides immitis* but lacks the characteristic and diagnostic reproductive spherule with daughter cysts. Instead, oval, indented mature fungal forms with a visible cell wall and blue centers are present with surrounding inflammation and necrosis. *Coccidioides* infection may cause subclinical disease or, in a small fraction of cases, acute illness ("San Joachim Valley Fever") with fevers, chest pain, erythema nodosum, and pulmonary involvement.

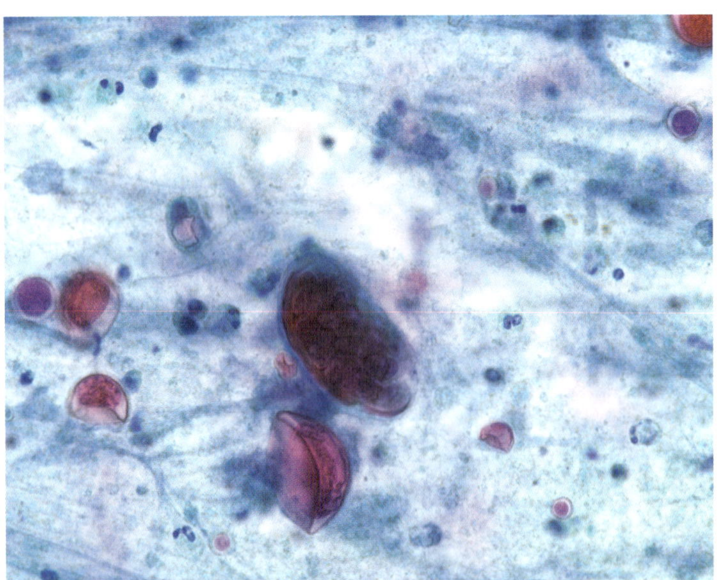

Figure 4.7e — *Coccidioides immitis*, Fine Needle Aspiration [Pap Stain; High Power]. The variably sized fungal spherules seen in this image are characteristic of *Coccidioides* infection. The spherules with multiple 2 to 5 micron endospores are characteristic of this organism. Humans acquire the infection by inhalation of arthroconidia, which in vivo morph into the multinucleated sphere containing numerous endospores.

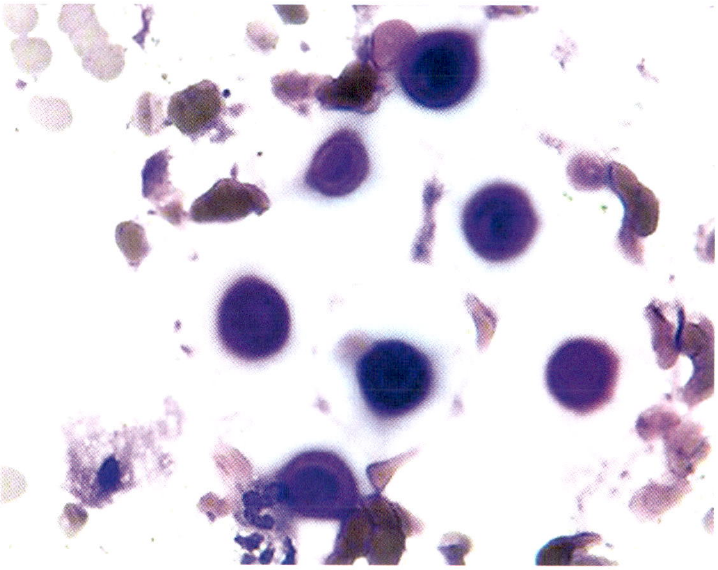

Figure 4.8a — *Cryptococcus neoformans*, Fine Needle Aspiration [Diff-Quik Stain; High Power]. The organisms of *cryptococcal* infection are 4 to 7 micron yeast with a thick, mucoid capsule that is evident on this Diff-Quik stained aspirate. Adjacent neutrophils are present at the bottom of the image. The yeast appears "indented" in some areas. Cryptococcal infection may present as a mucoid pneumonia in immunocompromised patients.

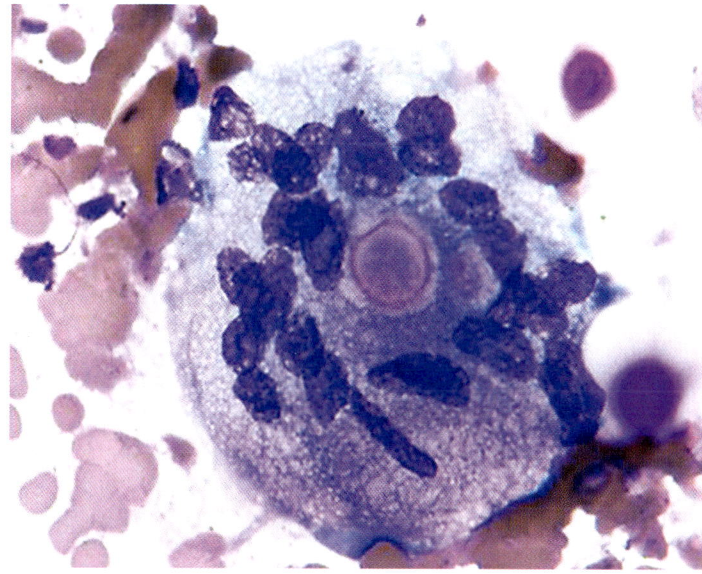

Figure 4.8b — *Cryptococcus neoformans*, Fine Needle Aspiration [Diff-Quik Stain; High Power]. *Cryptococcus* is often found intracellularly, particularly within histiocytes/multinucleated giant cells. The organism appears as a magenta oval to round body with surrounding pale clearing caused by the mucoid capsule. The yeasts can be pleomorphic in size, and the differential diagnosis includes Histoplasmosis, Blastomyces, and Pneumocystis, among others.

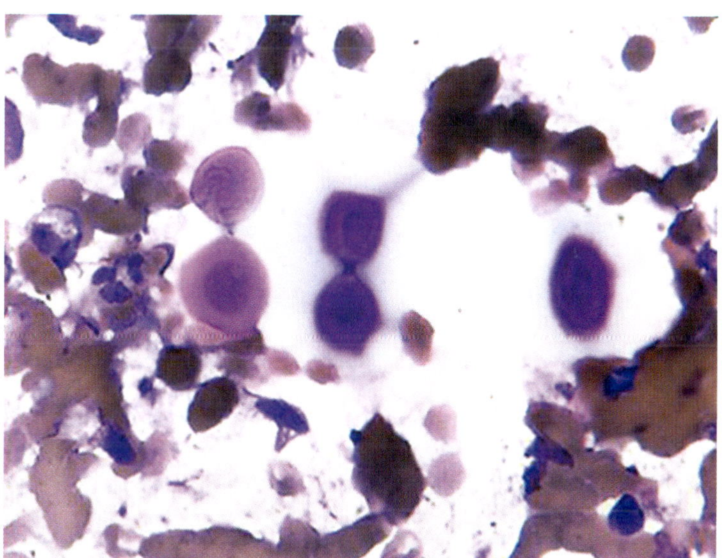

Figure 4.8c — *Cryptococcus neoformans*, Fine Needle Aspiration [Diff-Quik Stain; High Power]. The yeasts of *Cryptococcus* are variably sized, as seen in this image, and often found in clusters. The mucoid capsule is a key diagnostic feature. The capsule will be positive with mucicarmine staining, or other special stains targeting mucin. Occasional Cryptococcal strains are "capsule-deficient" and lack this characteristic feature, which makes diagnosis more difficult.

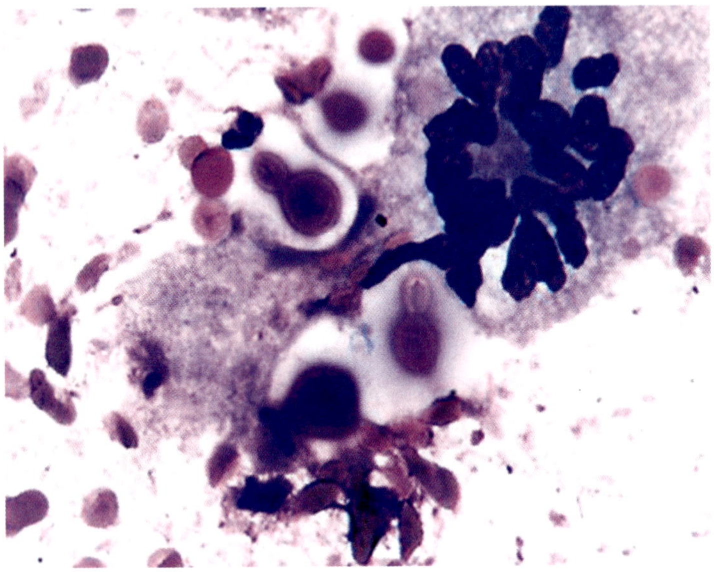

Figure 4.8d — *Cryptococcus neoformans*, Fine Needle Aspiration [Diff-Quik Stain; High Power]. *Cryptococcus* reproduce by budding, described as "narrow based." This Diff-Quik image shows two budding *Cryptococcal* organisms as well as multiple single-celled ones. A multinucleated giant cell is also present (upper right). Fontana-Masson staining will highlight Cryptococcal organisms, as they are melanin-producers.

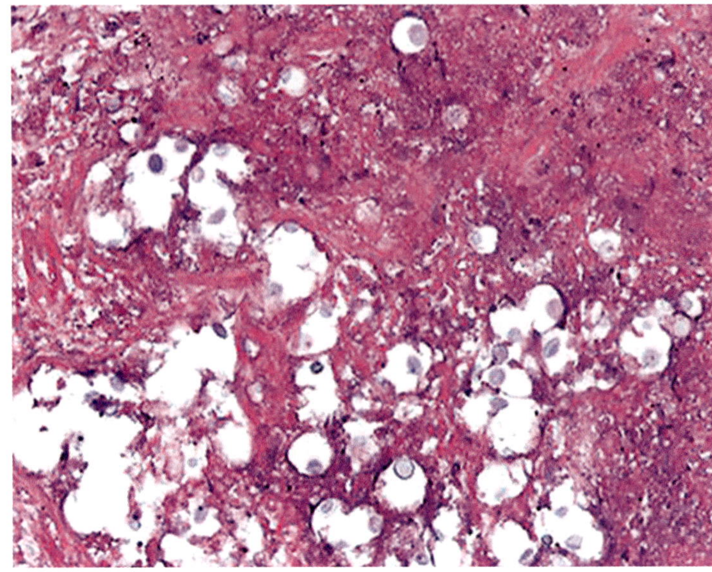

Figure 4.8e — *Cryptococcus neoformans*, Fine Needle Aspiration [H&E Stain; High Power]. On cell block sections, *Cryptococcus* will often appear to have a white or "negative space" around the yeast due to the mucoid capsule. In tissue sections, the organisms may be found with associated granulomatous inflammation and fibrosis. Often the lung is the first site of infection; however, from there the organisms can spread to the central nervous system, skin, or other sites.

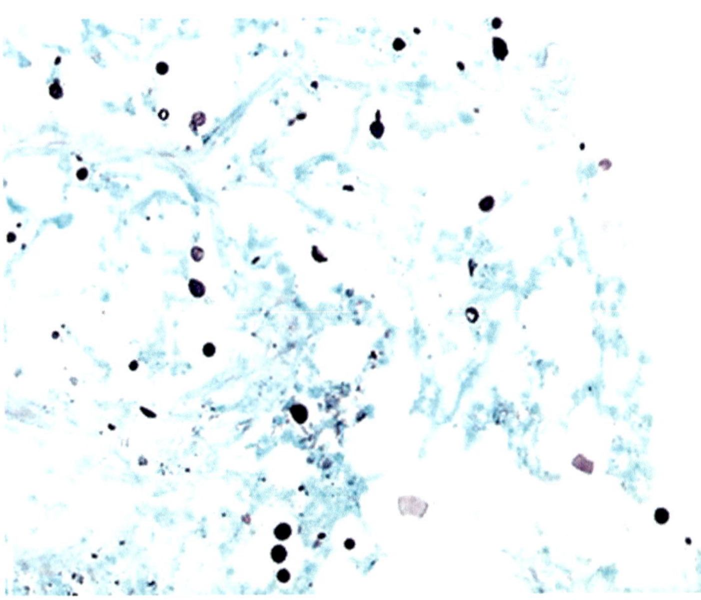

Figure 4.8f — *Cryptococcus neoformans*, Fine Needle Aspiration [Gomori Methenamine Silver Special Stain; High Power]. In addition to Fontana-Masson or mucicarmine stains, a Gomori methenamine silver stain will also help identify the yeasts. This image shows the rounded yeasts of *Cryptococcus* with occasional narrow-based budding. The mucoid capsule is implied by the negative space around the yeast. Other diagnostic tests include serum or cerebrospinal fluid antigen tests, which are often directed against capsular antigens (and may be falsely negative if the organism is of a capsule-deficient strain).

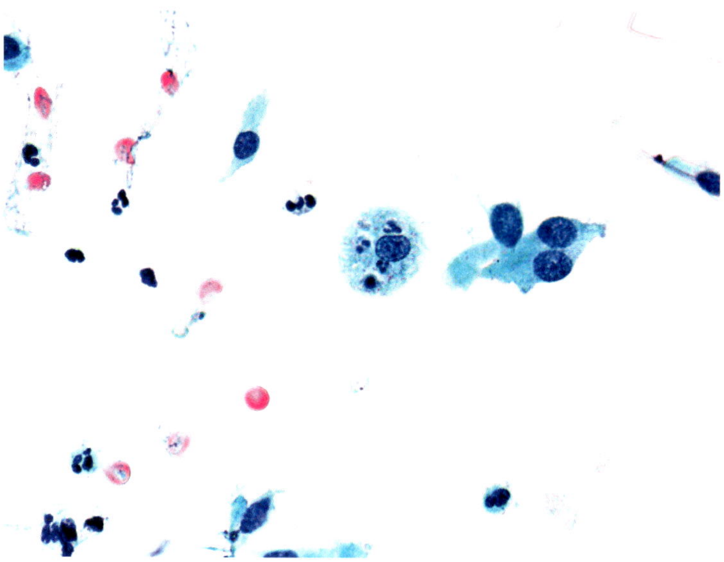

Figure 4.9a — *Histoplasma capsulatum*, Bronchoalveolar Lavage [Pap Stain; High Power]. Careful attention to the central histiocyte in this bronchoalveolar lavage fluid reveals multiple, clustered, small intracytoplasmic bodies with a surrounding clear zone created by the presence of a capsule. Adjacent to the macrophage are several benign ciliated respiratory epithelial cells and scattered neutrophils. Small (2–4 micron) intracytoplasmic yeast in clusters with a surrounding capsule are features of *Histoplasma capsulatum* var. *capsulatum.* This organism is found worldwide, often in old buildings or caves with associated bird and/or bat droppings, and is acquired via inhalation of microconidia.

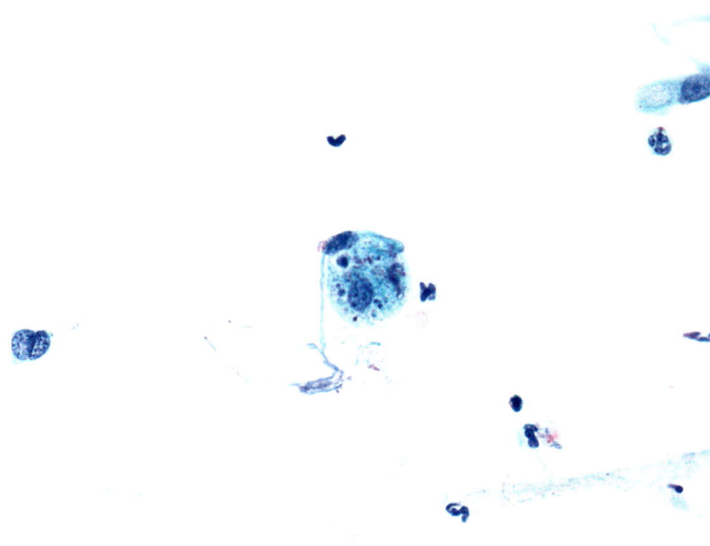

Figure 4.9b — *Histoplasma capsulatum*, Bronchoalveolar Lavage [Pap Stain; High Power]. The central intra-alveolar macrophage contains several yeast of *Histoplasma.* The yeast could be mistaken for intracytoplasmic debris, but the presence of the surrounding capsule is a good morphologic clue for the diagnosis. *Histoplasma* infection may present as either an acute or chronic pulmonary infection, disseminated disease, or may be asymptomatic. The organism is an intracellular pathogen, and may survive inside histiocytes for days or weeks and disseminate.

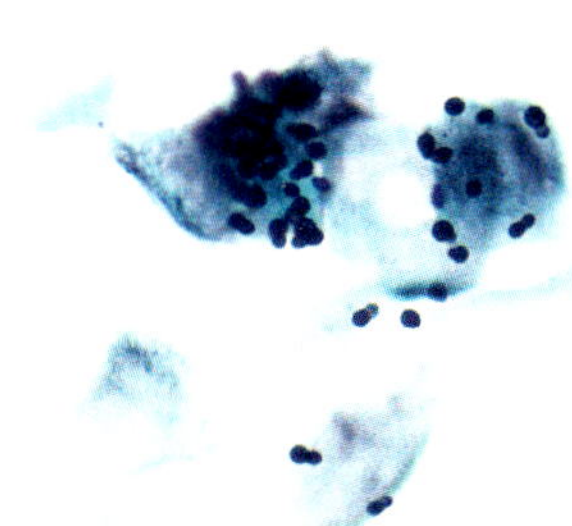

Figure 4.9c — *Histoplasma capsulatum*, Bronchoalveolar Lavage [Gomori Methenamine Silver Special Stain; High Power]. The organisms in *Histoplasma* infection may be abundant. A Gomori methenamine silver stain highlights the organisms of *Histoplasma* and the typical narrow-based budding of the spherical to oval yeast. Acute pulmonary histoplasmosis often shows a lympho-histiocytic inflammatory infiltrate with scattered granulomata, while chronic infections more commonly present with a single necrotizing granuloma with calcification.

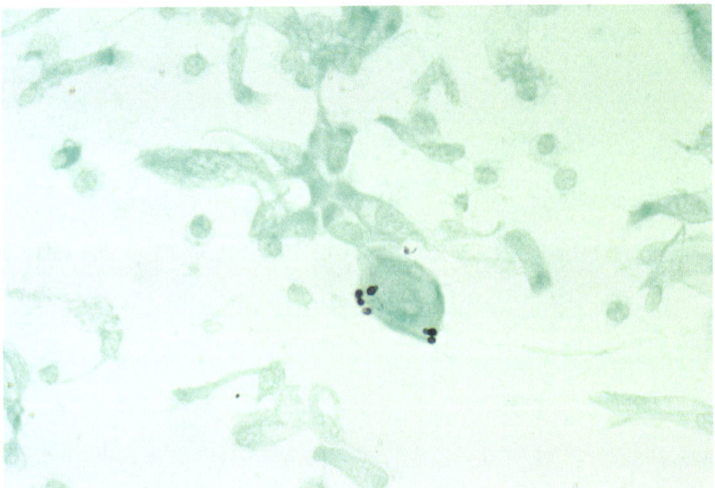

Figure 4.9d — *Histoplasma capsulatum*, Bronchoalveolar Lavage [Gomori Methenamine Silver Special Stain; High Power]. Again, the small, intracellular yeast of *Histoplasma* infection are easily seen with a Gomori methenamine silver stain. The small size and intracellular nature of the yeast contrasts *Histoplasma* with other common pathogenic fungi. Leishmaniasis or toxoplasmosis also may be seen as small intracellular forms. However, these organisms are negative by Gomori methenamine silver stain.

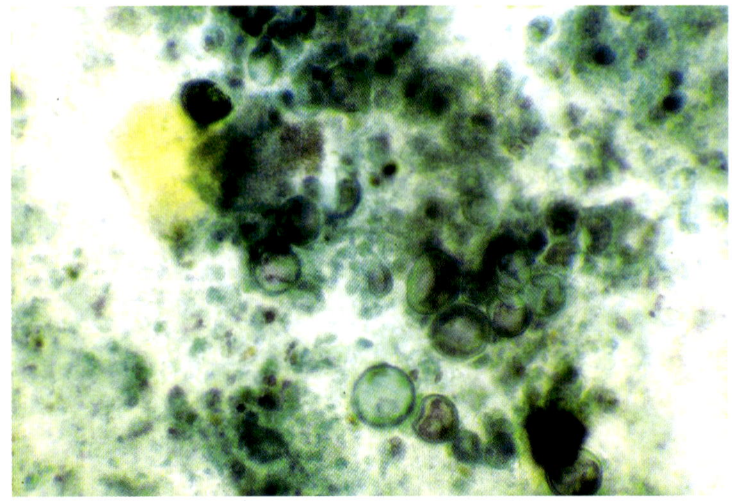

Figure 4.10a — *Blastomyces dermatitidis*, Fine Needle Aspiration [Pap Stain; High Power]. *Blastomyces* is a dimorphic fungus endemic to portions of North America. While infected patients may demonstrate symptoms similar to those of patients infected with *Histoplasma capsulatum*, the morphology of these two organisms differ substantially. *B. dermatitidis* forms spherical, double-contoured yeast that are 12 microns in size and reproduces via broad-based buds. By contrast, *Histoplasma capsulatum* are primarily intracellular organisms with narrow-based budding of smaller (2–4 micron) yeast.

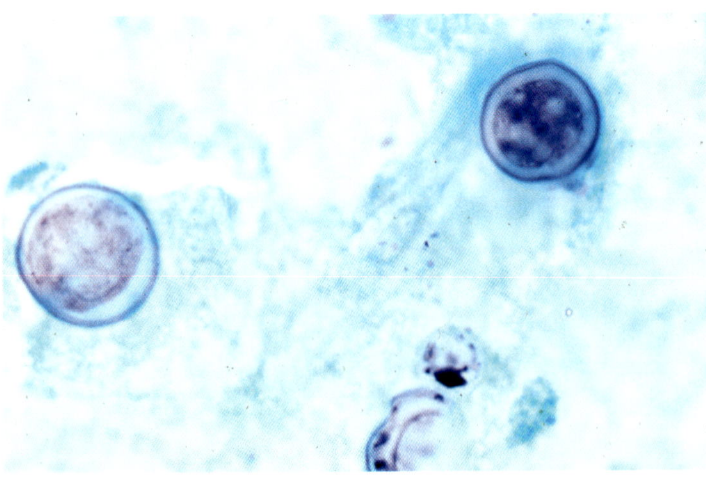

Figure 4.10b — *Blastomyces dermatitidis*, Fine Needle Aspiration [Pap Stain; High Power]. Here the "double contour" morphology of *B. dermatitidis* can be appreciated. Note the relatively large and uniform size of the organisms. Fungal organisms may not be well preserved on preparations and the differential diagnosis often includes acellular contaminants. If a cell block can be created, silver stains such as Grocott's methenamine silver stain can be used to support the fungal nature of such structures.

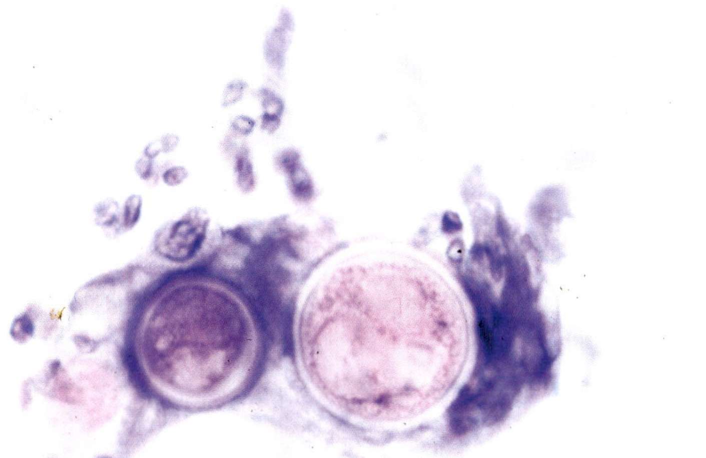

Figure 4.10c — *Blastomyces dermatitidis*, Fine Needle Aspiration [Diff-Quik Stain; High Power]. Note the spherical rings with the double contour morphology. As a dimorphic fungus, the phase transition to the pathogenic yeast form occurs at body temperature. In culture at room temperature, the fungus exists as a mold. Patient symptoms include bone pain, chest pain, cough, fatigue, and fever.

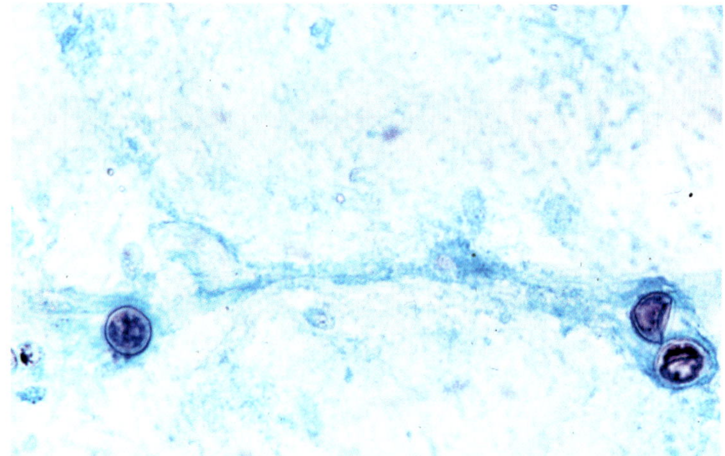

Figure 4.10d — *Blastomyces dermatitidis*, Fine Needle Aspiration [Pap Stain; Medium Power]. Several yeast forms can be seen here in a background of granular debris, likely necrotic. Note the similar size of the yeast forms and the pink color with which they appear after Pap staining. Skin lesions may develop secondary to pulmonary blastomycosis when airborne conidia are inhaled in endemic regions. Other patients may have subclinical infections.

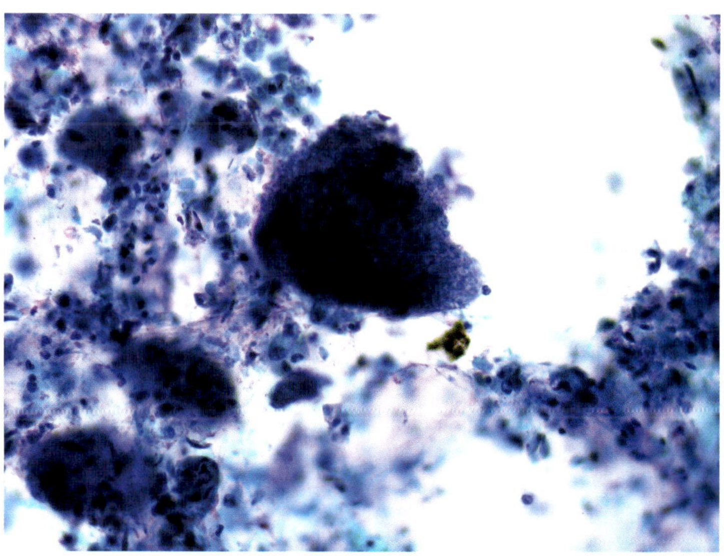

Figure 4.11a — *Pneumocystis jirovecii*, Bronchoalveolar Lavage [Pap Stain; Medium Power]. In bronchoalveolar lavage specimens, *Pneumocystis* may be found in aggregates composed of amassed fungal organisms. The organisms are surrounded by cellular debris and inflammatory cells, characteristic of this infection. *Pneumocystis jirovecii*, the new name for the organism previously known as *Pneumocystis carinii*, causes a diffuse pneumonia in immunocompromised patients (which is still sometimes referred to by the older term *Pneumocystis carinii* pneumonia, commonly abbreviated PCP). Patients most at risk are those with a blood CD4+ T-cell level below 200 cells/μL.

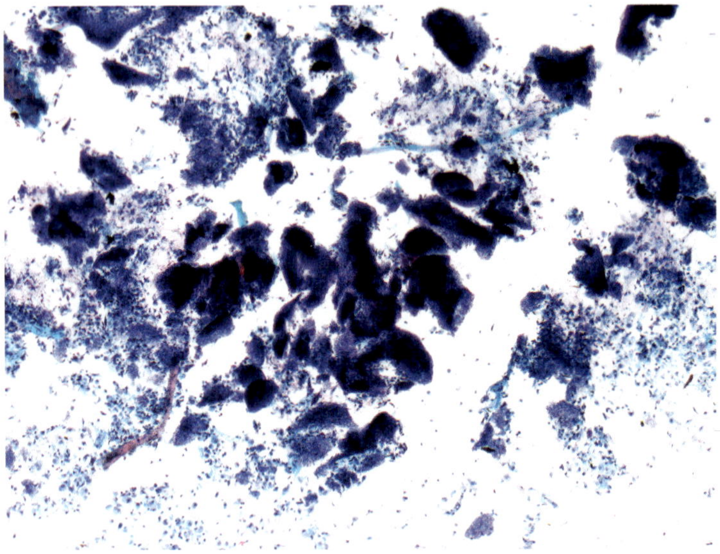

Figure 4.11b — *Pneumocystis jirovecii*, Bronchoalveolar Lavage [Pap Stain; Low Power]. At low power, the large, geometric fungal aggregates stand out from the background mucus, inflammatory cells, and debris. In vivo, the fungus aggregates and proliferates in alveolar spaces, and retains the shape imposed by alveolar walls. This growth pattern also results in a characteristic interstitial pneumonia pattern on chest x-ray.

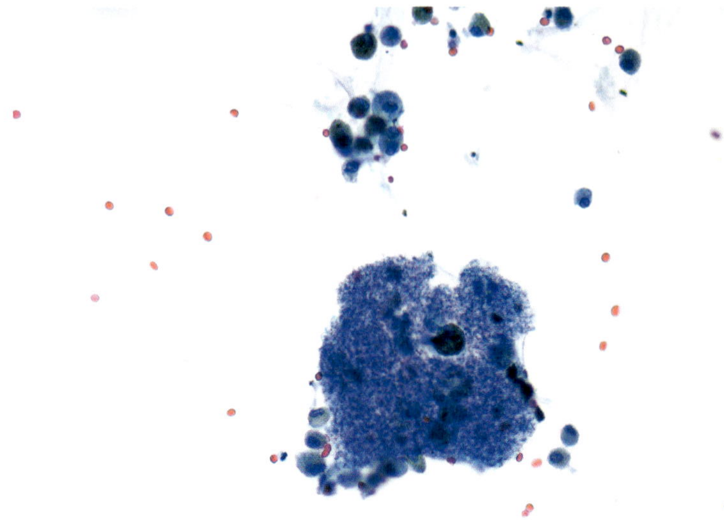

Figure 4.11c — *Pneumocystis jirovecii*, Bronchoalveolar Lavage [Pap Stain; High Power]. At this magnification, the individual rounded to cup-shaped fungal cysts (4–6 microns) within the granular aggregate are distinguishable, particularly around the edge. If any uncertainty exists, a Gomori methenamine silver stain will highlight the organisms. Treatment has shifted to prophylaxis, especially for HIV patients with CD4 less than 200.

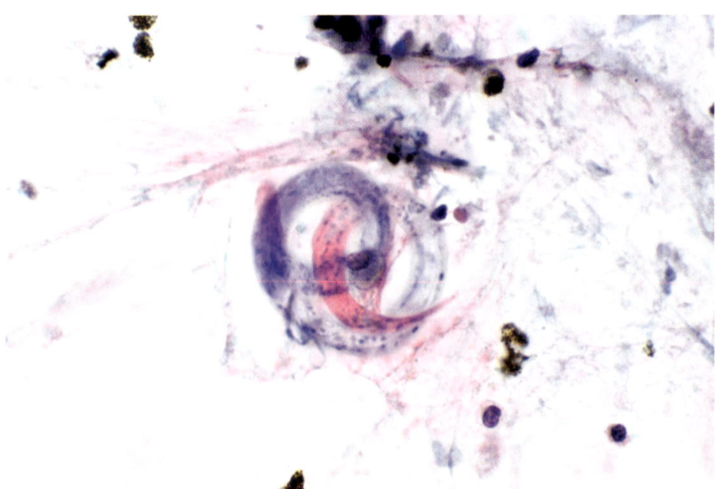

Figure 4.12 — *Strongyloides stercoralis*, Sputum [Pap Stain; High Power]. Strongyloides is most common in developing countries in which water or soil may become contaminated with fecal material. Filariform larvae penetrate the skin and enter the bloodstream. Once reaching the lung, they enter alveolar spaces. It is thought that the larvae are coughed up and swallowed; in the small intestines, adult forms produce eggs that become rhabditoid larvae. These forms can survive in the external environment and transform into adults or infective filariform larvae.

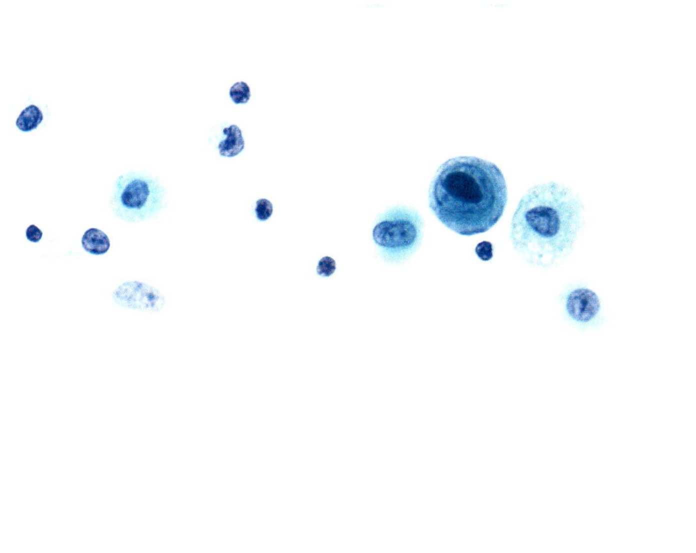

Figure 4.13a — Cytomegalovirus, Bronchoalveolar Lavage [Pap Stain; High Power]. One cell in this image, to the right of center, has a markedly enlarged nucleus with a prominent oval nuclear inclusion and darkened basophilic cytoplasmic inclusions—characteristic of cytomegalovirus infection. The surrounding cells are primarily mononuclear inflammatory cells. Cytomegalovirus infection is most dangerous in immunocompromised patients, where it may present as a reactivation of a latent infection or as a primary infection.

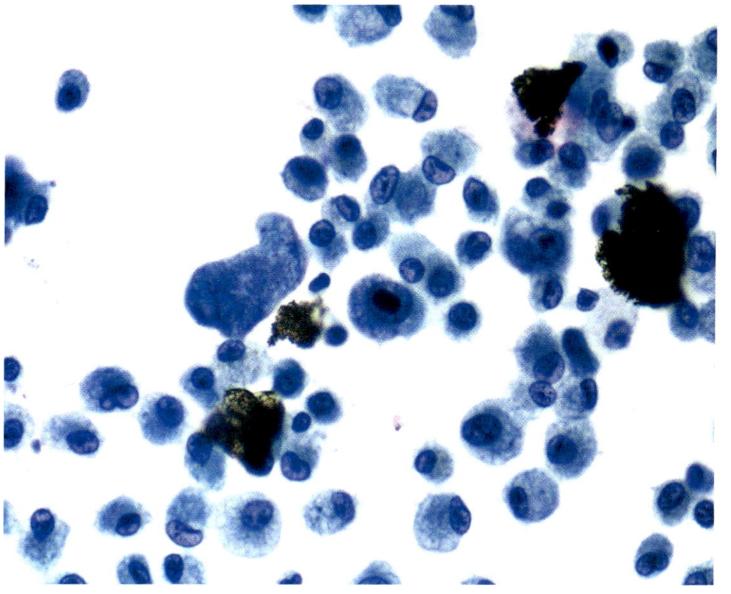

Figure 4.13b — Cytomegalovirus, Bronchoalveolar Lavage [Pap Stain; High Power]. A slightly enlarged central cell has a prominent oval basophilic nuclear inclusion with a surrounding slight clearing. Also present are numerous hemosiderin-laden macrophages and other mononuclear cells. Cytomegalovirus pneumonia in immunocompromised patients is life threatening, even with antiviral therapies.

5

Benign Lung Neoplasms

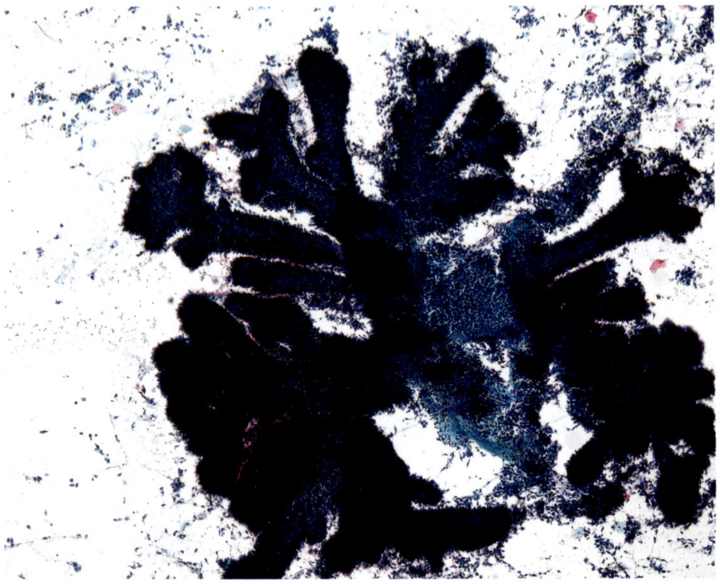

Figure 5.1a — Papillomatosis, Bronchial Brushing [Pap Stain; Low Power]. Three-dimensional bifurcating papillary stalks are immediately noticeable in this large microfragment of tissue. Single cells exfoliated from these branching fronds are also numerous. These neoplasms may be solitary or multiple and are more likely in children and adolescents, but may occur in adults also. As squamous papillomas arise in both major and minor bronchi, their exophytic polypoid-like protrusions into the bronchial lumen allow for this florid architectural branching.

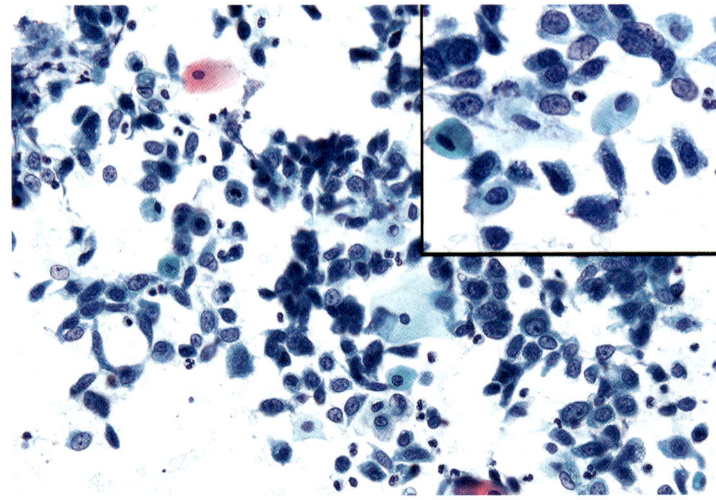

Figure 5.1b — Papillomatosis, Bronchial Brushing [Pap Stain; High Power]. High power magnification shows cells that have exfoliated as single forms and in loose clusters. Cells have the appearance of squamous metaplasia with a modest amount of opaque cytoplasm and rounded nuclei. Admixed with these metaplastic squamous cells are histiocytes and an occasional ciliated bronchial cell. The inset shows evenly dispersed nucleoplasm and smooth nuclear outlines. Though not present in this field, koilocytic change typical of low-grade squamous intraepithelial lesions would not be unusual because of the well-established association of pulmonary squamous papilloma with low-risk human papillomavirus, particularly human papillomavirus-6 and human papillomavirus-11.

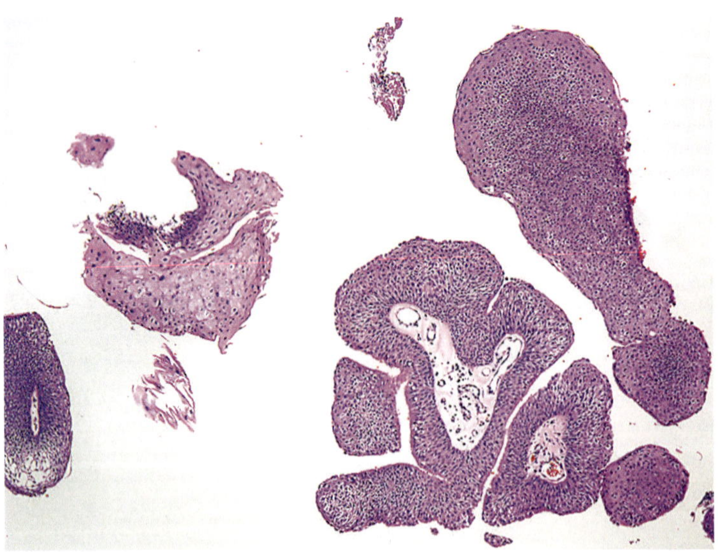

Figure 5.1c — Papillomatosis, Resection [H&E Stain; Low Power]. Tracheobronchial papillomatosis is an uncommon complication of laryngeal disease. The papillomas harbor human papillomavirus types 6 or 11, and are morphologically similar to the laryngeal lesions. This endobronchial biopsy shows characteristic fragments of acanthotic squamous epithelium covering a hyalinized fibrovascular core. The oriented fragments show orderly maturation. Bronchoscopically, the mucosa may appear velvety or shaggy; postobstructive inflammatory changes and even bronchiectasis may supervene.

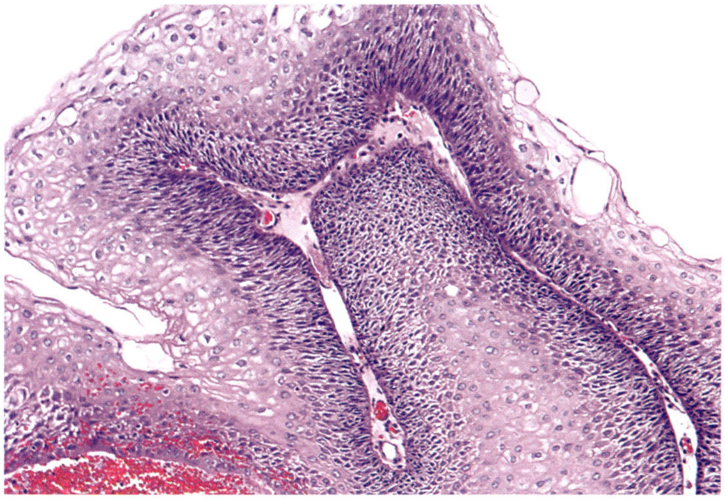

Figure 5.1d — Papillomatosis, Resection [H&E Stain; High Power]. The maturing cells at the surface of this papilloma show human papillomavirus cytopathic effect, with koilocytosis and nuclear hyperchromasia with "raisinoid" features. High grade dysplasia in a papilloma, associated with human papillomavirus-16 and -18, is associated with partial or failed maturation, and is graded according to the World Health Organization classification of preinvasive lesions.

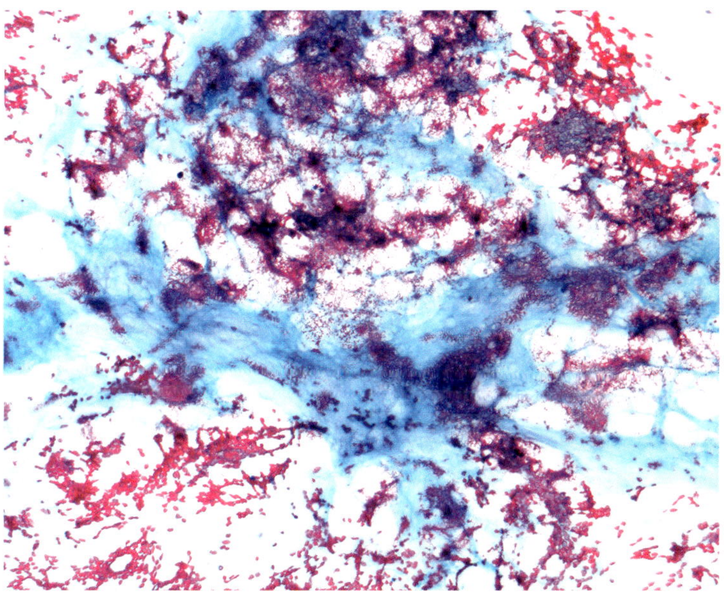

Figure 5.2a — Pulmonary Hamartoma, Fine Needle Aspiration [Pap Stain; Medium Power]. Pulmonary hamartoma is the most common benign neoplasm of the lung. Most are solitary, incidental findings, but multiple lesions have been described, particularly in patients with Carney syndrome. Hamartomas may be endobronchial or intra-parenchymal and radiographically are smoothly contoured, leading to their description as a "coin" lesion. When present radiographically, speckled (so-called "popcorn") calcifications are diagnostically useful. Hyaline-type cartilage and adipose tissue are the two most common components of hamartomas, and as seen here cartilage may be abundant, or minimal in amount, as seen in the next image.

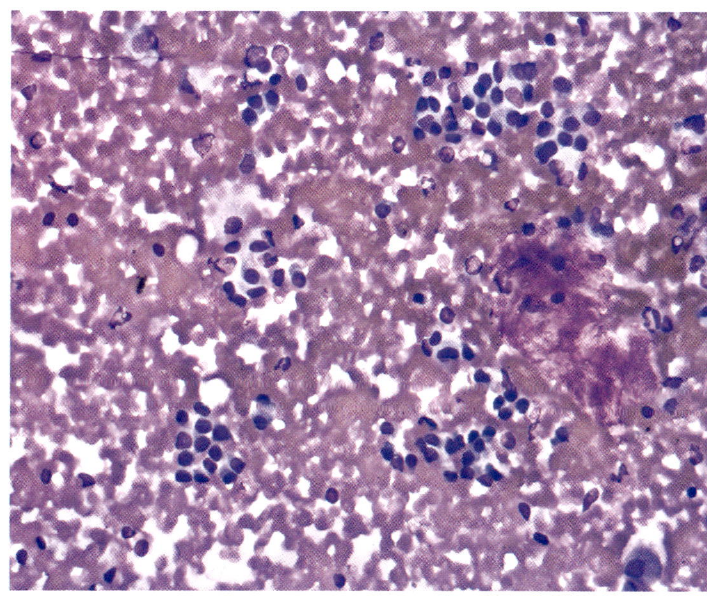

Figure 5.2b — Pulmonary Hamartoma, Fine Needle Aspiration [Diff-Quik Stain; High Power]. Most hamartomas are 3 cm or less in diameter, though larger lesions have been reported. Cellularity is variable and can be dispersed in loose or tight clusters and as single cells. The cellular component is composed of cytologically bland isomorphic cells, but in some cases high cellularity is possible, simulating the possibility of low-grade malignancy such as carcinoid tumor. These cells are derived from bronchiolar or alveolar cells and typically lack cilia. A concentrated search for a mesenchymal component usually allows for a specific diagnosis. In contrast to the prior image, only a small wispy fragment of chondromyxoid stroma is present in this case.

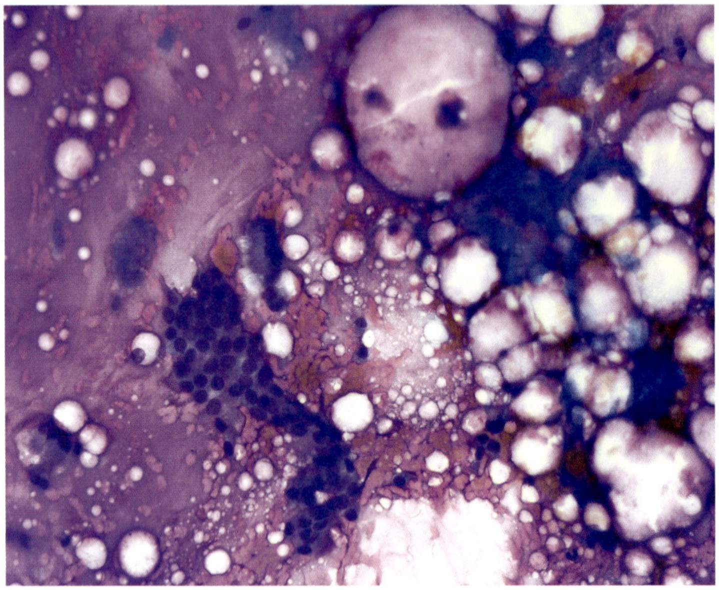

Figure 5.2c — Pulmonary Hamartoma, Fine Needle Aspiration [Diff-Quik Stain; High Power]. This image shares all three components of a pulmonary hamartoma: mature adipose tissue (most noticeable on the right), a cluster of monotonous epithelial cells (center), and myxoid/chondromyxoid stroma (upper left). The stroma is more opaque and chondroid in centrally located hamartomas, and more myxoid or myxohyaline in peripheral lesions.

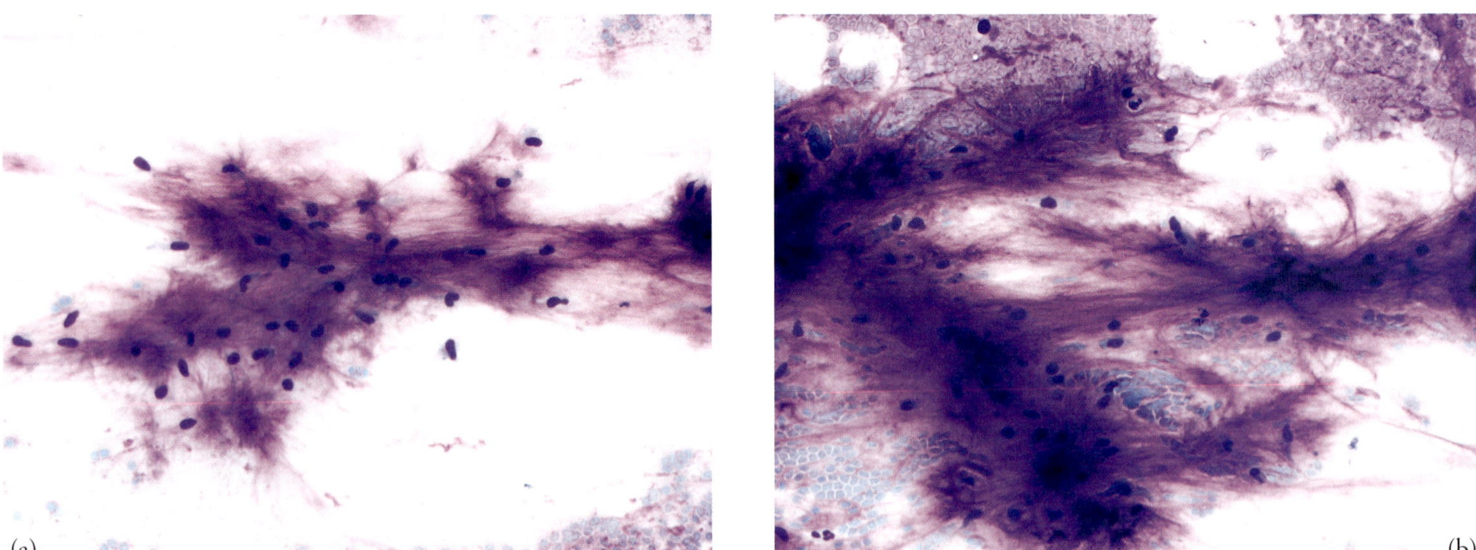

Figure 5.3(a, b) — Hamartoma, Fine Needle Aspiration [Diff-Quik Stain; Medium Power]. The smears show abundant magenta-colored, fibrillary matrix material surrounding bland-appearing epithelioid cells with a thin rim of blue cytoplasm. If this were taken from the salivary gland, it would be strongly suggestive of a pleomorphic adenoma. There is also significant overlap with chondrosarcoma (discussed in Chapter 7). Examination of other fields or fine needle aspiration passes may reveal secondary components more suggestive of hamartoma.

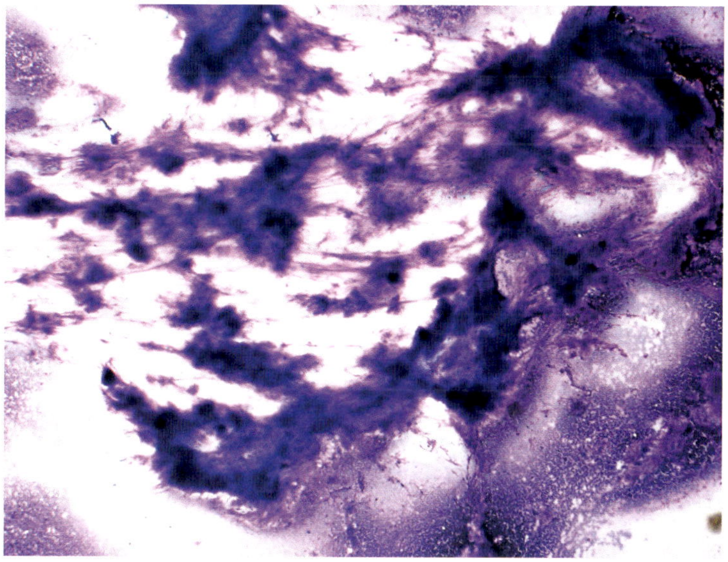

Figure 5.3c — Hamartoma, Fine Needle Aspiration [Diff-Quik Stain; Low Power]. This field contains a large amount of acellular magenta-colored, fibrillary matrix that has the quality of matrix material seen in a pleomorphic adenoma. Given that this sampling was taken from a hamartoma, the matrix material is likely chondroid in origin. Chondroid matrix material can have many different appearances. This highlights the challenge of definitively identifying the origin of background material. For instance, the misidentification of mucinous material as chondromyxoid could lead one far down the incorrect diagnostic path.

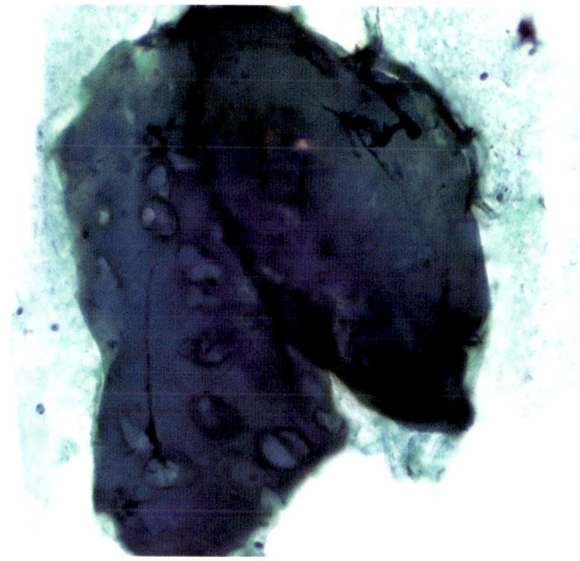

Figure 5.3d — Hamartoma, Fine Needle Aspiration [Pap Stain; High Power]. This fragment of cartilage appears denser and less myxoid than the cartilaginous matrix seen in the previous images. It is also more definitively identifiable as cartilaginous material, given the presence of Swiss cheese-like holes within the matrix. If seen on a separate pass from the same lesion as in the previous images, this would cause one to consider a hamartoma rather than a pleomorphic adenoma. Unfortunately, this could also represent contamination from the normal cartilage if the needle has passed through a large airway, in which case the differential diagnosis remains between hamartoma and pleomorphic adenoma.

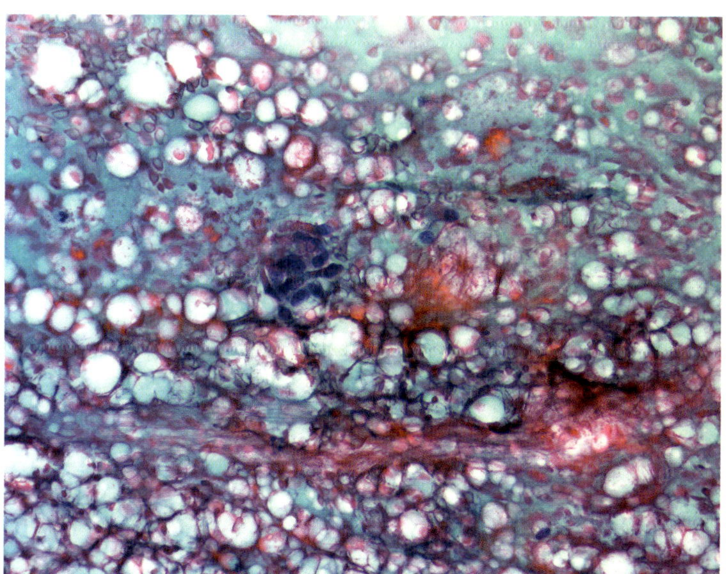

Figure 5.4a — Hamartoma, Fine Needle Aspiration [Pap Stain; Medium Power]. This colorful field demonstrates intermixed lipid and myxoid material with rare, bland-appearing cuboidal epithelial cells present in the center of the field. It is thought that these epithelial cells may represent entrapped respiratory or alveolar epithelium that has undergone metaplasia and/or hyperplasia. Hamartomas contain a variable mixture of components and the fine needle aspiration findings are representative of the components present, as well as which components are sampled.

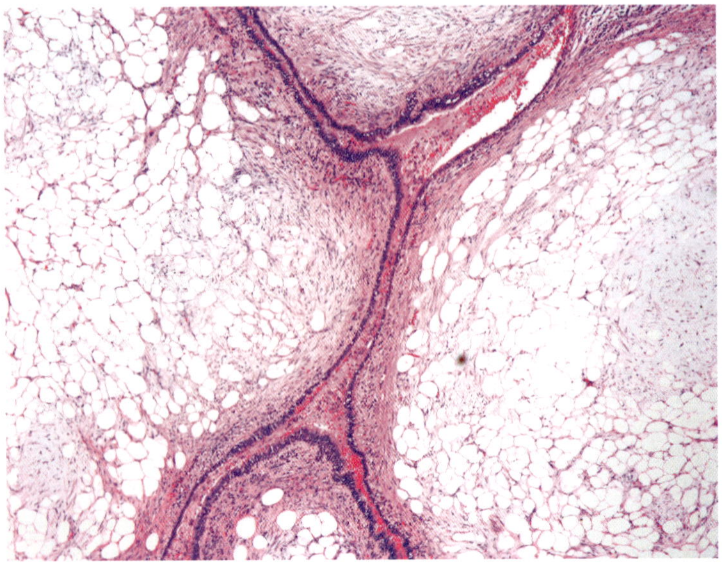

Figure 5.4b — Hamartoma, Biopsy [H&E Stain; Low Power]. At low power, the characteristic lobulated architecture of hamartoma is apparent. Nodules of adipose tissue and myxoid stroma are separated by entrapped bronchiolar epithelium. Although disorganized, the histomorphology is otherwise that of normal tissues.

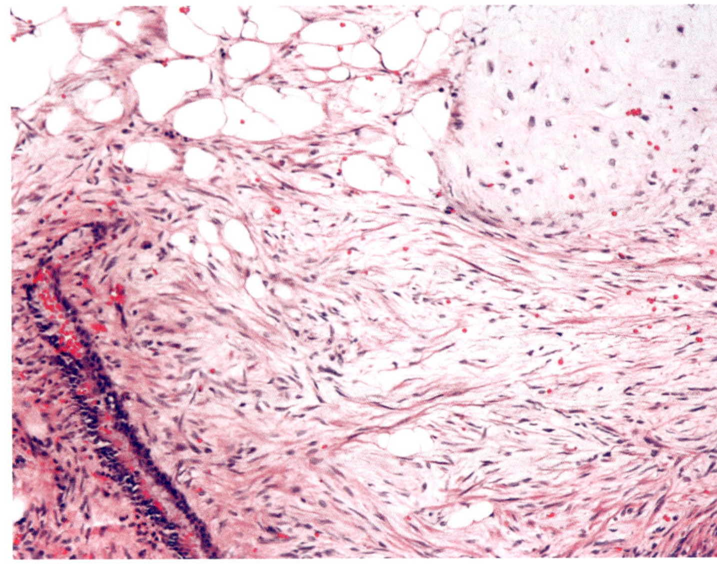

Figure 5.4c — Hamartoma, Biopsy [H&E Stain; High Power]. This mesenchymal neoplasm is composed of mature chondroid tissue admixed with fibrous and adipose tissue. The epithelium at the lower left represents entrapped bronchiolar epithelium. Other examples may contain varying proportions of a range of mesenchymal elements, including bone, smooth muscle, and myxoid stroma. Hamartomas are distinguished from benign pulmonary soft tissue tumors by the presence of two or more mesenchymal components. Carney Triad-associated chondromas are encapsulated and lack entrapped epithelium; osseous metaplasia is often present. Primary or metastatic sarcoma should be considered if significant nuclear atypia is present.

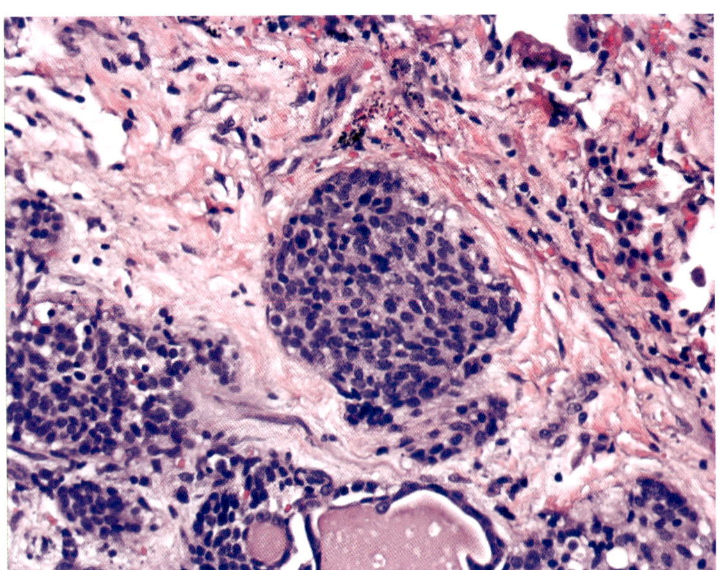

Figure 5.5 — Tumorlet, Biopsy [H&E Stain; High Power]. Tumorlets are well-circumscribed nests of neuroendocrine cells, ≤3 mm, embedded in fibrous stroma, typically adjacent to small bronchioles. The component cells may be round, oval, or spindled, and have a moderate amount of eosinophilic cytoplasm; salt and pepper-type chromatin is characteristic. Tumorlets are usually an incidental finding in abnormal lungs biopsied or resected for a wide variety of chronic lung diseases. A diagnosis of "diffuse idiopathic pulmonary neuroendocrine cell hyperplasia" is appropriate when tumorlets are numerous and diffuse throughout the lungs. In small biopsies, tumorlets may mimic meningothelial nodules (EMA- and PR-positive, negative for neuroendocrine markers) and granulomas (CD68-positive, negative for keratins, and neuroendocrine markers). The fine needle aspiration of tumorlets has rarely been described in literature; most likely they are rarely sampled due to their small size.

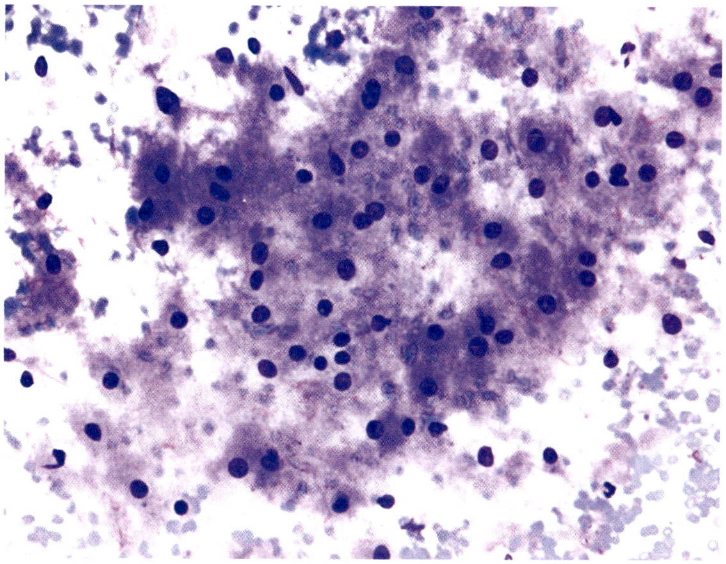

Figure 5.6a — Granular Cell Tumor, Fine Needle Aspiration [Diff-Quik Stain; High Power]. Granular cell tumor of the lower respiratory tract is rare, occurring in patients in the fourth to fifth decades of life. It arises primarily as an endobronchial plaque or exophytic mass near the bifurcation of the major bronchi. Due to this, most cytologic citations have been from bronchial brushing specimens. Smears are variable cellular and sometimes hypocellular as a result of the desmoplasia induced by this neoplasm. Polygonal cells are characterized by an enormous amount of cytoplasm with blurry cell borders. Due to cell fragility, bare nuclei are common. Romanowsky staining of this air-dried smear fails to demonstrate the prototypical cytoplasmic granularity in this syncytial aggregate.

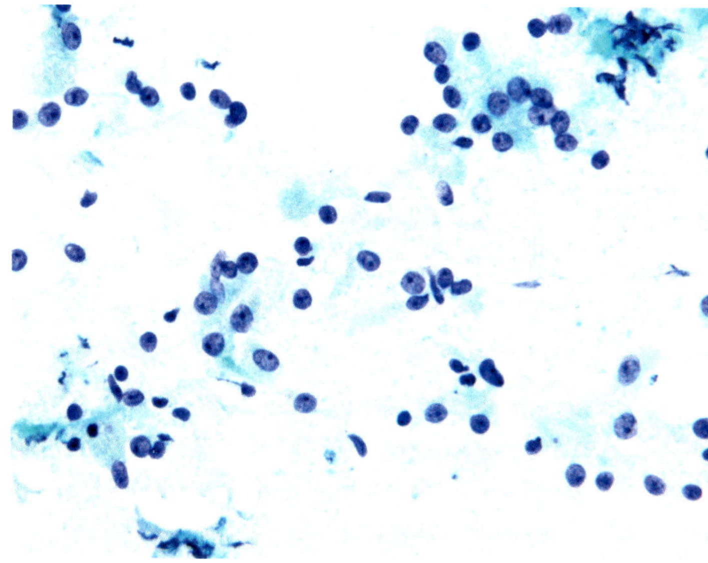

Figure 5.6b — Granular Cell Tumor, Fine Needle Aspiration [Pap Stain; High Power]. With alcohol-fixed preparations, cytoplasmic granularity is slightly better perceived. Despite large nuclei and discrete single nucleoli, the granular cell tumor is a benign neoplasm. Necrosis and mitotic figures are absent. By immunohistochemistry, granular cell tumor is positive for S-100, SOX-10, and inhibin, and negative for keratin, HMB-45 and Melan-A.

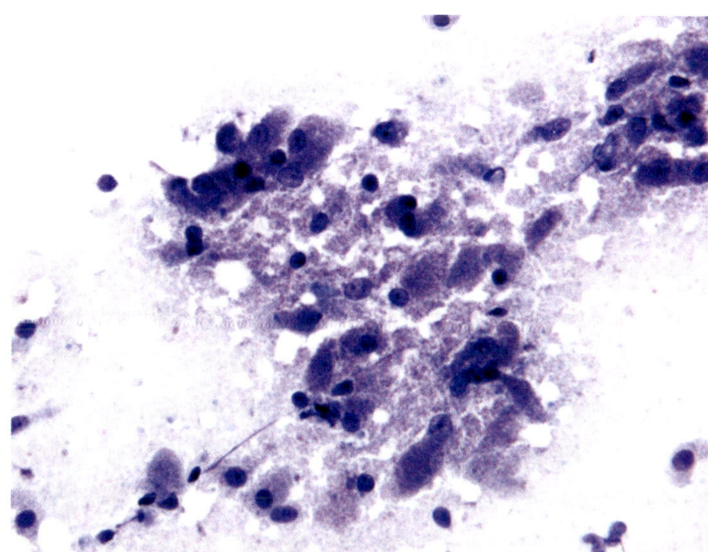

Figure 5.6c — Granular Cell Tumor, Fine Needle Aspiration [Pap Stain; High Power]. Coarse granules are easily recognized in this example. Cytoplasmic granules are not confined to cells that are easily ruptured, but also "spill" into the smear background. Unlike most histiocytic proliferations that may enter into the differential diagnosis, such as malakoplakia or mycobacterial infection, granular cell tumor lacks cytoplasmic vacuoles.

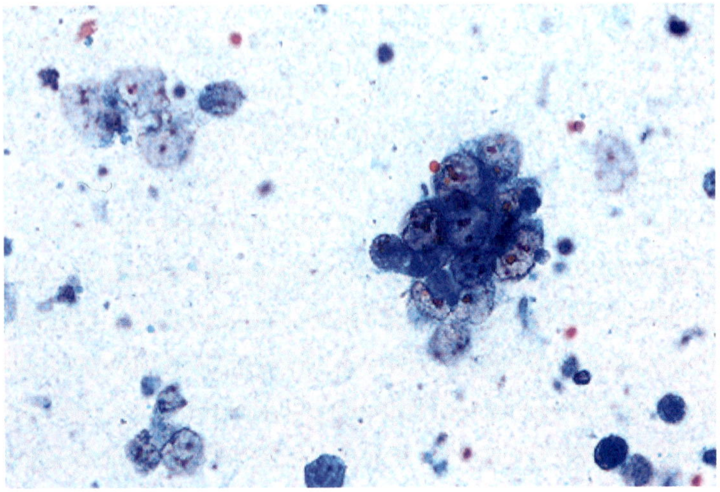

Figure 5.6d — Granular Cell Tumor, Fine Needle Aspiration [Pap Stain; High Power]. The cells of a granular cell tumor in Pap-stained smears are present singly and in small aggregates and have open chromatin and conspicuous nucleoli with the eponymous granular cytoplasm. The granules are coarse and variably sized, and the background is gritty. The differential diagnosis of a granular cell tumor includes smooth muscle tumors, histiocytic tumors, melanoma, and alveolar soft part sarcoma (particularly in children).

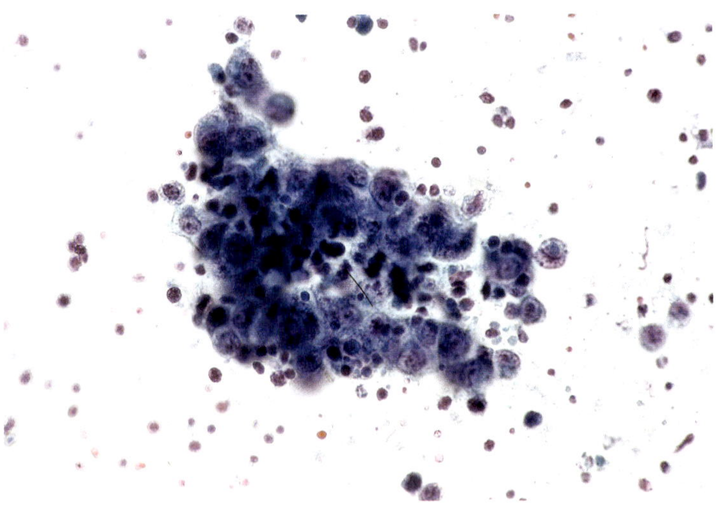

Figure 5.7a — Granular Cell Tumor, Fine Needle Aspiration [Pap Stain; High Power]. This is another example of a granular cell tumor. The tumor cells are present in a loose aggregate with scattered lymphocytes and a histiocytoid look to the tumor cells themselves. Granular cell tumors are usually benign; however, large size, rapid growth, and nodal metastasis are characteristic of malignancy in granular cell tumors. Immunohistochemically, the tumor cells express CD68 and also express S100 diffusely, which suggests a nerve sheath origin; indeed, these tumors are considered of Schwann cell origin.

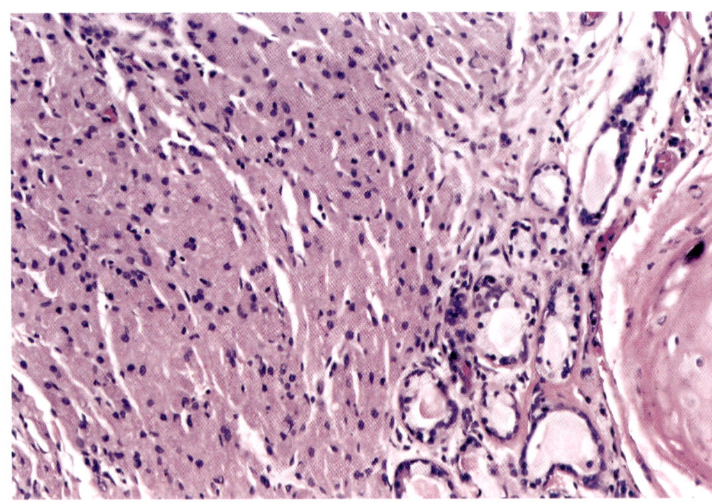

Figure 5.7b — Granular Cell Tumor, Biopsy [H&E Stain; High Power]. To the right is a fragment of cartilage and submucosal glands, but the remainder of the field is filled by sheets of eosinophilic cells. The cells have round to oval nuclei with visible nucleoli and abundant pink cytoplasm with a granular appearance. This is the typical appearance for a granular cell tumor. Although more common in the oral cavity and skin, tumors in visceral sites have been reported. In the lung, granular cell tumors may be associated with the airways and may present as an endobronchial lesion.

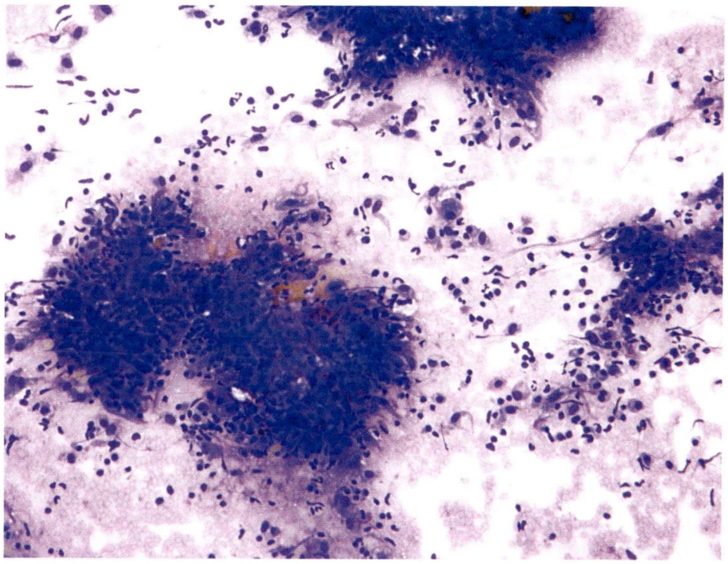

Figure 5.8a — Inflammatory Myofibroblastic Tumor, Fine Needle Aspiration [Diff-Quik Stain; Medium Power]. Inflammatory myofibroblastic tumor is a mesenchymal neoplasm of children and adults composed of spindled myofibroblastic and fibroblastic cells admixed with an inflammatory infiltrate. The latter is typically composed of plasma cells, lymphocytes, and eosinophils, but not neutrophils. The lung is one of the least affected organs as most examples occur in an intra-abdominal location. Adult patients are typically less than 50 years of age. Patients may be asymptomatic or present with nonspecific constitutional symptoms such as chronic cough, fever, and chest pain. These are intra-parenchymal nodules, and as such fine-needle aspirates are the usual cytologic specimen. Smears are hypercellular and consist of cell aggregates of variable quantity and size with irregular ragged edges. Myofibroblastic cells seem to peel off the edges of these aggregates, and mix with inflammatory cells. Necrosis is usually absent, and mitoses are infrequent.

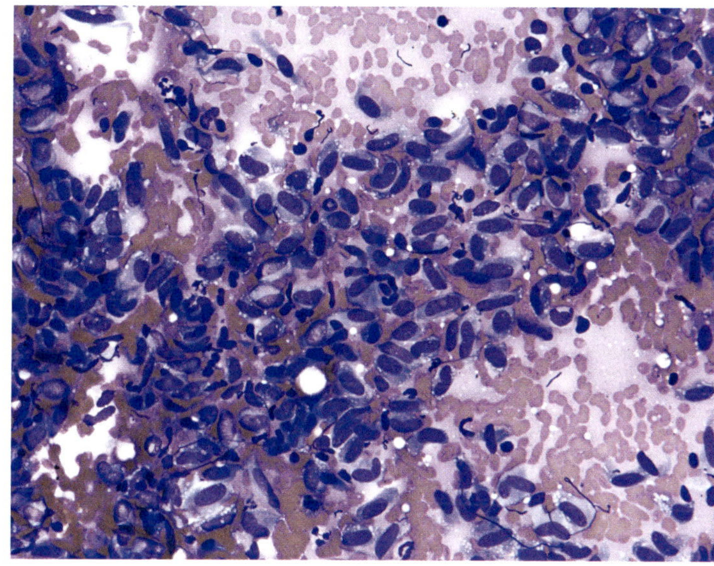

Figure 5.8b — Inflammatory Myofibroblastic Tumor, Fine Needle Aspiration [Diff-Quik Stain; High Power]. This image of an almost pure population of single and loosely clustered homogeneous spindle-shaped cells evokes a differential diagnosis of a mesenchymal neoplasm, in particular nonpleomorphic spindle cell proliferations such as synovial sarcoma, solitary fibrous tumor, schwannoma, and well-differentiated leiomyosarcoma. Immunohistochemical staining using an appropriate panel of antibodies should easily exclude these entities. Since some cells have blunt-edged elongated nuclei that are slightly indented on one side, one might also consider the possibility of a granuloma. However, the extremely loose arrangement of these cells is distinctly unusual for nonnecrotic granulomas in which the epithelioid histiocytes are typically tightly clustered.

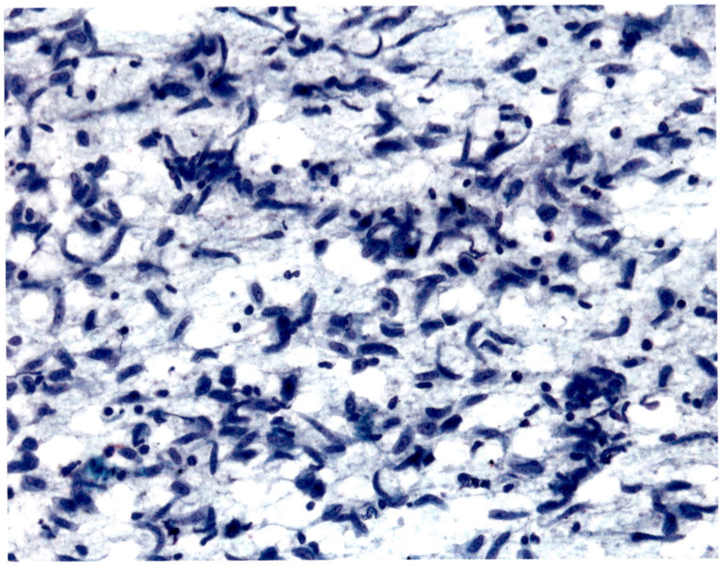

Figure 5.8c — Inflammatory Myofibroblastic Tumor, Fine Needle Aspiration [Pap Stain; High Power]. In contrast to the prior image, these fibroblasts/myofibroblasts show distinct tapering of nuclei with curvilinear forms and bipolar or unipolar cytoplasmic extensions. An almost equal distribution of lymphocytes and mesenchymal cells is present. Alcohol-fixed smears allow for the detailed delineation of single micronucleoli and vesicular nuclei in spindle cells.

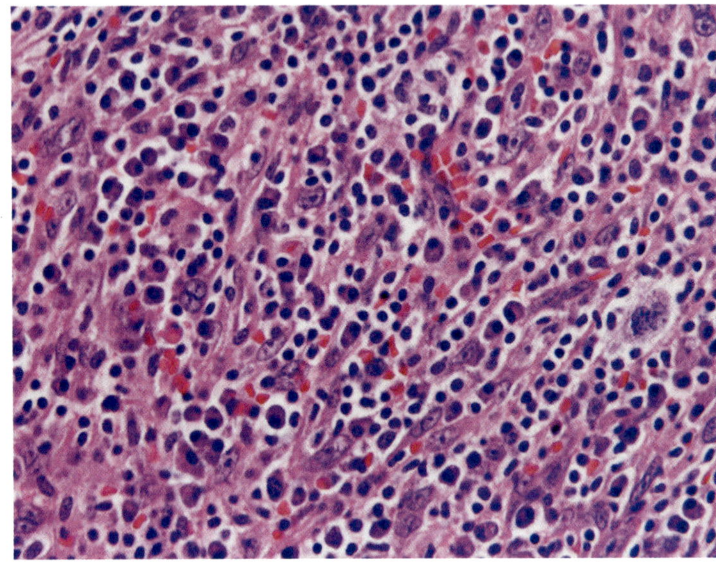

Figure 5.8d — Inflammatory Myofibroblastic Tumor, Fine Needle Aspiration [H&E Stain; High Power]. In some examples from formalin-fixed paraffin-embedded cell blocks, the spindled myofibroblasts are partially masked by a dense plasmacytic and lymphocytic inflammatory infiltrate. Inflammatory myofibroblastic tumor is positive with smooth muscle actin, and less so with muscle specific actin (HHF35) stain and desmin consistent with myofibroblastic differentiation. About one third of cases also express pan-keratin staining. Chromosomal rearrangement involving the *ALK* gene translates into positive staining with the ALK antibody in less than 50% of pulmonary examples in adults.

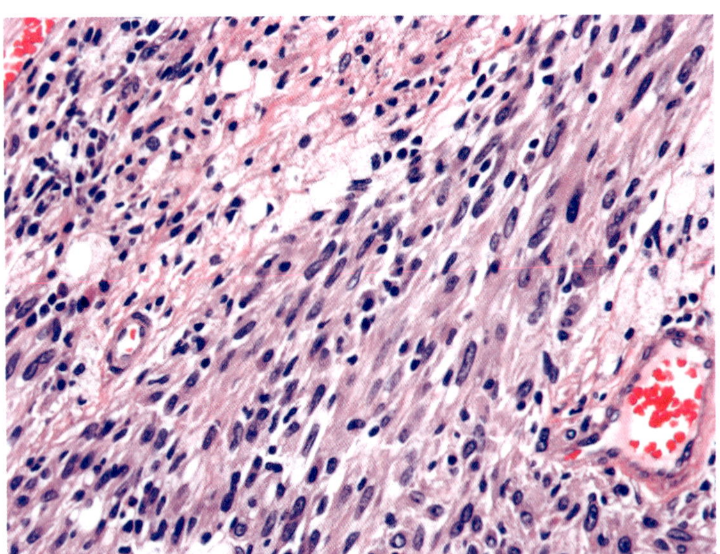

Figure 5.9a — Inflammatory Myofibroblastic Tumor, Lobectomy [H&E Stain; High Power]. The tumor cells of inflammatory myofibroblastic tumor are spindled, with pale eosinophilic cytoplasm, indistinct borders, and vesicular nuclei with tapering ends. The cells are most often in fascicles, although a storiform pattern is sometimes seen. Mitotic rate is variable, but does not correlate with biologic behavior. Zones of foamy cells, as in this example, are sometimes present. A superimposed reactive chronic inflammatory infiltrate is of variable density, and may focally obscure the spindle cells; plasma cells often predominate, and germinal centers are sometimes present.

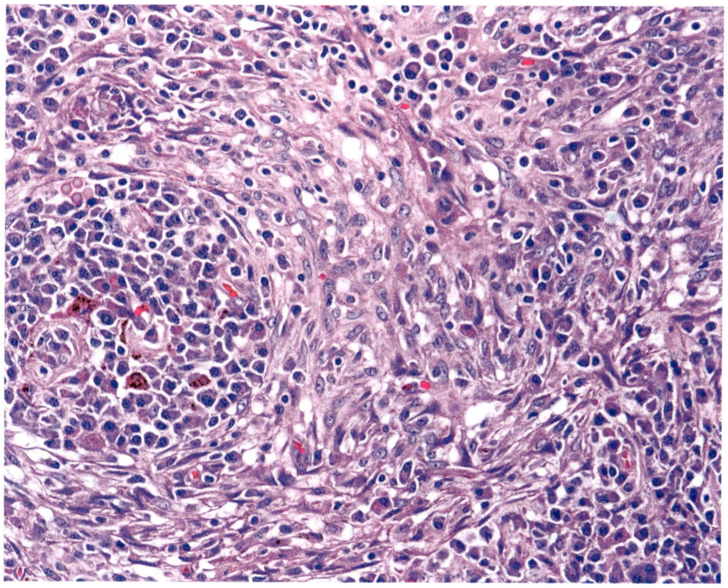

Figure 5.9b — Inflammatory Myofibroblastic Tumor, Lobectomy [H&E Stain; High Power]. Background spindle cells are obscured by a nodular and diffuse lymphoplasmacytic infiltrate (Hematoxylin and eosin stain, high power). An immunostain for ALK1 is positive in about 50% of instances, most commonly in children and young adults; in such cases, a break-apart fluorescence in situ hybridization study will demonstrate the fusion gene, also observed in anaplastic large-cell lymphoma and some B-cell lymphomas. Sarcoma with muscle differentiation should be excluded (marked nuclear atypia; atypical mitoses), and lymphoma becomes a consideration when the lymphoplasmacytic infiltrate is dense, monomorphous, and/or atypical; in such circumstances, flow cytometry and immunohistochemical phenotyping of the infiltrate may be indicated.

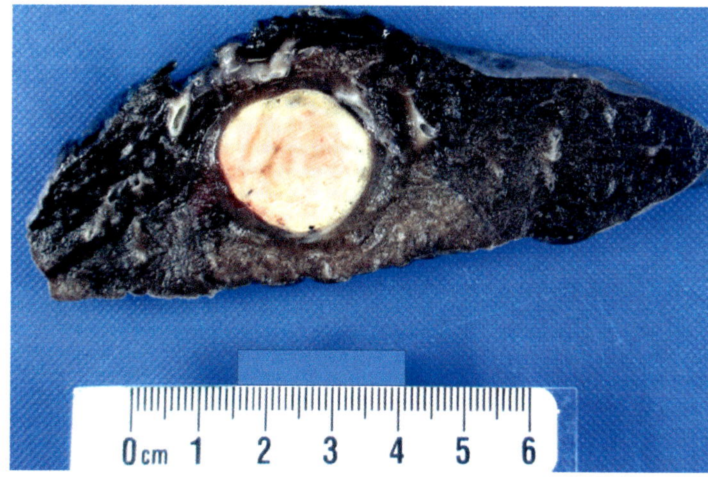

Figure 5.9c — Inflammatory Myofibroblastic Tumor, Lobectomy [Gross Examination]. This inflammatory myofibroblastic tumor was an incidental finding during an employment physical examination. The lesion is well circumscribed and tan-yellow, with a whorled cut surface.

6

Malignant Lung Neoplasms

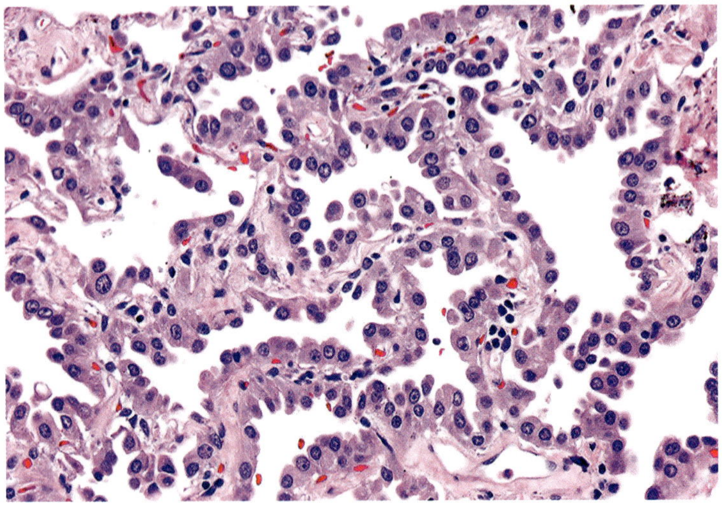

Figure 6.1 — Atypical Adenomatous Hyperplasia, Biopsy [H&E Stain; High Power]. This preinvasive neoplastic glandular proliferation is made up of cuboidal to low columnar cells with cytoplasmic snouts, which proliferate along alveolar septal surfaces. There is only mild nuclear atypia, with rare to no mitoses, and without associated septal thickening. Double nuclei, slight stratification, and cytoplasmic vacuolation may be present, and some examples have intranuclear pseudoinclusions. An important differential diagnostic consideration is reactive pneumocyte hyperplasia, in which the cells are more uniform, with associated inflammation and fibrosis in a clinical context of recent injury. Atypical adenomatous hyperplasia closely resembles nonmucinous adenocarcinoma in situ and lepidic-pattern invasive adenocarcinoma, and cannot be confidently distinguished from these on a small biopsy.

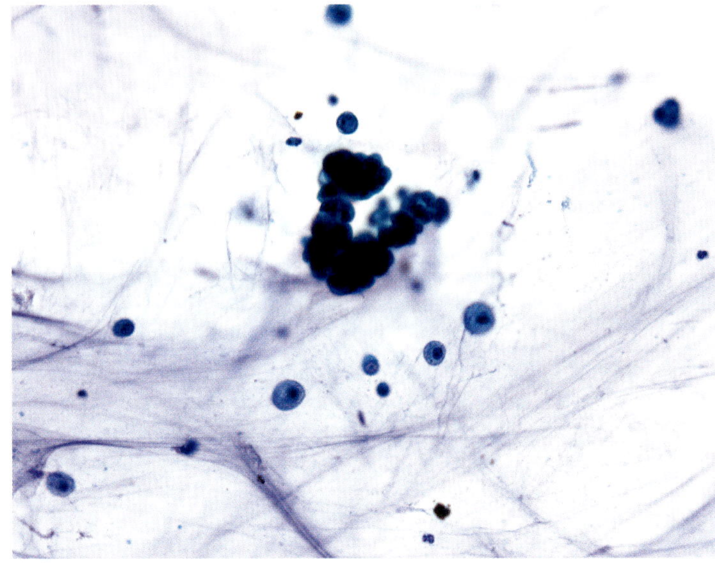

Figure 6.2a — Adenocarcinoma, Well-Differentiated, Sputum [Pap Stain; Medium Power]. This specimen is representative of what used to be known as "bronchoalveolar carcinoma," a well-differentiated adenocarcinoma of the lung that is associated with a lepidic growth pattern on histology; it is no longer classified as a distinct entity according to International Association for the Study of Lung Cancer (IASLC)/the American Thoracic Society (ATS). Furthermore, World Health Organization classification of bronchoalveolar carcinoma requires histology in order to exclude invasion. Cytologic specimens demonstrate cytomorphologic features distinct from other adenocarcinomas of the lung. As seen here, the neoplastic cells are cuboidal, small, and have round uniform nuclei. The cells form a three-dimensional papillary structure, but other patterns include flat sheets and acinar arrays.

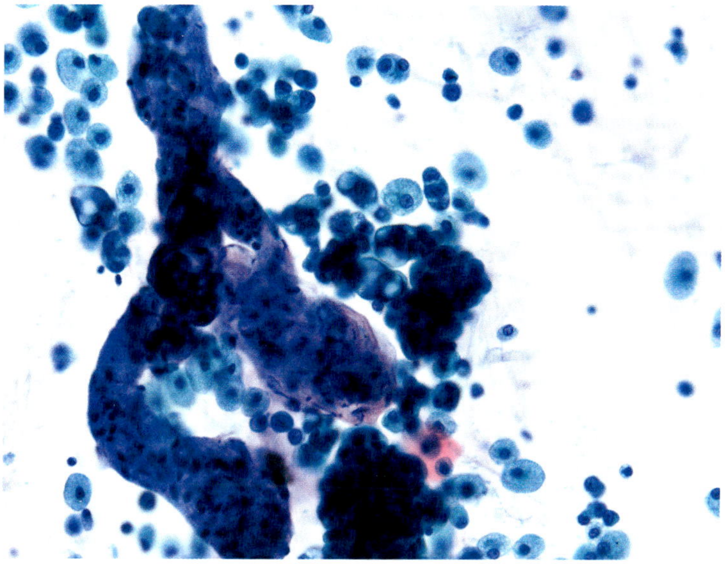

Figure 6.2b — Adenocarcinoma, Well-Differentiated, Sputum [Pap Stain; Medium Power]. Well-differentiated adenocarcinoma with a lepidic growth pattern may be mucinous or, more commonly, nonmucinous. This field demonstrates a mucinous adenocarcinoma in which some neoplastic cells contain large mucinous vacuoles. This reduces the nuclear-to-cytoplasmic ratio and makes the cells appear bland. Due to growth within airways, the mucin-producing cells have created a mucin plug in the shape of the airway that contains neoplastic cells. Note the muciphages in the background, with bubbly cytoplasm, which may be difficult to distinguish from discohesive individual neoplastic cells at first glance.

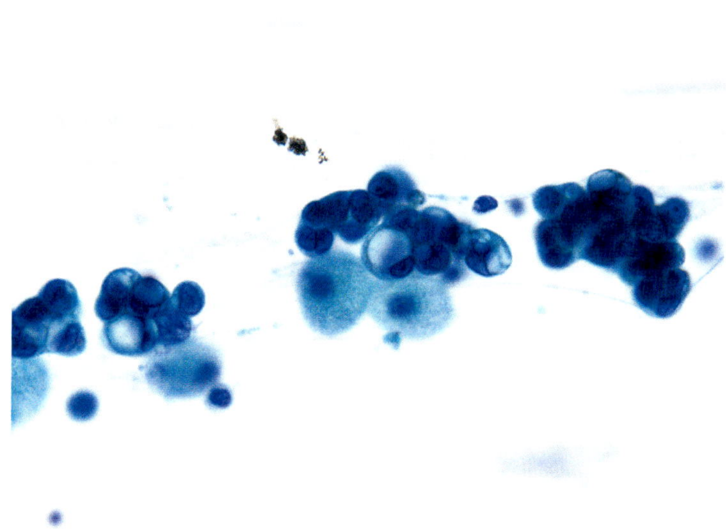

Figure 6.2c — Adenocarcinoma, Well-Differentiated, Sputum [Pap Stain; High Power]. Some cells contain large mucin vacuoles while other cells have high nuclear-to-cytoplasmic ratios; however, the nuclei share similar features: moderately hyperchromatic, with moderate to marked nuclear border irregularities and a distinct nucleolus. The cells form loose clusters.

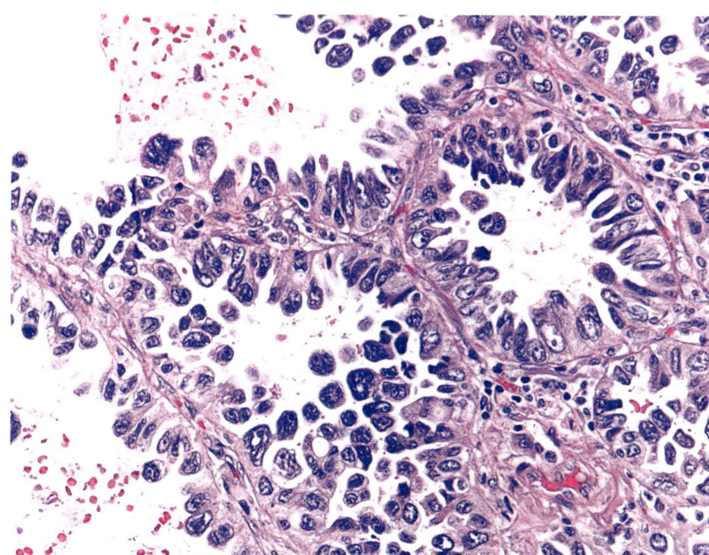

Figure 6.2d — Lepidic-Predominant Adenocarcinoma, Wedge Resection [H&E Stain; High Power]. The neoplastic cells are nonmucinous, with a "hobnail" appearance reminiscent of type II pneumocytes or Clara cells, and moderate to marked nuclear atypia; other examples are quite bland cytologically. Lepidic-pattern adenocarcinoma grows along the surfaces of alveolar septa. TTF-1 and napsin A are routinely positive. This appearance may be seen as a pure pattern in adenocarcinoma in situ and in minimally invasive adenocarcinoma, or as one of several patterns in invasive adenocarcinoma ("adenocarcinoma with a lepidic component"). The World Health Organization recommended terminology in small biopsies (including cytology specimens) with identifiable lepidic growth pattern is "adenocarcinoma (lepidic pattern)."

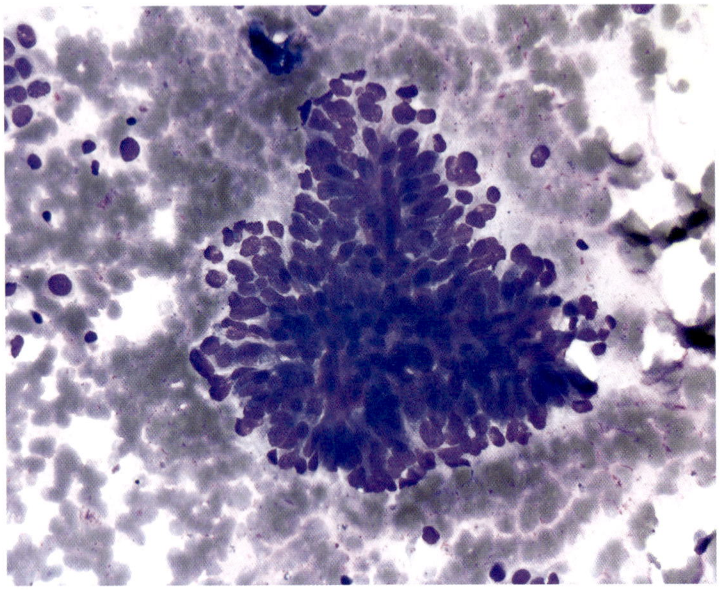

Figure 6.3a — Adenocarcinoma, Papillary Growth Pattern, Fine Needle Aspiration [Diff-Quik Stain; Medium Power]. The malignant cells have elongated nuclei with nuclear grooves and are attached to a true papillary stalk, as defined by the presence of a fibrovascular core. Lung adenocarcinomas can have a papillary growth pattern, though the differential includes metastases of a papillary lesion, such as papillary thyroid carcinoma, urothelial carcinoma, and papillary renal cell carcinoma.

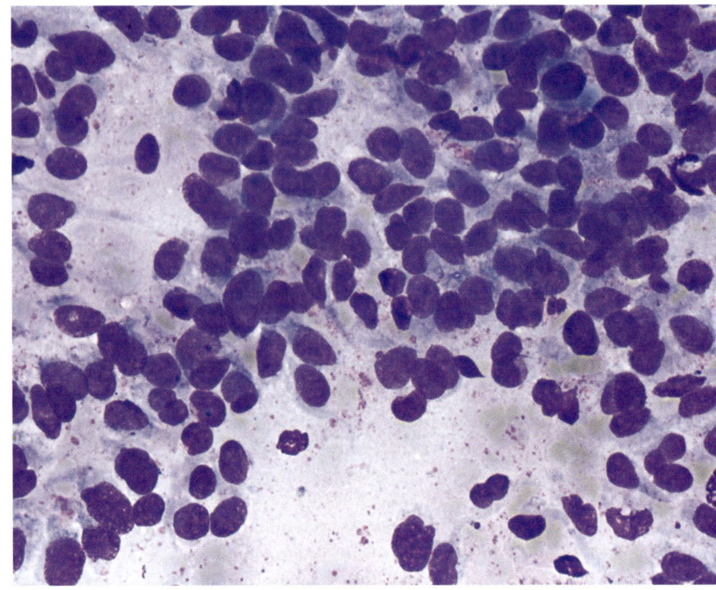

Figure 6.3b — Adenocarcinoma, Papillary Growth Pattern, Fine Needle Aspiration [Diff-Quik Stain; High Power]. Subclassifying the growth pattern of lung adenocarcinoma on cytology is not typically possible or necessary. While this field contains malignant cells from a papillary adenocarcinoma, the absence of fibrovascular cores in this field makes this distinction impossible. However, the features of adenocarcinoma are present: enlarged nuclei with irregular nuclear borders, anisonucleosis, and nuclear overlap. The cytoplasmic boundaries are difficult to discern, but most nuclei are eccentrically placed, a feature of glandular differentiation.

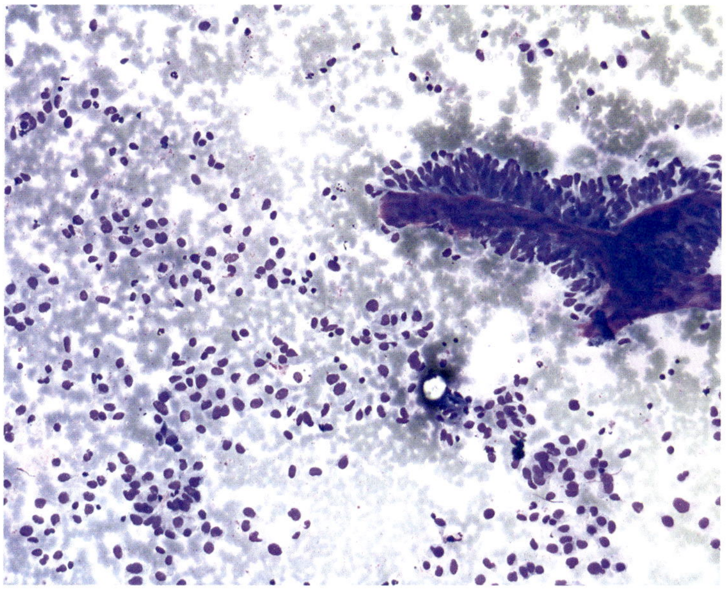

Figure 6.3c — Adenocarcinoma, Papillary Growth Pattern, Fine Needle Aspiration [Diff-Quik Stain; Low Power]. The papillary fragment with a fibrovascular core indicates the papillary nature of this lesion. By contrast, the left-hand side of the field contains predominantly singly dispersed tumor cells with similar features as those seen on the papillary fragment. While it is likely that these cells have become dissociated from the papillary fragment, a papillary growth pattern is often seen as a mixed pattern in lung adenocarcinoma. Other growth patterns may not be sampled or, if sampled, may not be discernible by cytology.

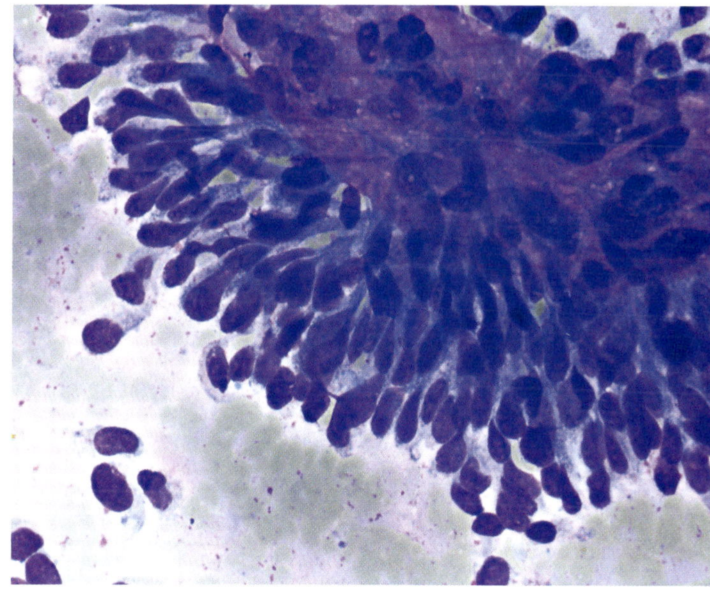

Figure 6.3d — Adenocarcinoma, Papillary Growth Pattern, Fine Needle Aspiration [Diff-Quik Stain; High Power]. The malignant cells attached to the papillary stalk are monotonous appearing and show little nuclear size variation. However, the cellular nature of this lesion—as well as the presence of a fibrovascular stalk—leaves little doubt that it is neoplastic. The cells have a flask-shaped appearance, perhaps due to forces exerted during the aspiration procedure or creation of the smear. Some cells have become detached from the fragment.

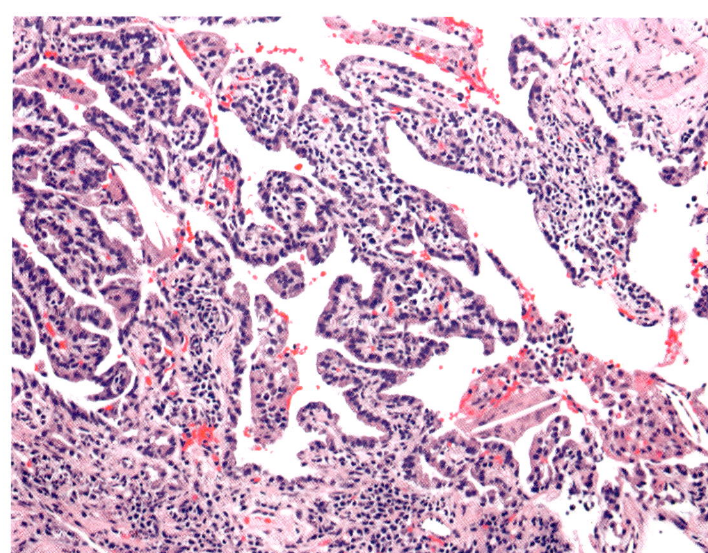

Figure 6.4a — Adenocarcinoma, Papillary Growth Pattern, Lobectomy [H&E Stain; Low Power]. This adenocarcinoma is composed of papillae with variably sclerotic fibrovascular cores. In inflated specimens, the papillary features can be readily identified; if inflation is poor, compressed papillae can mimic lepidic growth.

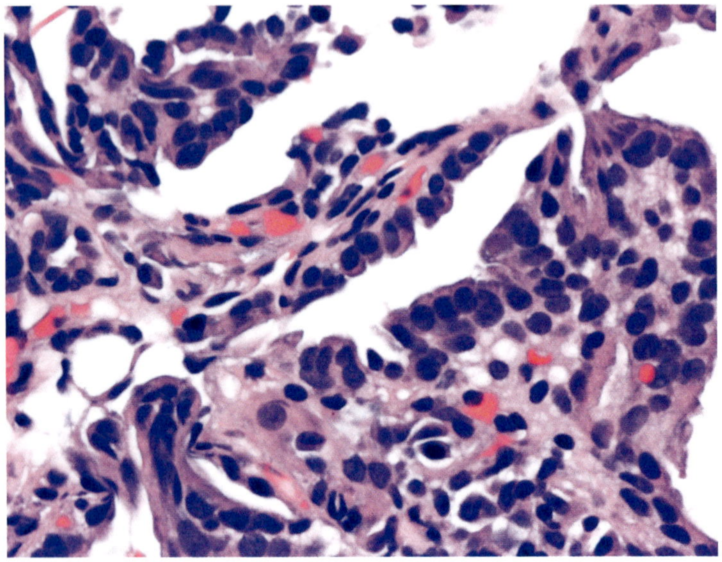

Figure 6.4b — Adenocarcinoma, Papillary Growth Pattern, Lobectomy [H&E Stain; High Power]. The neoplastic cells are arrayed in an orderly fashion along the papillae. There is only mild atypia, although crowding and overlapping are occasionally present. Some examples have intranuclear pseudoinclusions.

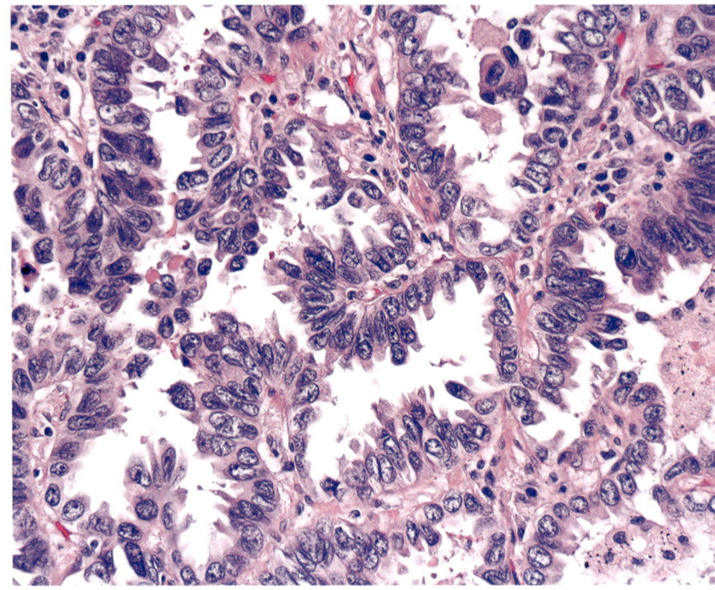

Figure 6.4c — Adenocarcinoma, Papillary Growth Pattern, Lobectomy [H&E Stain; High Power]. Exophytic finger-like fronds with fibrovascular cores are characteristic of the papillary pattern of pulmonary adenocarcinoma. The nuclei show moderate to marked pleomorphism and significant atypia, with frequent nucleoli. Most adenocarcinomas of lung origin have a mix of patterns, and papillary architecture is a common component. Expression of napsin A and TTF-1 is characteristic, and allows distinction from papillary adenocarcinoma originating in the gastrointestinal (CK20 and CDX2+) or GYN (PAX8 and ER+) tracts.

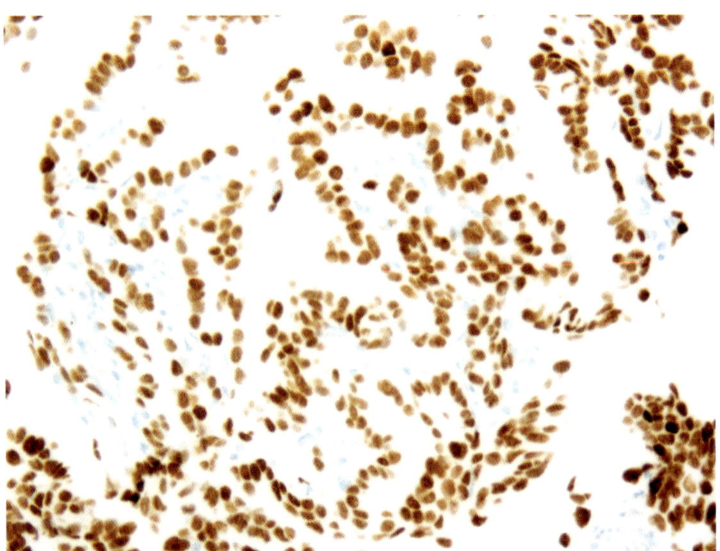

Figure 6.4d — Adenocarcinoma, Papillary Growth Pattern, Lobectomy [TTF-1 Immunohistochemical Stain; Low Power]. Expression of TTF-1 is strong and uniform in tumor cell nuclei. The major histologic differential consideration is metastatic papillary thyroid cancer, which can be excluded with history, imaging, and a thyroglobulin stain.

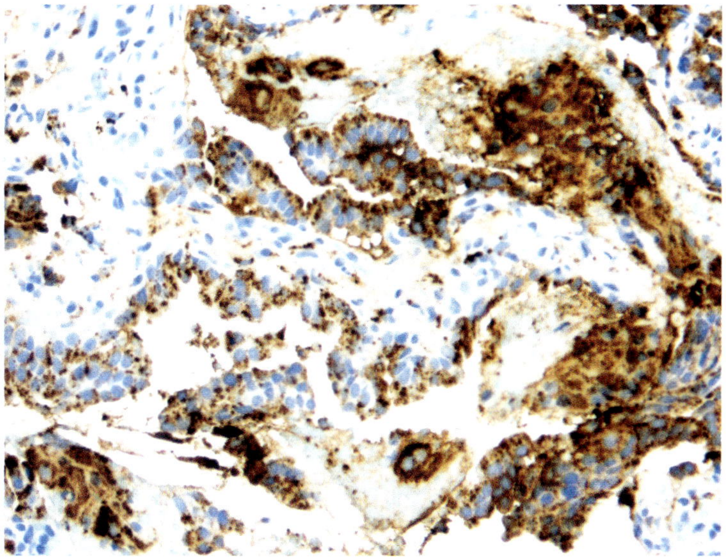

Figure 6.4e — Adenocarcinoma, Papillary Growth Pattern, Lobectomy [Napsin A Immunohistochemical Stain; Low Power]. There is strong and uniform staining for napsin A in the characteristic granular cytoplasmic pattern. Napsin A is relatively specific, but does stain some tumors of renal origin, including some papillary tumors. A panel of stains, including TTF-1 and renal-associated antigens (CA-IX, PAX8) is therefore optimal, depending on the specific patient context.

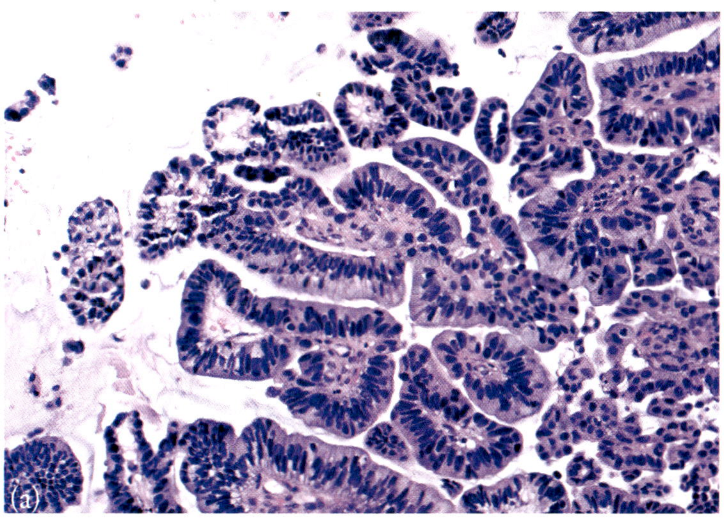

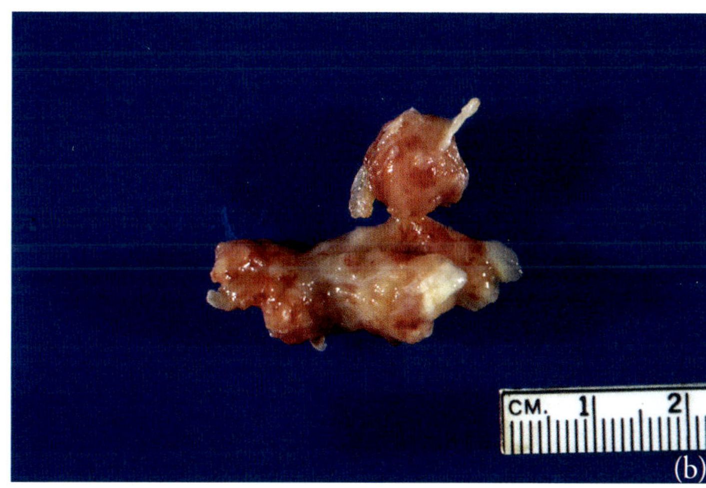

Figure 6.5(a, b) — Polypoid Endobronchial Adenocarcinoma, Excision [H&E Stain; Medium Power and Gross Examination]. Polypoid endobronchial adenocarcinoma is a descriptive term for adenocarcinomas that demonstrate an exophytic and polypoid growth within a large bronchus. This is an uncommon event. The histology is usually that of a well-differentiated papillary adenocarcinoma. Gross examination reveals the polypoid shape of this lesion.

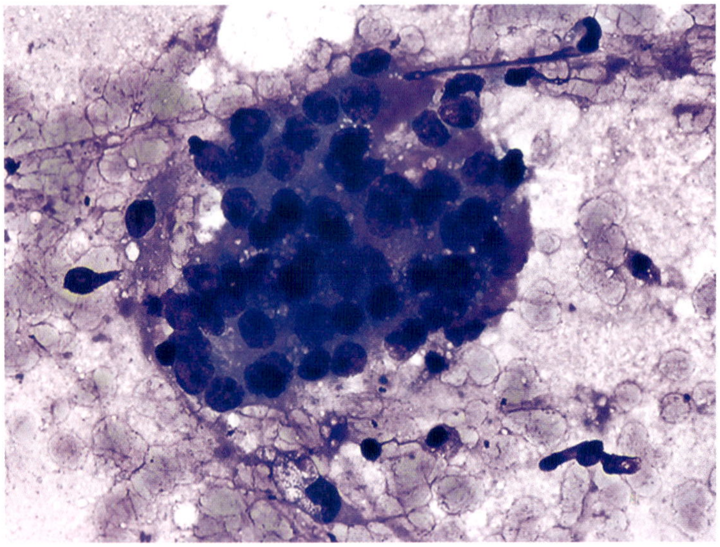

Figure 6.6a — Well-Differentiated Adenocarcinoma, Fine Needle Aspiration [Diff-Quik Stain; High Power]. This is a corresponding Diff-Quik preparation from the same patient as the previous image. Note the arrangement of the nuclei in rosette and/or acinar formations. Because the chromatin pattern is not as readily identifiable on this preparation as compared to a Pap stain, it is more challenging to exclude a carcinoid tumor. The creation of cell block material for immunohistochemical studies could prove helpful, since low-grade neuroendocrine neoplasms typically express synaptophysin and/or chromogranin.

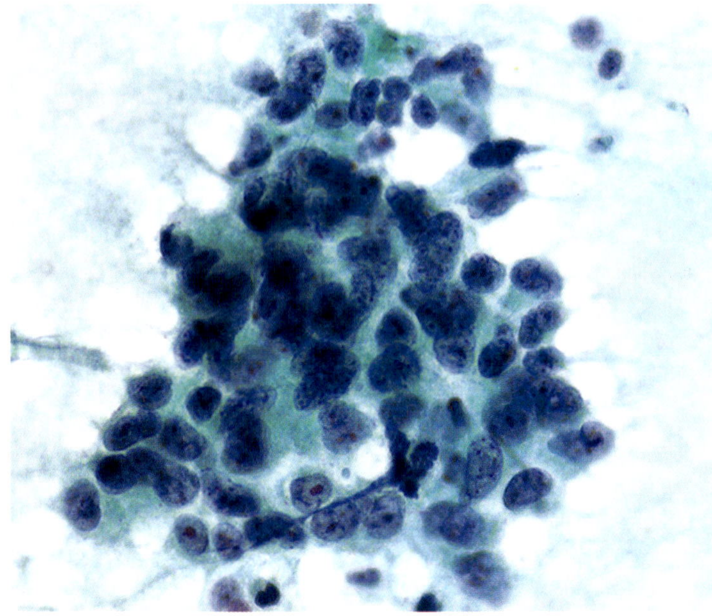

Figure 6.6b — Well-Differentiated Adenocarcinoma, Fine Needle Aspiration [Pap Stain; High Power]. The nuclei form small rosettes or acinar-like structures, an indication of gland formation. The presence of small rosettes in a well-differentiated neoplasm should always cause at least brief consideration of a neuroendocrine neoplasm, such as a carcinoid tumor. In this case, the nuclei have markedly atypical features, such as enlargement, irregular borders, and significant overlap, which favors an adenocarcinoma. However, the chromatin pattern is predominantly coarse and many cells have prominent nucleoli—a feature not typically seen in neuroendocrine neoplasms.

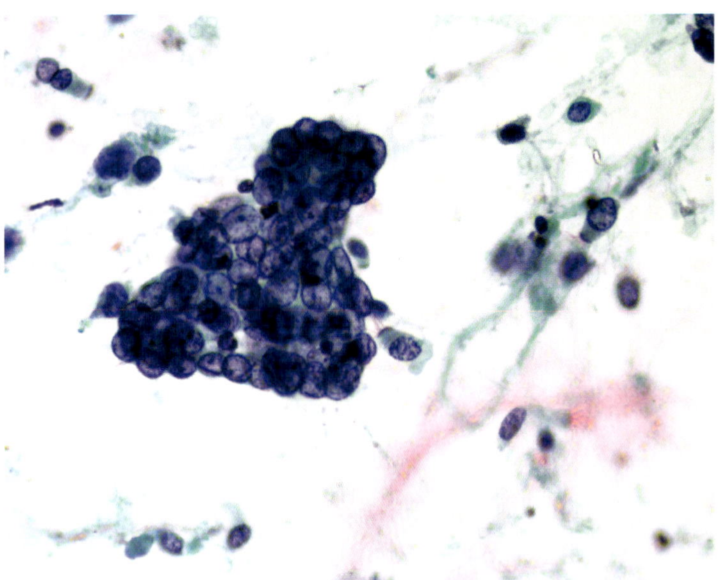

Figure 6.7a — Adenocarcinoma, Fine Needle Aspiration [Pap Stain; High Power]. This adenocarcinoma has a peculiar morphology, with optically clear chromatin and very little cytoplasm. The nuclei appear to mold against each other and may cause consideration of a small cell carcinoma. However, the cells are arranged in a three-dimensional shape with the nuclei lining the edges, suggesting a glandular differentiation. The cells also have nuclear size variation, ranging up to a 3:1 ratio, and are found predominantly in a tissue fragment rather than individually. These favor an adenocarcinoma over a small cell carcinoma.

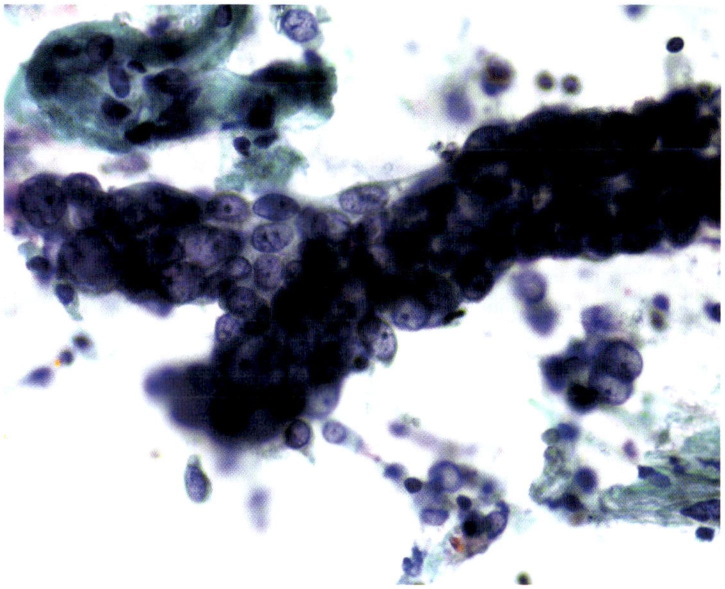

Figure 6.7b — Adenocarcinoma, Fine Needle Aspiration [Pap Stain; High Power]. The malignant cells form a papillary fragment, but the fragment lacks a fibrovascular core and thus is not a true papillae. The nuclei are enlarged, dark, and have distinct nucleoli. The nuclei are disorganized within the structure and are overlapping, vary greatly in size, and have irregular borders.

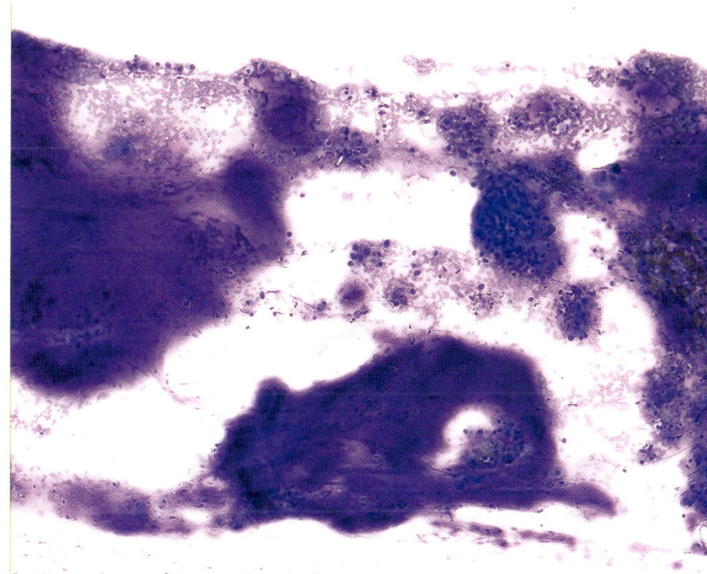

Figure 6.8a — Mucinous Acinar/Colloid Adenocarcinoma, Fine Needle Aspiration [Diff-Quik Stain; Low Power]. The current World Health Organization classification of adenocarcinomas having a plentiful amount of mucin is subdivided into invasive mucinous and colloid adenocarcinoma. The former term was newly introduced to replace mucinous bronchioloalveolar carcinoma. It differs from the colloid variant by preserving air spaces and growing primarily in a lepidic pattern along alveolar septa. With the colloid variant, mucin pools fill the alveolar space and replace the parenchymal architecture. Since spatial relationships between cells, stroma, and pulmonary architecture are lost in aspirate smears, it is doubtful that this subtle distinction between both invasive mucinous and colloid variants can be appreciated cytologically. Typical of all forms of colloid adenocarcinoma is the copious amount of mucin discharged onto glass slides. This stains metachromatically in air-dried smears and varies in thickness depending on the amount expelled. Mixed with this opaque stroma are variable-sized cell clusters.

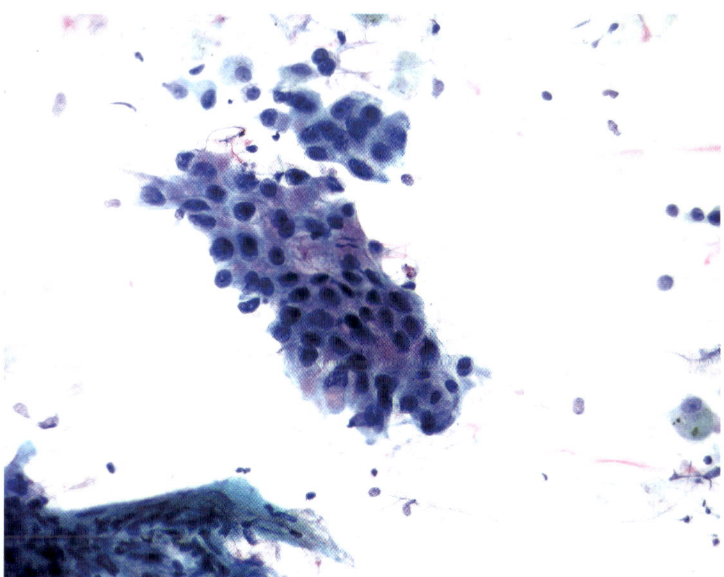

Figure 6.8b — Mucinous Acinar/Colloid Adenocarcinoma, Fine Needle Aspiration [Pap Stain; High Power]. Colloid adenocarcinoma is rare as a pure subtype. Typical of lung adenocarcinomas, it is mostly a peripheral-based mass with no special imaging characteristics. Because there is so much mucinous stroma, smears are typically paucicellular. In this example, background mucin has a wispy diaphanous quality in contrast to the thick, opaque character in the prior image. Polygonal cells show variable degrees of disorder when seen in tight clusters, and some cells contain cytoplasmic mucin. The amount of intracellular mucin varies from being absent to having enormous goblet cell shapes.

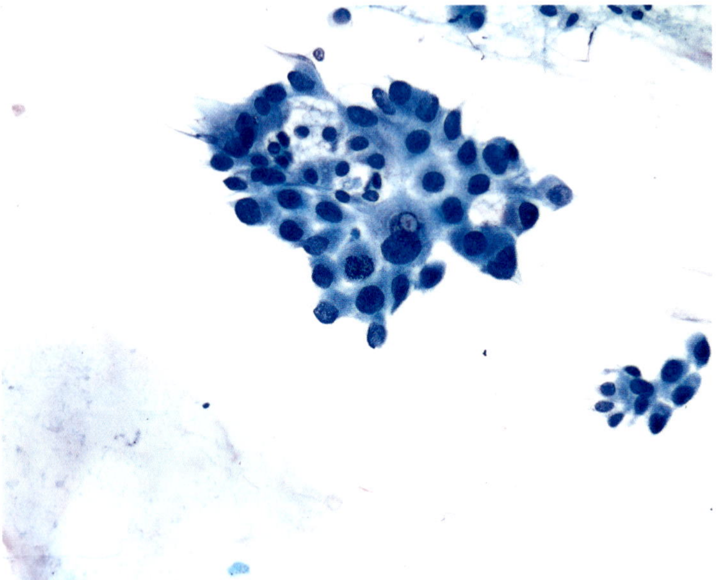

Figure 6.8c — Mucinous Acinar/Colloid Adenocarcinoma, Fine Needle Aspiration [Pap Stain; High Power]. This cluster exemplifies the cytologic uniformity and nuclear blandness of malignant cells. Only slight anisonucleosis is present, allowing one to confuse these cells as either reactive pneumocytes or bronchial cells that have lost their cilia. An almost transparent globule of mucin is seen at the lower left of this image. Colloid adenocarcinoma routinely expresses intestinal-type immunohistochemical markers such as cytokeratin 20, cytokeratin 7, and CDX2. TTF-1 staining is weak at best. Because of this, one must clinically exclude a metastatic lesion from the gastrointestinal tract, pancreas, and possibly ovary.

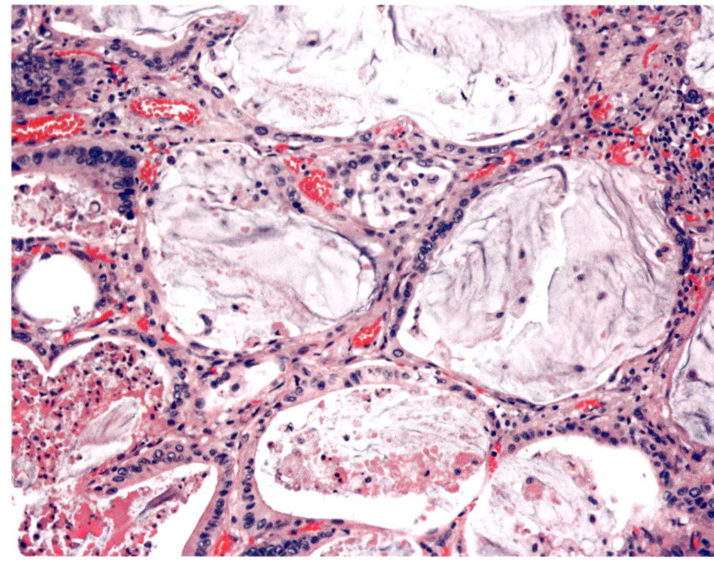

Figure 6.9a — Adenocarcinoma, Colloid Type, Lobectomy [H&E Stain; High Power]. This special subtype of adenocarcinoma is defined histologically by the filling of air spaces with pools of mucin, often acellular, or with interrupted strips of neoplastic glandular epithelium along septal surfaces or floating in the mucin. The neoplastic cells in this image are mildly to moderately atypical, with only slightly increased nuclear:cytoplasmic ratios and focal crowding. Colloid adenocarcinomas tend to be weakly and heterogeneously PET-avid, probably due to the large zones of acellular mucin. The major differential consideration is metastasis from the gastrointestinal tract, breast, ovary, or pancreas.

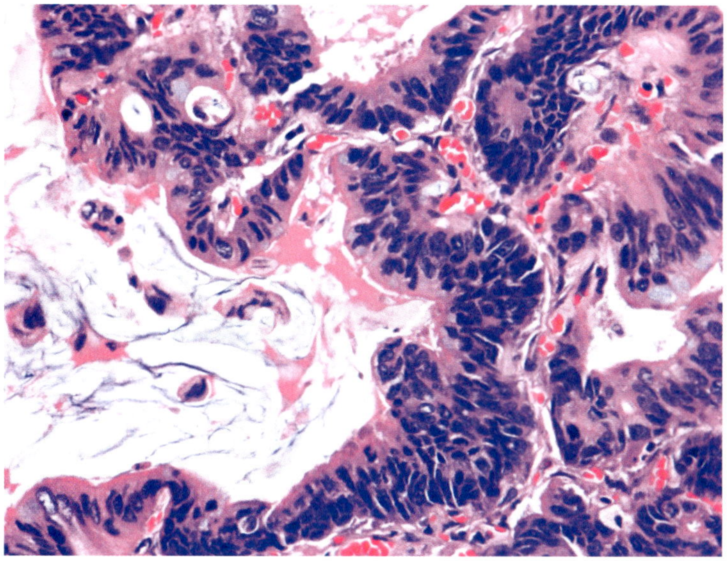

Figure 6.9b — Adenocarcinoma, Colloid Type, Gastrointestinal-Like Area, Lobectomy [H&E Stain; High Power]. The neoplastic epithelium in this field strongly resembles tumors of gastrointestinal origin (especially the colon, appendix, and pancreas). Further confounding interpretation is the fact that colloid adenocarcinoma of the lung expresses gastrointestinal markers (CK20, CDX2, MUC2), and is often negative or weak/focal+ for CK7, TTF-1, and napsin A. History and imaging findings are therefore important in establishing the correct diagnosis.

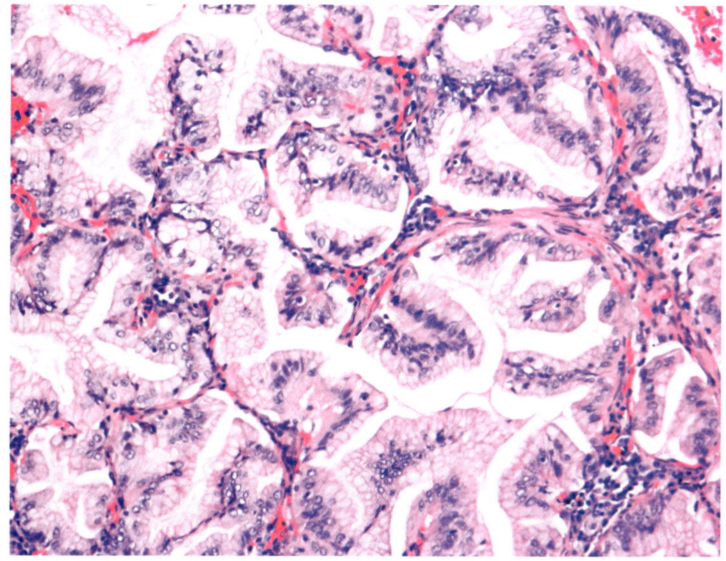

Figure 6.9c — Invasive Mucinous Adenocarcinoma, Lobectomy [H&E Stain; Low Power]. This entity, newly defined in the 2015 World Health Organization classification of lung tumors, is composed of a dominant (greater than 90%) population of cells with abundant cytoplasmic mucin. Surrounding alveoli may be mucin-filled, causing these tumors to appear larger than they are, grossly and by imaging studies; and fine needle aspiration may yield paucicellular mucin. Growth patterns include varying proportions of any or all of those observed in nonmucinous tumors, except solid—papillary, micropapillary, acinar, and lepidic; adenocarcinoma in situ and minimally invasive adenocarcinoma also occur. This image shows acinar and papillary patterns.

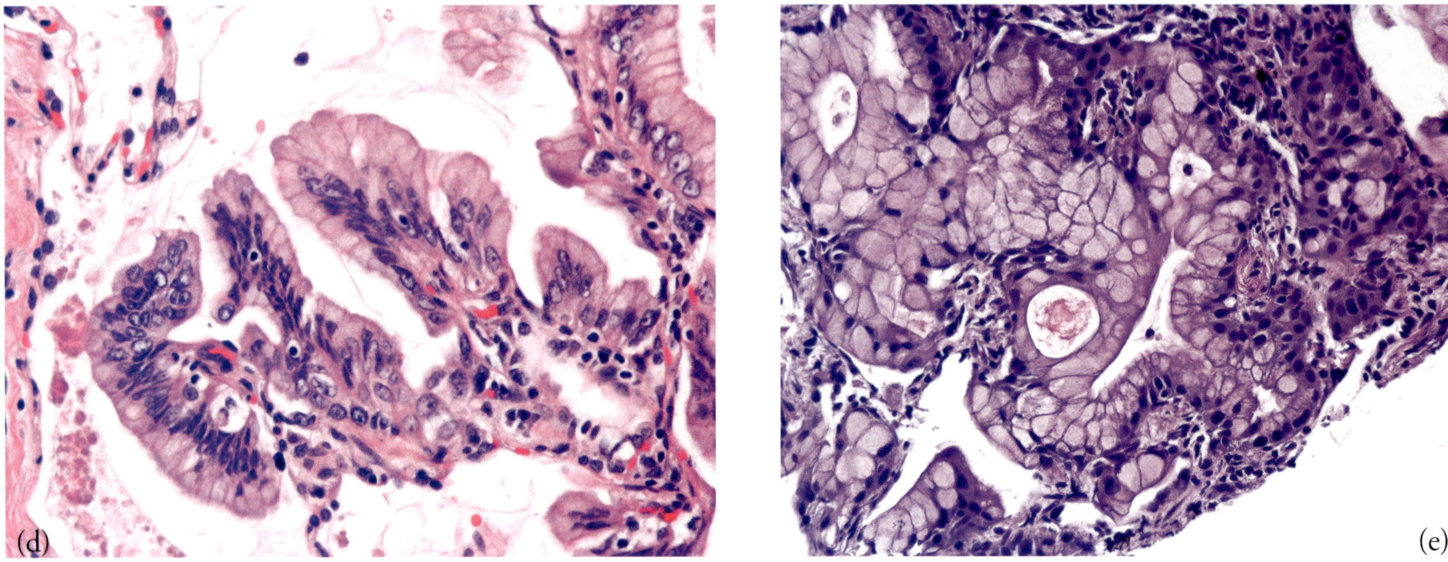

Figure 6.9(d, e) — Invasive Mucinous Adenocarcinoma, Wedge Resection [H&E Stain; High Power]. This neoplasm is composed of a uniform population of goblet cells and/or columnar cells with abundant intracytoplasmic mucin and small, basally oriented nuclei with minimal to mild atypia. Adjacent alveolar spaces may be filled with mucin. Often predominantly lepidic, these lesions may also have acinar, papillary, and micropapillary growth patterns. Differential diagnostic considerations include mucinous adenocarcinoma in situ and minimally invasive mucinous adenocarcinoma, both of which require tissue sections for diagnosis; and colloid carcinoma (more mucus than cells; occasional strips of variably mucinous columnar cells). Mucinous lung tumors of all types typically co-express CK7 and CK20, with variable expression of CDX2, and are often negative for TTF-1 and napsin A. Thus, metastasis from the gastrointestinal and pancreatobiliary tracts should be carefully excluded.

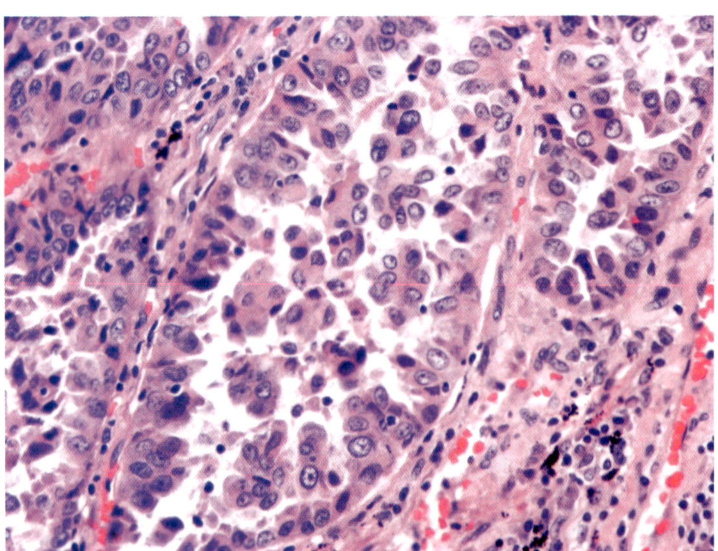

Figure 6.10a — Adenocarcinoma, Micropapillary, Lobectomy [H&E Stain; High Power]. This neoplastic gland contains multiple "micropapillae," small detached tufts of neoplastic glandular cells that lack a fibrovascular core. This pattern occurs most often as a component of a mixed-pattern adenocarcinoma, but rarely does it occur in pure form. Micropapillae may be associated with psammoma bodies and intranuclear pseudoinclusions, features that can be striking on fine needle aspiration biopsies. Micropapillary adenocarcinoma can arise as a primary lesion in numerous organs (e.g., breast, urinary bladder); distinguishing primary from metastatic disease may thus require a panel of immunohistochemical stains.

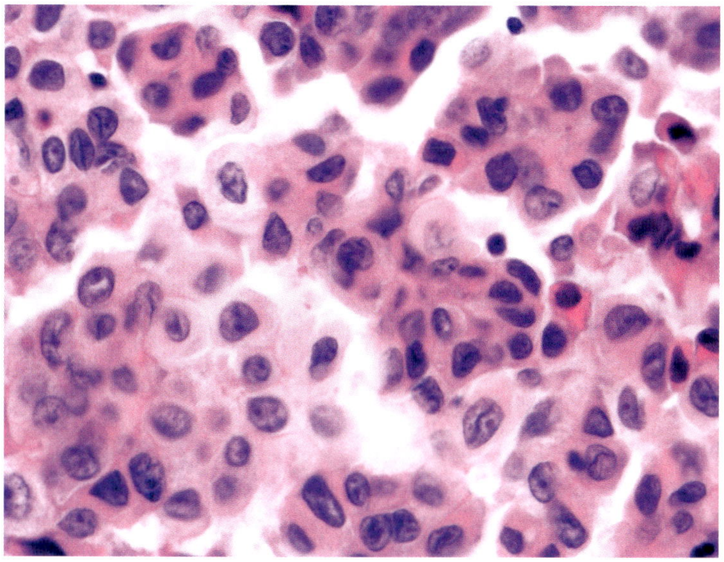

Figure 6.10b — Adenocarcinoma, Micropapillary, Lobectomy [H&E Stain; High Power]. These micropapillae show marked nuclear grooving, pleomorphism, and prominent nucleoli, with moderately abundant eosinophilic cytoplasm. The micropapillary pattern of glandular neoplasia tends to be associated with a strong propensity for stromal and vascular invasion; pure or predominantly micropapillary tumors are thus often regionally and distantly metastatic at presentation.

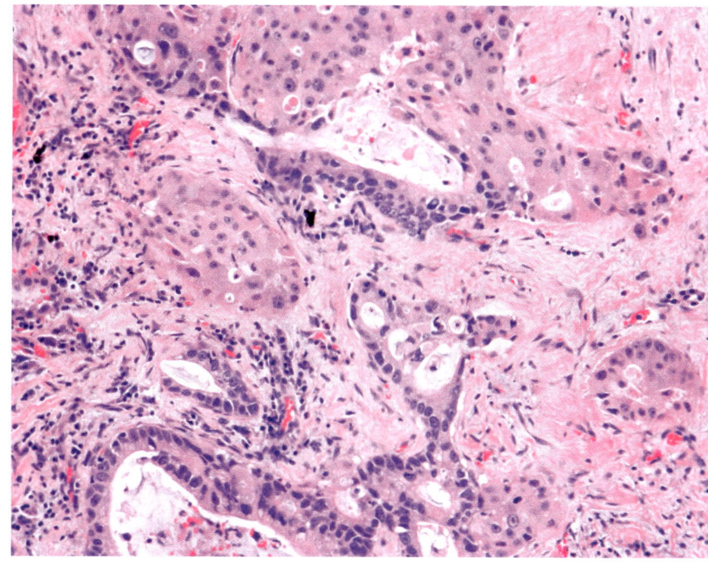

Figure 6.11a — Adenocarcinoma With Mixed Acinar and Solid Patterns, Wedge Resection [H&E Stain; Low Power]. Adenocarcinoma of the lung most often has a mix of growth patterns. This image shows a solid pattern at the top, with an acinar pattern at the bottom. Note the mucin vacuole at the top left, in the solid portion. Thorough sampling of adenocarcinoma will allow accurate determination of the dominant subtype and the percent of all other patterns present; the World Health Organization recommends that final reporting include all patterns, in 5% increments.

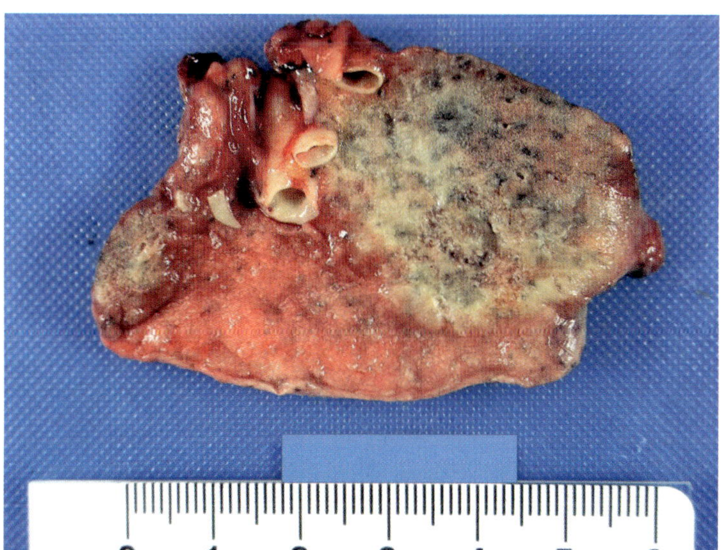

Figure 6.11b — Adenocarcinoma With Solid and Acinar Patterns, Wedge Resection [Gross Examination]. This wedge resection shows a peripheral yellow-gray lesion with indistinct infiltrative borders. The tumor broadly abuts the pleura; elastin staining of multiple sections across the tumor-pleura interface may be required to fully evaluate for foci of invasion of the visceral pleural elastic lamina (PL1 or PL2 disease).

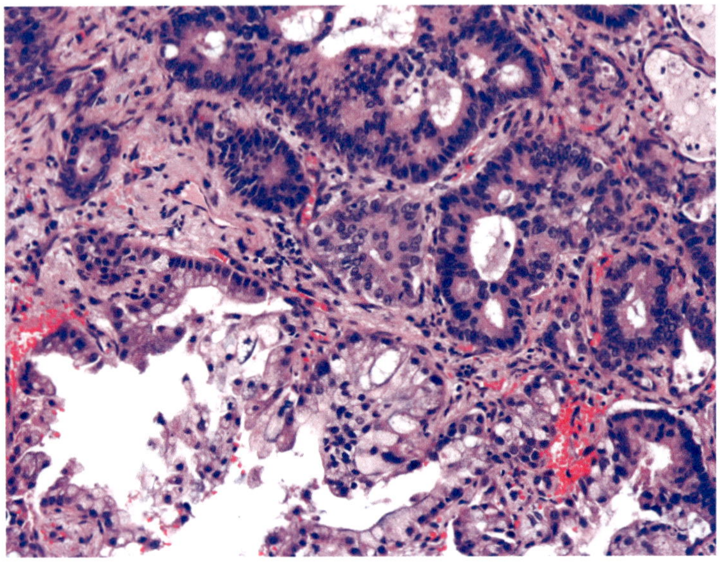

Figure 6.12 — Adenocarcinoma, Mixed Mucinous and Nonmucinous Type, Lobectomy [H&E Stain; High Power]. Invasive mucinous adenocarcinoma, acinar pattern, is present at the bottom, while the top half of the image shows nonmucinous adenocarcinoma with cribriform pattern, considered a variant of the acinar pattern. If both mucinous and nonmucinous cytologies exceed 10% of the tumor as a whole, the lesion is designated "mixed mucinous and nonmucinous adenocarcinoma," with all growth patterns reported, in standard fashion.

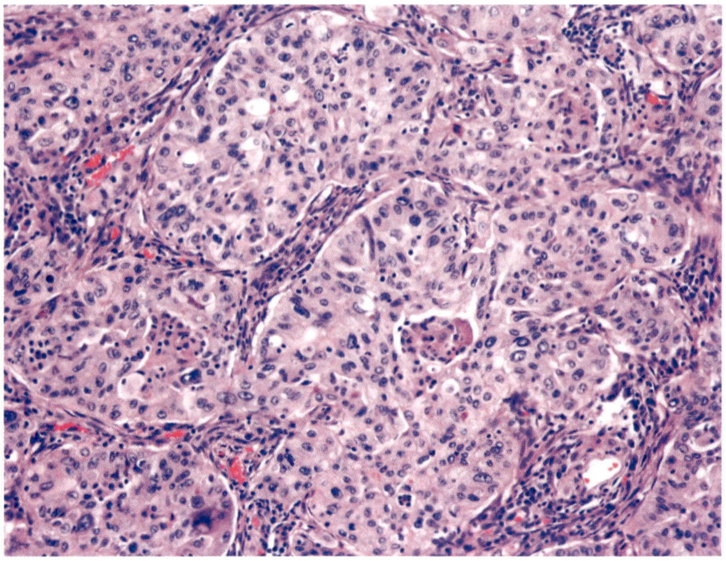

Figure 6.13a — Adenocarcinoma, Solid Pattern, Lobectomy [H&E Stain; Low Power]. This tumor had a uniformly solid growth pattern; studies suggest such tumors tend to be more aggressive. Note the nested pattern and the absence of specific cytoplasmic differentiation. Squamous cell carcinoma is a differential consideration.

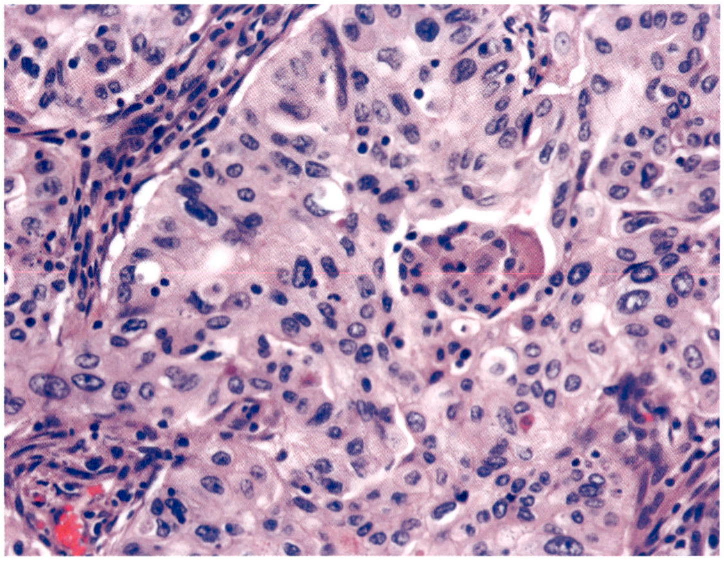

Figure 6.13b — Adenocarcinoma, Solid Pattern, Lobectomy [H&E Stain; High Power]. Higher magnification shows disorganized nests of pleomorphic cells with nuclear anisocytosis, nuclear creases and irregularities, and frequent nucleoli.

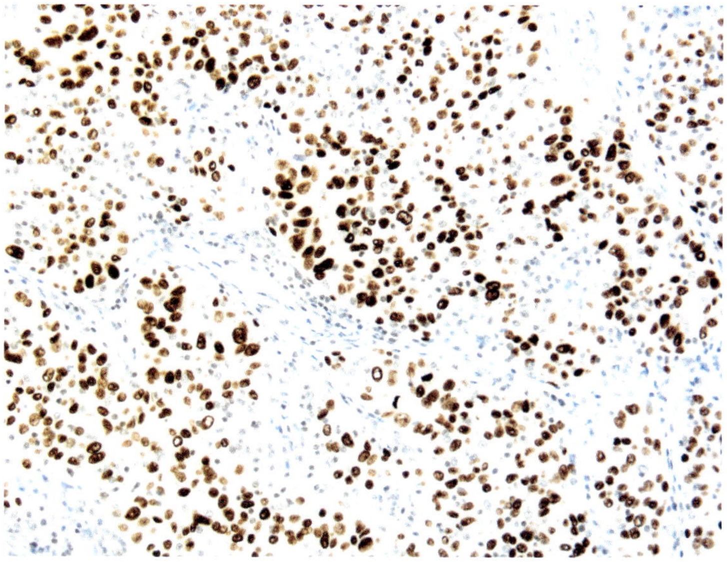

Figure 6.13c — Adenocarcinoma, Solid Pattern, Lobectomy [TTF-1 Immunohistochemical Stain; Low Power]. TTF-1 staining is strong and uniform. In the 2015 World Health Organization classification, TTF-1 or napsin A expression is sufficient to classify a solid-pattern tumor as adenocarcinoma, even in the absence of stainable mucin. TTF-1 expression is identifiable in about 75% of adenocarcinomas; napsin A is slightly more sensitive. Note that TTF-1 expression is not specific to pulmonary adenocarcinoma, but is also expressed in large cell neuroendocrine carcinoma and some carcinoid tumors, as well as thyroid carcinomas.

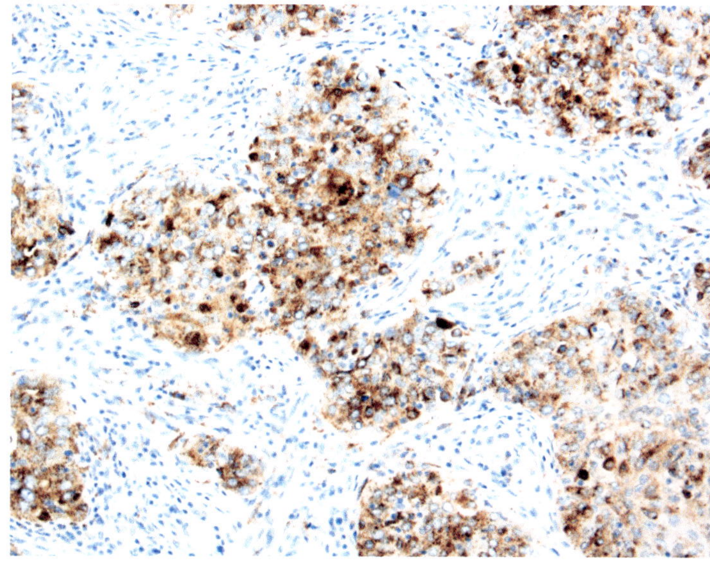

Figure 6.13d — Adenocarcinoma, Solid Pattern, Lobectomy [Napsin A Immunohistochemical Stain; Low Power]. There is diffuse granular cytoplasmic staining for napsin A. This protein is secreted, and often taken up by resident alveolar macrophages; at low power, solid aggregates of alveolar macrophages may therefore mimic solid adenocarcinoma with napsin A staining. Some non–small cell carcinomas lack specific growth patterns and are negative for napsin A, TTF-1, p40/p63, and CK5/6; these are designated "large cell carcinoma—null" on resection specimens, and "non–small cell carcinoma, NOS" on small biopsy specimens.

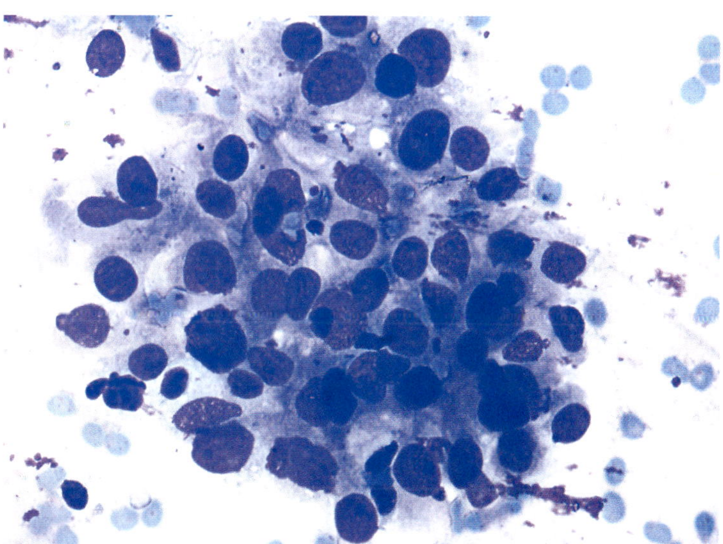

Figure 6.14a — Moderately Differentiated Adenocarcinoma, Fine Needle Aspiration [Diff-Quik Stain; High Power]. At high magnification, notice the eccentric placement of the nuclei. At the top left-hand side of the fragment, the nuclei are arranged outward from a central point, forming an acinar structure. This can also be appreciated in other areas of the fragment, such as at the lower right-hand corner. These features help identify this as an adenocarcinoma.

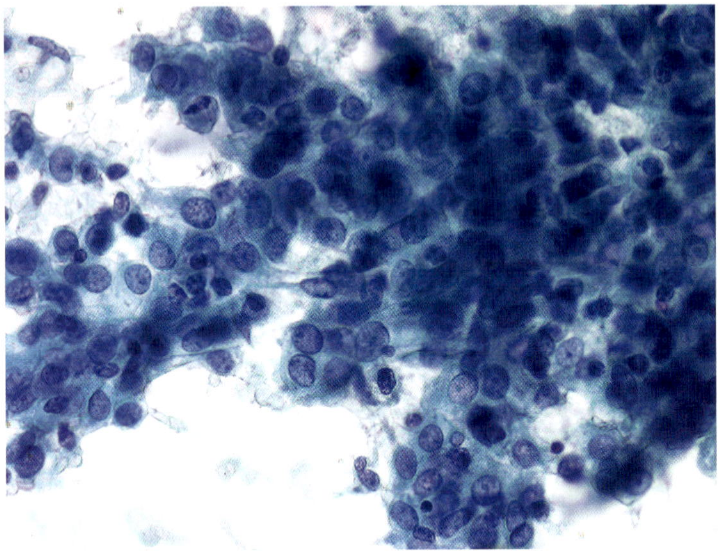

Figure 6.14b — Moderately Differentiated Adenocarcinoma, Fine Needle Aspiration [Pap Stain; High Power]. The malignant cells are present in a complex epithelial sheet and have prominent nucleoli, wispy cytoplasm, mildly irregular nuclear borders, and moderate anisonucleosis. The cells are disorganized within the epithelial fragment, resulting in a large amount of nuclear overlap. While there is no question that this is an adenocarcinoma, the determination of whether this is a primary lung lesion or metastatic lesion would require immunohistochemical studies.

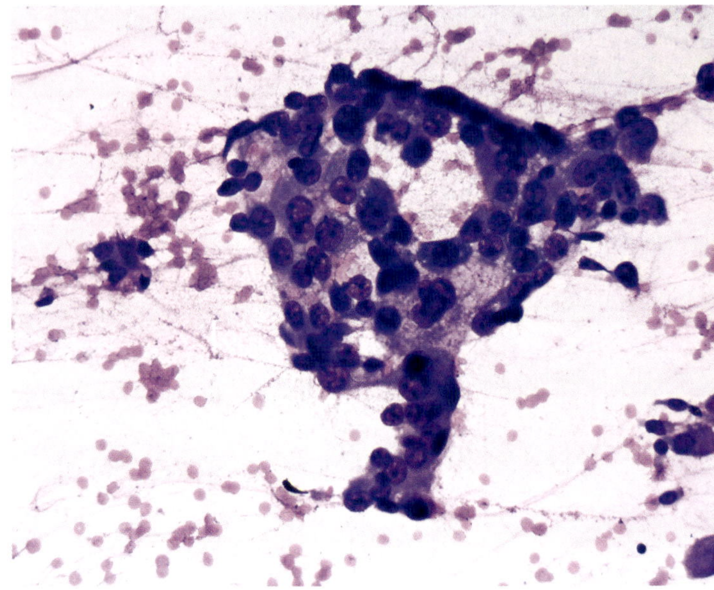

Figure 6.14c — Moderately Differentiated Adenocarcinoma, Fine Needle Aspiration [Diff-Quik Stain; High Power]. The malignant cells have round nuclei, mild nuclear border irregularities, and prominent nuclei. Most cells have an eccentrically placed nucleus and are hyperchromatic. The cells are arranged in a three-dimensional structure. Can you identify the benign ciliated epithelial cells in the background? The ciliated cells are smaller and have smaller nuclei and a different chromatin appearance as compared to the malignant cells. Comparing atypical cells to benign cells—especially their nuclear features—can help determine whether the atypia is secondary to reactive atypia or malignancy.

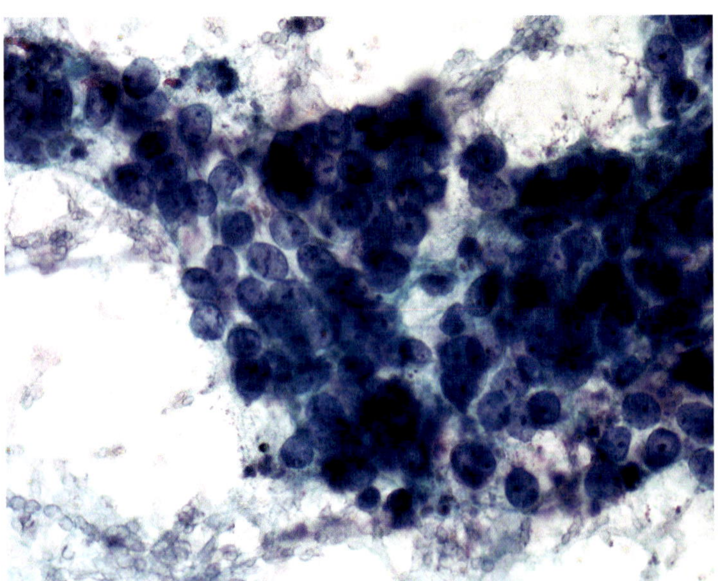

Figure 6.14d — Moderately Differentiated Adenocarcinoma, Fine Needle Aspiration [Pap Stain; High Power]. There is little variation in nuclear size among the malignant cells. Many cells have prominent nucleoli and greatly enlarged nuclei with minimal cytoplasm. In some areas, the tumor cells form three-dimensional structures and have significant overlap. While any adenocarcinoma can have prominent nucleoli, they are most often seen in renal cell carcinoma and prostate carcinoma. In this case, the patient had a lung primary.

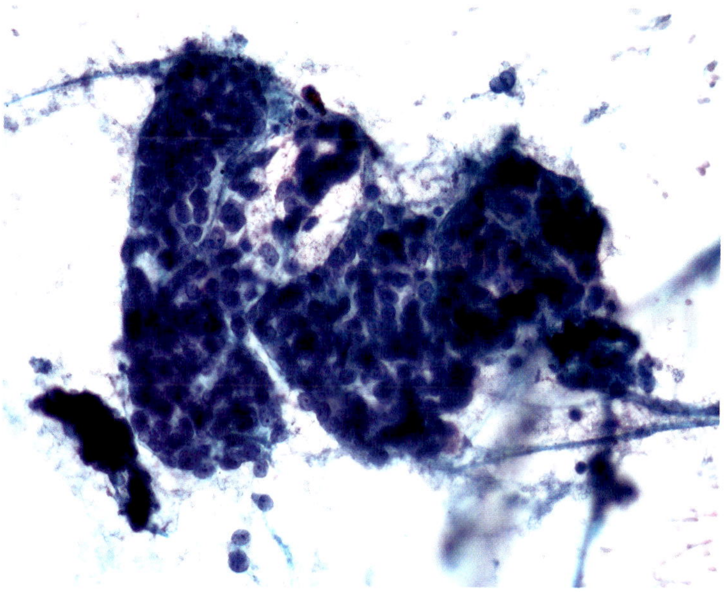

Figure 6.15a — Moderately Differentiated Adenocarcinoma, Fine Needle Aspiration [Pap Stain; Medium Power]. At lower magnification, the arrangement of cells within these tissue fragments can be better appreciated. The cells form three-dimensional sheets with smooth edges. Even though the nuclei overlap significantly, there are "empty" areas within the sheets in which the nuclei are absent, a suggestion that a glandular or acinar structure is present.

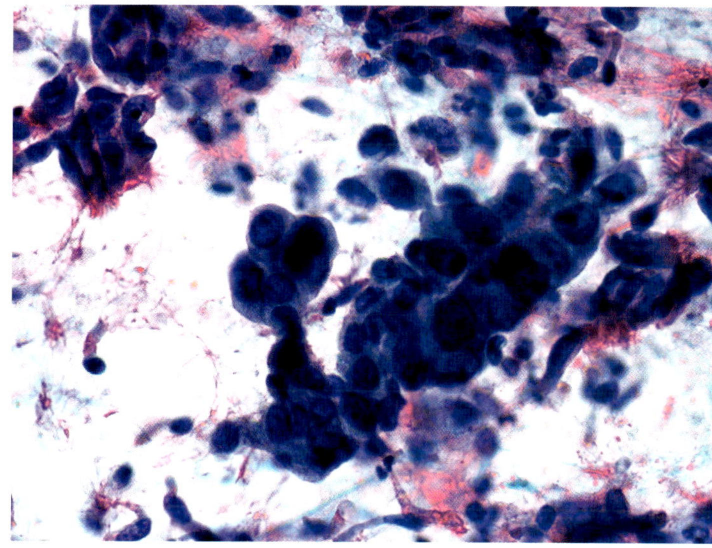

Figure 6.15b — Moderately Differentiated Adenocarcinoma, Fine Needle Aspiration [Pap Stain; High Power]. Compare the malignant cells in the center of the field to the numerous ciliated benign bronchial respiratory epithelial cells in the background. Some malignant nuclei are easily more than five times the size of the bystander cell nuclei. The ciliated cells show little variation in nuclear size, whereas there is anisonucleosis in the malignant cells. The malignant cells have prominent nucleoli. While the chromatin of the malignant cells is not significantly darker than that of the bystander benign cells, the malignant cells must be aneuploid to maintain the same amount of chromasia over such enlarged nuclei.

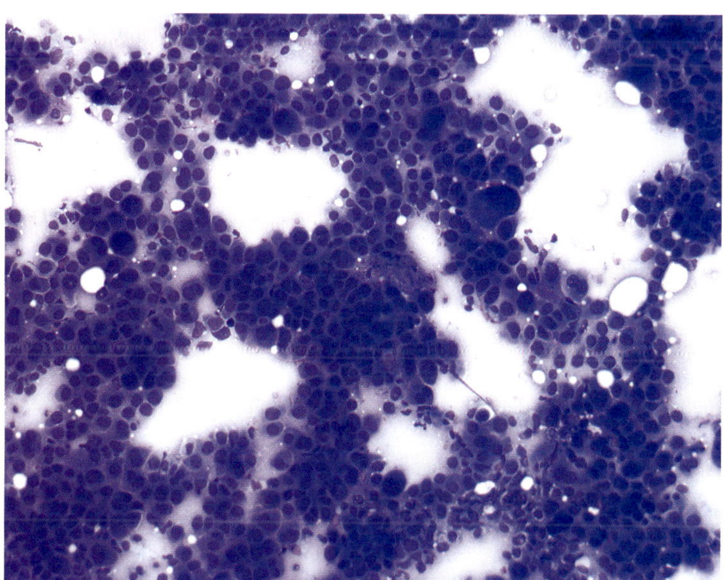

Figure 6.16a — Poorly Differentiated Adenocarcinoma, Fine Needle Aspiration [Diff-Quik Stain; Medium Power]. The field is packed with discohesive cells. The cells have abundant cytoplasm and dramatic nuclear size variations. The cellularity of the field suggests a neoplasm and the greatly enlarged nuclei possessed by some cells indicate a malignant process. However, the neoplasm does not have features to suggest a particular origin. Because the cells are discohesive and do not form tissue fragments, this could be a poorly differentiated carcinoma, melanoma, or sarcoma. Because poorly differentiated carcinomas may be negative for keratin, immunohistochemical studies are not always useful.

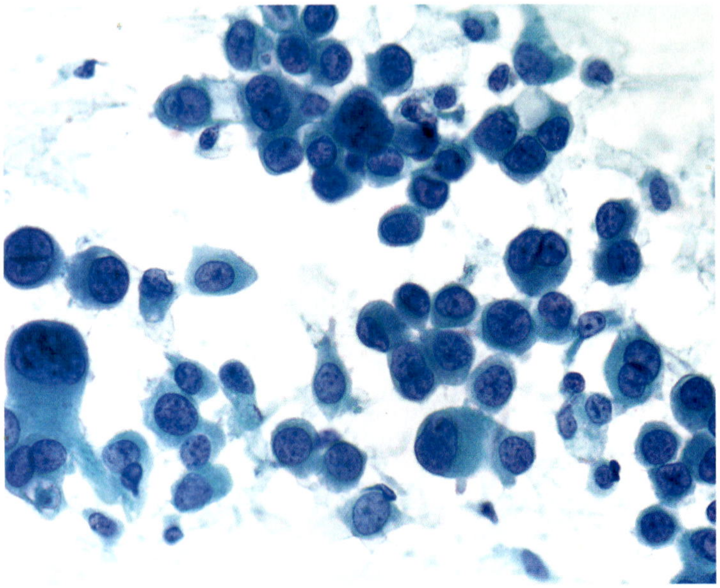

Figure 6.16b — Poorly Differentiated Adenocarcinoma, Fine Needle Aspiration [Pap Stain; High Power]. The malignant cells are discohesive; while most only contain one nucleus, some are binucleate. While the chromatin pattern is not overtly malignant, some cells have highly complex nuclear borders and elevated nuclear-to-cytoplasmic ratios. This could safely be diagnosed as a malignant neoplasm, and if cell block material is available, immunohistochemical studies may help confirm this as a carcinoma.

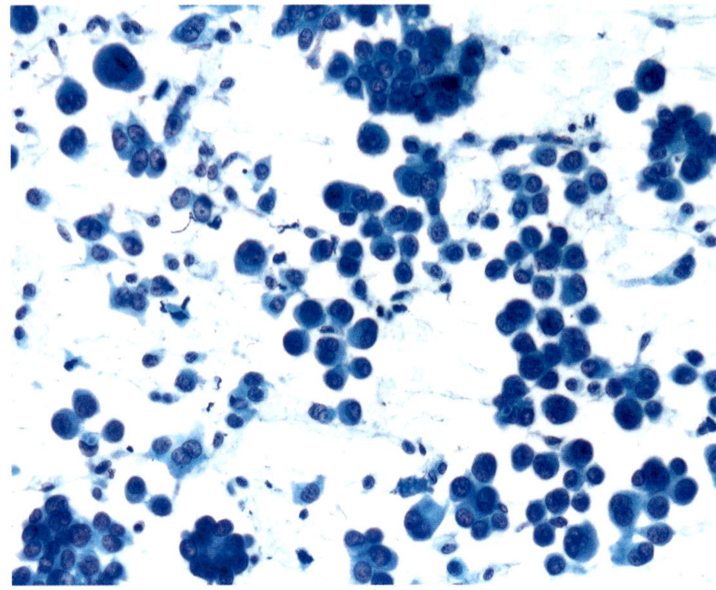

Figure 6.16c — Poorly Differentiated Adenocarcinoma, Fine Needle Aspiration [Pap Stain; High Power]. Careful examination of the specimen may reveal focal clues as to a tumor's origin. In this case, while most of the cells are discohesive, the malignant cells form a small fragment at the top of the field as well as a glandular structure at the bottom left-hand side of the field. At the very least, adenocarcinoma can be favored here if immunohistochemical studies cannot be performed or are not useful.

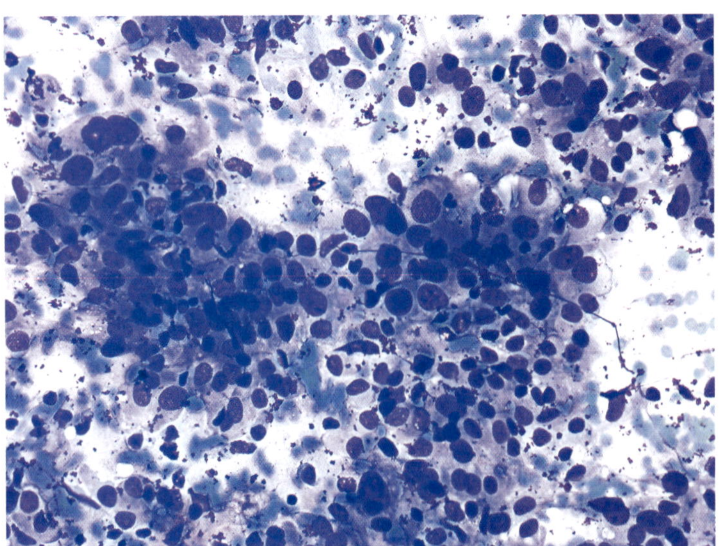

Figure 6.16d — Poorly Differentiated Adenocarcinoma, Fine Needle Aspiration [Diff-Quik Stain; Medium Power]. The cells are large and the size of the nucleus varies greatly between cells. Most cells have an eccentrically placed nucleus and delicate cytoplasm, features of adenocarcinoma. Squamous cell carcinomas tend to have centrally placed nuclei and dense cytoplasm. Prominent nucleoli are also seen, a feature more often seen in adenocarcinomas but also sometimes seen in squamous cell carcinomas. Definite gland formation is not seen, though the cells form three-dimensional fragments that almost form acinar arrangements.

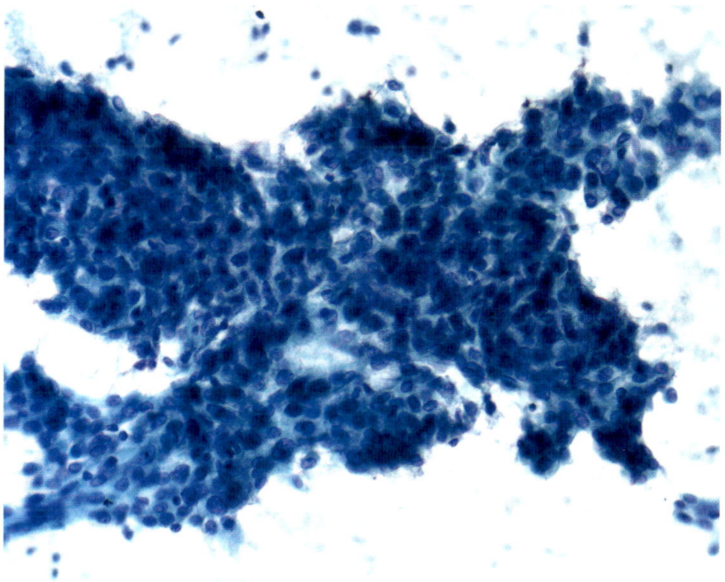

Figure 6.17a — Poorly Differentiated Adenocarcinoma, Fine Needle Aspiration [Pap Stain; Medium Power]. The anisonucleosis seen here—with some nuclei being more than four times larger than adjacent nuclei—is a common finding in adenocarcinomas. The chromatin is dark but has a granular appearance, and the nuclear borders are moderately irregular. In squamous cell carcinomas, variation in nuclear size is also accompanied by pyknotic nuclei and/or markedly irregular nuclear borders.

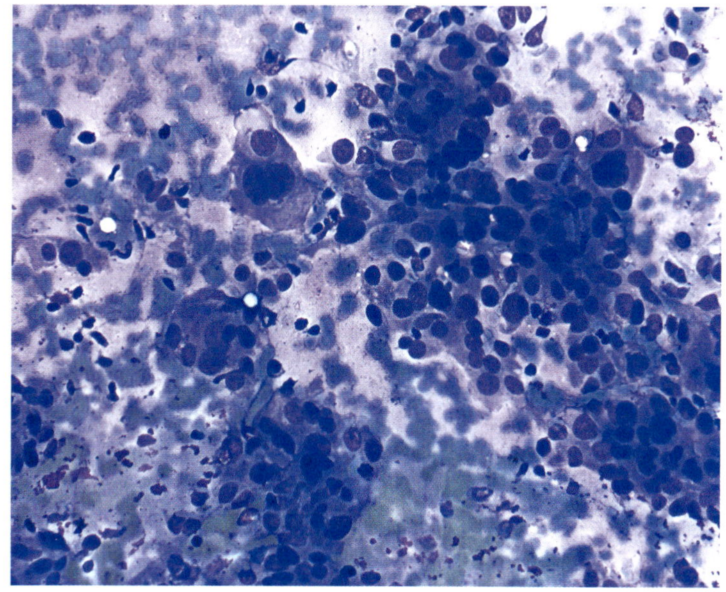

Figure 6.17b — Poorly Differentiated Adenocarcinoma, Fine Needle Aspiration [Diff-Quik Stain; Medium Power]. Here the adenocarcinoma shows some signs of glandular differentiation, with more distinct gland-like formations seen at the top of the field. However, in other areas the adenocarcinoma cells are present singly and have marked anisonucleosis, features found in poorly differentiated adenocarcinomas. Many cells contain an appreciable amount of cytoplasm, possibly due to mucin production.

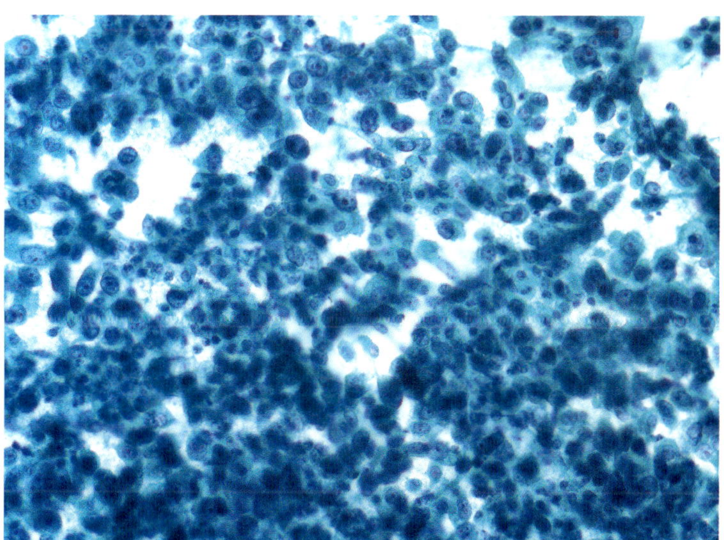

Figure 6.17c — Poorly Differentiated Adenocarcinoma, Fine Needle Aspiration [Pap Stain; Medium Power]. The cells are discohesive or form small fragments. There is granular debris in the background that suggests this is a necrotic tumor, and this may also explain how the individual cells have become detached. The cells have eccentric nuclei and elongated cytoplasm. Some cells are columnar but lack cilia and have the prominent nucleoli seen in other malignant cells. The discohesive nature of the cells, rare binucleate forms, and prominent nucleoli may cause one to consider the possibility of melanoma—however, the nuclei are too pleomorphic to make melanoma very likely.

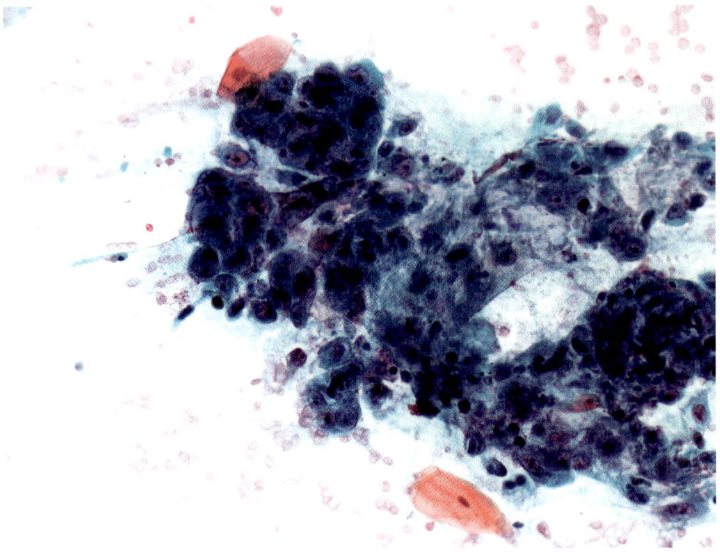

Figure 6.18 — Non-Small Cell Carcinoma, Sputum [Pap Stain; High Power]. The malignant cells form a sheet and have prominent nucleoli, marked nuclear size variation, high nuclear-to-cytoplasmic ratios, and irregular nuclear borders. The cells are poorly differentiated, and in the absence of keratinization, gland formation, and mucin, it is challenging to determine whether this represents a squamous cell carcinoma, an adenocarcinoma, or an adenosquamous carcinoma. The use of immunohistochemical studies on cell block material, if enough residual sputum remains, can help narrow the differential diagnosis.

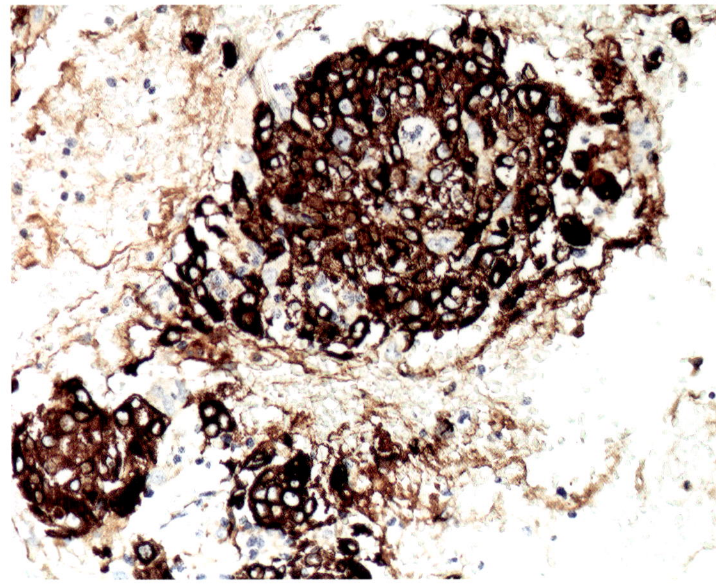

Figure 6.19a — Adenocarcinoma, Fine Needle Aspiration [CK7 Immunohistochemical Stain; High Power]. A cell block was created from dedicated passes of a patient's lung tumor, allowing for immunohistochemical studies to be performed. Most lung adenocarcinomas are positive for CK7, but the pattern is nonspecific, as adenocarcinomas from many other sites express CK7, as well as some lung squamous cell carcinomas. CK7 may be helpful to prove that a poorly differentiated neoplasm is a carcinoma.

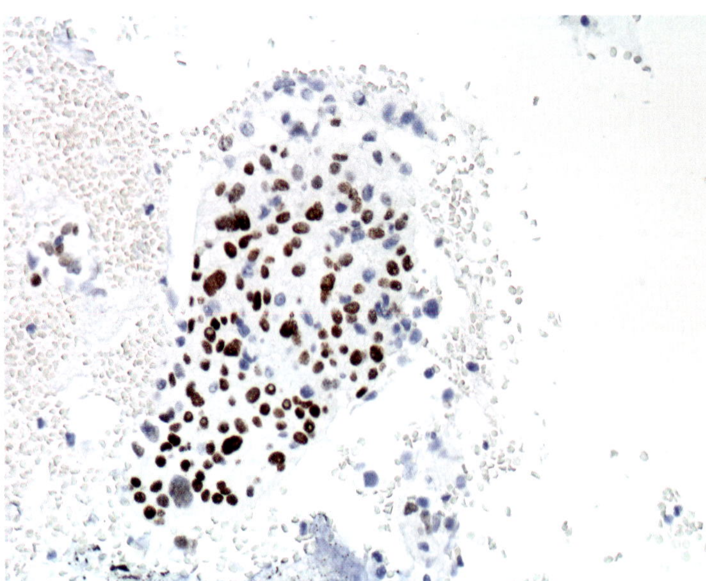

Figure 6.19b — Adenocarcinoma, Fine Needle Aspiration [TTF-1 Immunohistochemical Stain; High Power]. The carcinoma cells present in this fragment stain positively for TTF-1. While not all cells are positive, typically lung adenocarcinomas stain diffusely and strongly for TTF-1 in a nuclear pattern. Lung squamous cell carcinomas and mesotheliomas are usually negative for TTF-1.

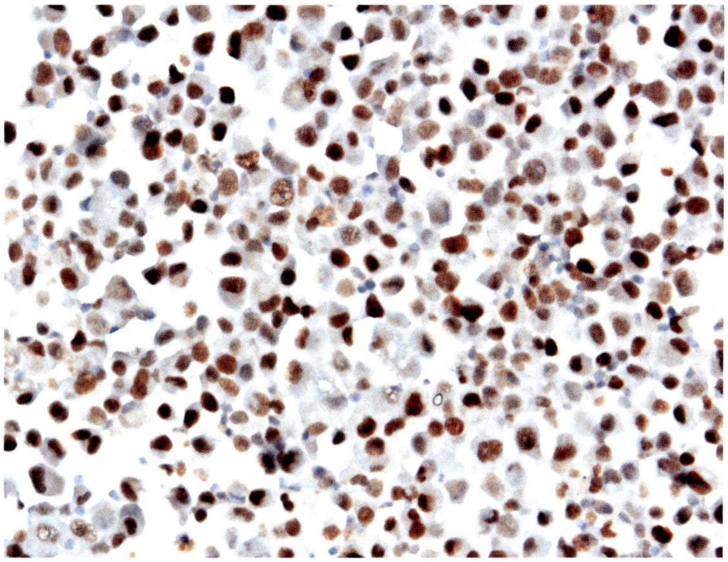

Figure 6.19c — Adenocarcinoma, Fine Needle Aspiration [TTF-1 Immunohistochemical Stain; High Power]. In this case, the dispersed cell population is seen in a poorly differentiated neoplasm. TTF-1 should only be interpreted as positive if there is nuclear staining—cytoplasmic staining can occasionally be seen nonspecifically, such as in liver tissue. While TTF-1 is a sensitive stain for lung primary adenocarcinomas (75%) and small cell carcinomas (90%) it is nonspecific and is usually positive in some other neoplasms, such as those derived from thyroid follicular cells, and is sometimes positive in carcinomas from other sites.

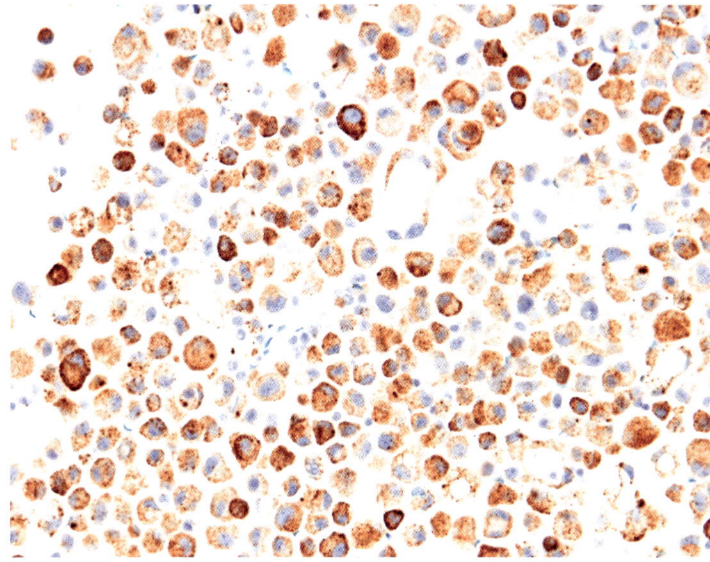

Figure 6.20 — Adenocarcinoma, Fine Needle Aspiration [Napsin-A Immunohistochemical Stain; High Power]. Napsin A is a less sensitive but more specific marker than TTF-1 for lung adenocarcinomas. The staining pattern is typically cytoplasmic and granular. Napsin A is typically not expressed in small cell carcinomas or squamous cell carcinomas of the lung. It is typically used to prove that an adenocarcinoma has a lung origin, but can also be expressed in renal cell carcinomas, especially papillary renal cell carcinoma (79% positive in one study).

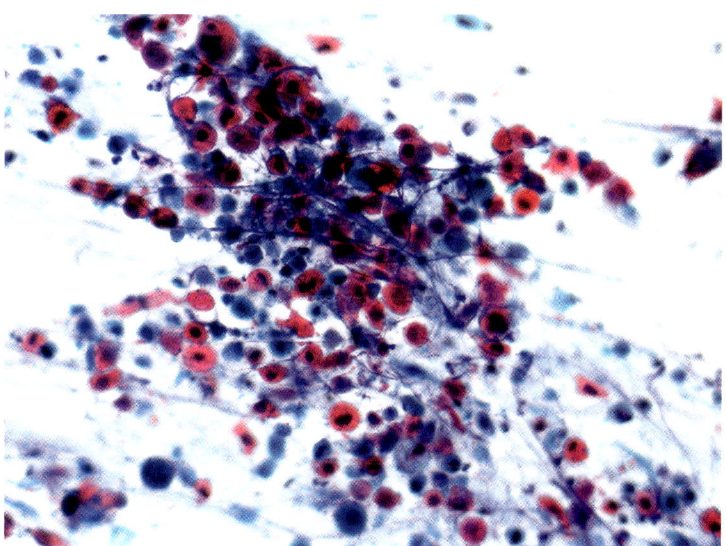

Figure 6.21a — Well-Differentiated Squamous Cell Carcinoma, Sputum [Pap Stain; Medium Power]. This image is rather "busy" with numerous cells encompassing nearly the entire field. Approximately half of the cells have distinct orangeophilic, keratinized cytoplasm, identifying these as squamous cells. These cells have enough atypical features to warrant a diagnosis of well-differentiated squamous cell carcinoma. The nuclei are hyperchromatic, with many nuclei additionally being quite large (inflammatory cells may be used for internal size comparison). These large, hyperchromatic nuclei additionally exhibit high nuclear to cytoplasmic ratios. The individual, dyshesive keratinized cells also identify this specimen as a well-differentiated squamous cell carcinoma.

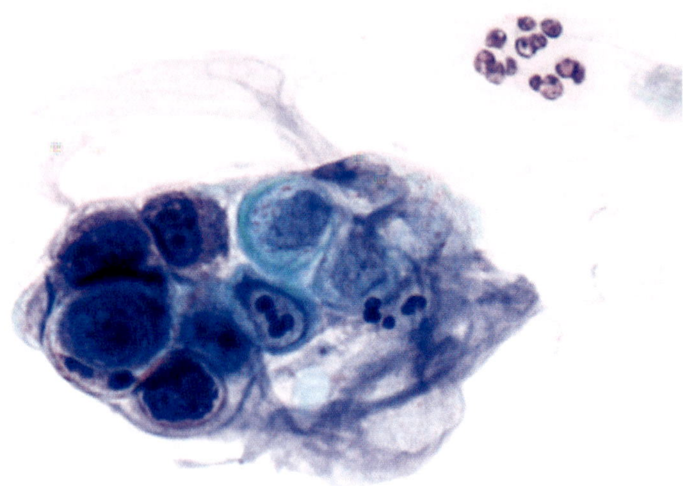

Figure 6.21b — Well-Differentiated Squamous Cell Carcinoma, Sputum [Pap Stain; High Power]. A single cluster of atypical cells exhibits nuclear molding in addition to a high nuclear:cytoplasmic ratio and nuclear hyperchromasia, all features of malignancy. The few neutrophils present in an otherwise clean background provide a helpful size comparison. The cytoplasm, particularly prominent in the cell in the upper right of the cluster, has the deep turquoise hue and dense, "hard" character of keratin production. Given that this cluster came from a sputum sample, and all malignant cells had similar features, the ultimate diagnosis was well-differentiated squamous cell carcinoma.

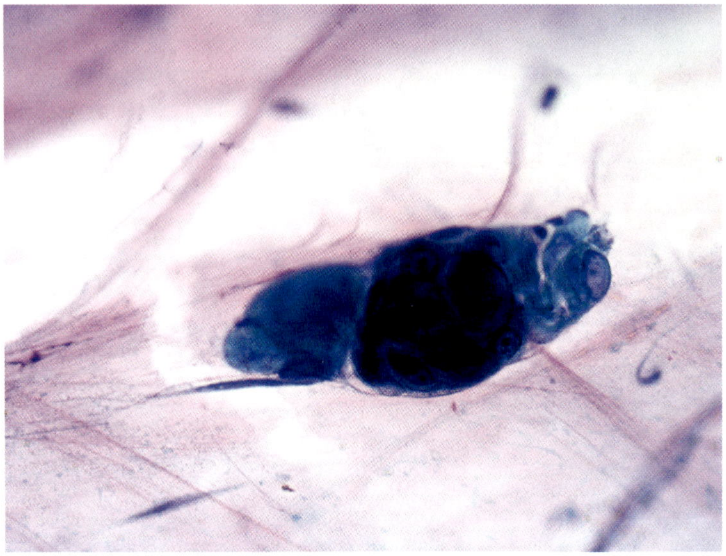

Figure 6.21c — Well-Differentiated Squamous Cell Carcinoma, Sputum [Pap Stain; High Power]. The single cluster of atypical cells hovers over a background of rosy streaked mucous strands. Within the cluster, numerous hyperchromatic, angulated, molded atypical nuclei with a faint rim of blueish cytoplasm aggregate into a tight ball-like structure in the center, flanked on the left by dense, turquoise cytoplasm consistent with keratinized cytoplasm that identifies the structure as having squamous differentiation and keratinization, which suggests a well-differentiated process. The nuclear features identify the process as malignant.

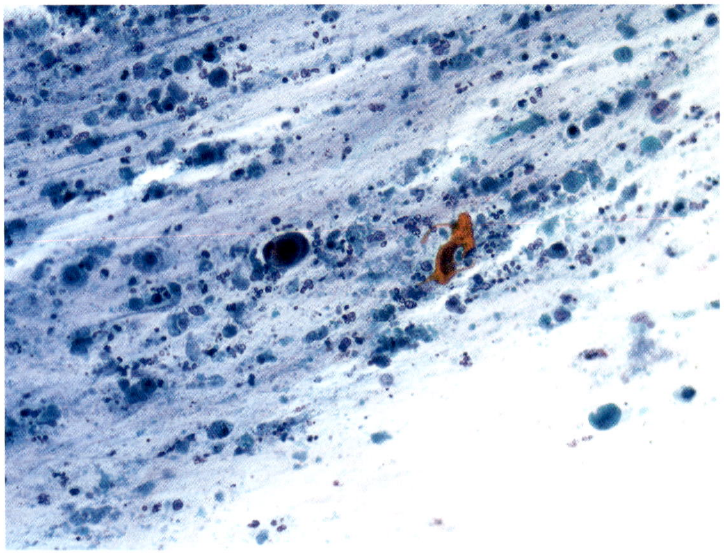

Figure 6.21d — Well-Differentiated Squamous Cell Carcinoma, Sputum [Pap Stain; Medium Power]. First to catch the eye is the central, almost arachnoid-appearing, isolated orangeophilic keratinized cell with pronounced curvilinear dendrites. This atypical and irregular keratinized cell provides strong evidence of a malignant squamous process. Further evidence of malignancy is the atypical cells with hyperchromatic nuclei and increased nuclear:cytoplasmic ratios. These cells, in combination with the irregularly shaped anucleate swaths of cytoplasm with that "hard" blue-turquoise squamous appearance of keratin production seen on Pap stain and the background of necrotic debris and inflammatory cells all support a diagnosis of squamous cell carcinoma. Squamous cell carcinoma of the lung is often associated with a history of smoking.

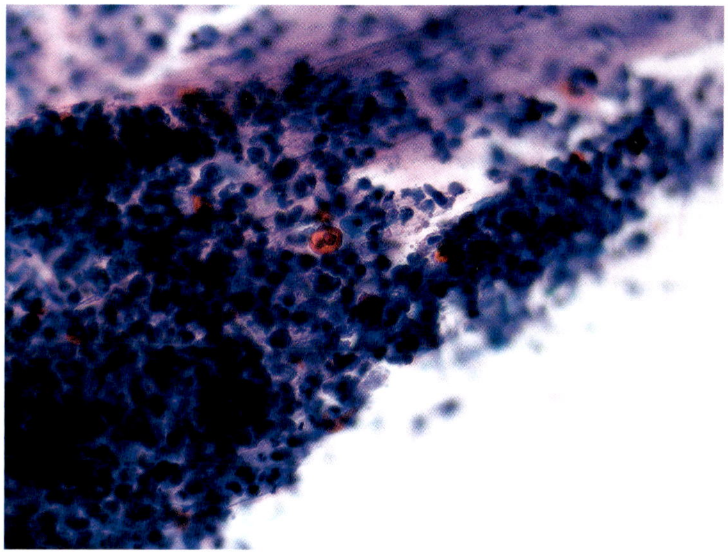

Figure 6.22a — Well-Differentiated Squamous Cell Carcinoma, Sputum [Pap Stain; High Power]. Immediately striking in this image are the orangeophilic, keratinized, atypical cells scattered across the field. A closer examination reveals the rest of the cellular cohort to be composed of atypical cells with high nuclear:cytoplasmic ratios and hyperchromatic nuclei with irregular borders. A few cells have more abundant blue cytoplasm with the homogenous, dense appearance typical of squamous differentiation. The cells are mostly dyshesive and held in association by the delicate, filamentous sputum matrix, seen streaking across the upper right of the image, and accompanied by scattered neutrophils and other inflammatory cells. These inflammatory cells provide a good internal size control. The more dyshesive cell collection is to be expected in a sputum, since these cells will have been shed autonomously and thereby tend to be the looser cells in the tumor.

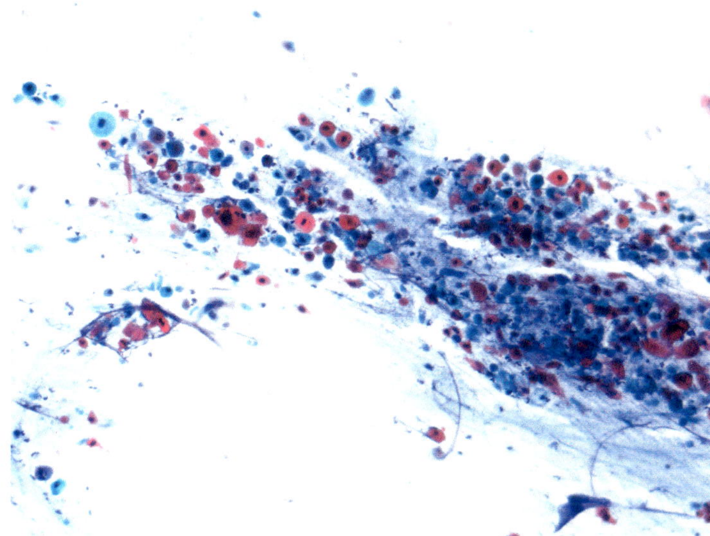

Figure 6.22b — Well-Differentiated Squamous Cell Carcinoma, Sputum [Pap Stain; Medium Power]. This medium power view of a sputum specimen shows a collection of squamous cells, many keratinized, with marked nuclear pleomorphism and hyperchromasia confined within the visible mucoid matrix of the sputum itself. Anucleate surface squames are also seen. Squamous cell carcinoma of the lung often arises more centrally, associated with a bronchus and may present with obstructive symptoms. There is often squamous metaplasia and dysplasia of the bronchial epithelium adjacent to the tumor.

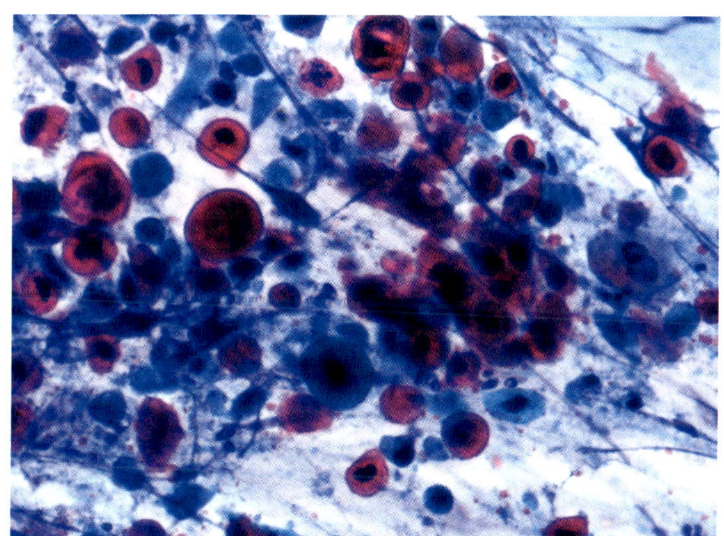

Figure 6.22c — Well-Differentiated Squamous Cell Carcinoma, Sputum [Pap Stain; High Power]. The tumor in this image shows abundant keratinized cells and surface anucleate cells, showing the typical pleomorphism and nuclear hyperchromasia expected in squamous cell carcinoma. The prominent keratinization suggests a well-differentiated tumor; a poorly differentiated tumor would contain only rare, if any, keratinized cells. Other subtypes of squamous cell carcinoma include basaloid, clear cell, papillary, and sarcomatoid (spindle cell).

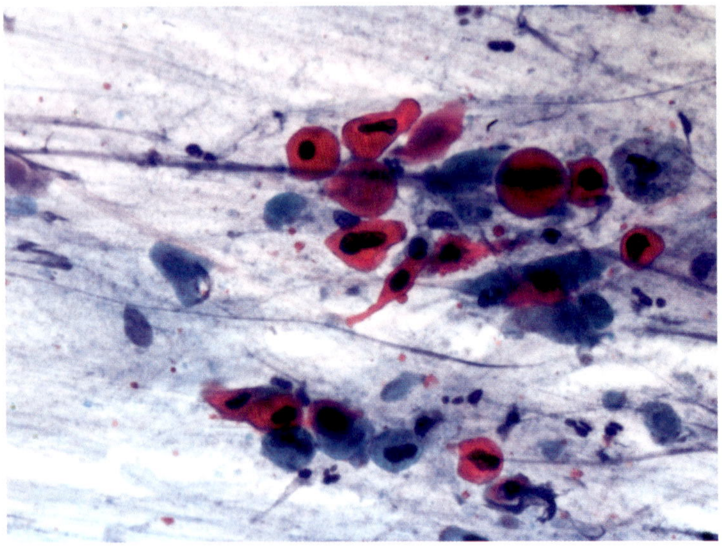

Figure 6.22d — Well-Differentiated Squamous Cell Carcinoma, Sputum [Pap Stain; High Power]. Differentiating malignant from reactive or metaplastic squamous epithelium can be difficult, but several features can help. Here the noticeable variation in cell size and shape, as well as the presence of keratin pearls, are indications of atypia. Additionally, the nuclei are hyperchromatic, enlarged, and have very irregular nuclear membranes. These features all point to a diagnosis of squamous cell carcinoma. Squamous cell carcinoma is the second most common subtype of lung cancer, after adenocarcinoma.

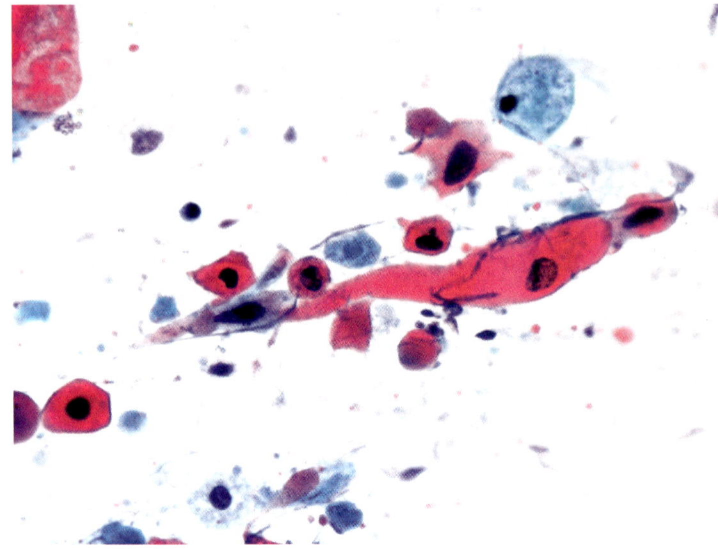

Figure 6.22e — Well-Differentiated Squamous Cell Carcinoma, Sputum [Pap Stain; High Power]. Here is the so-called "tadpole cell," an asymmetric cell with a streaming cytoplasmic "tail" on one side. These atypical and bizarre shapes are suggestive of squamous cell carcinoma. Additionally, the surrounding cells have markedly hyperchromatic nuclei with irregular nuclear borders and increased nuclear:cytoplasmic ratios. Recurring genetic alterations in pulmonary squamous cell carcinoma include FGFR1 amplification.

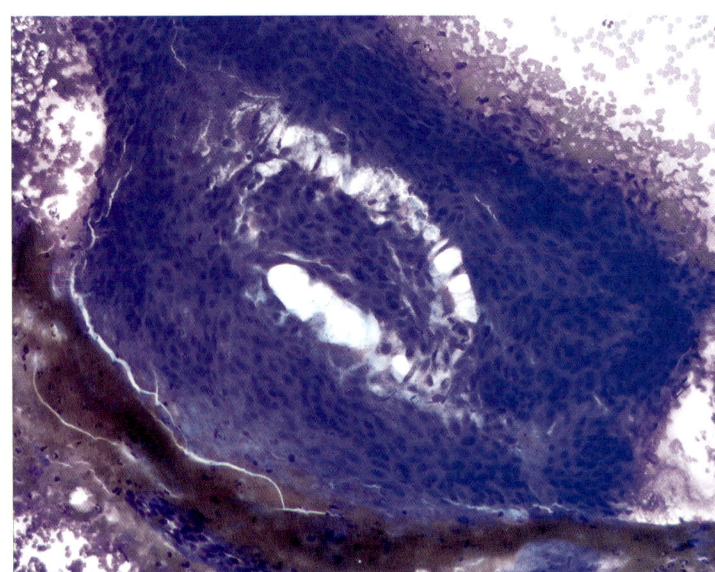

Figure 6.23 — Well-Differentiated Squamous Cell Carcinoma, Fine Needle Aspiration [Pap Stain; High Power]. Intercellular bridging, seen between the central cluster of cells and the surrounding ring, is caused by cell to cell cytoplasmic adhesions. This feature is a good diagnostic clue to squamous differentiation. Fine needle aspiration is often superior to bronchoalveolar lavage in obtaining diagnostic material in lung carcinomas.

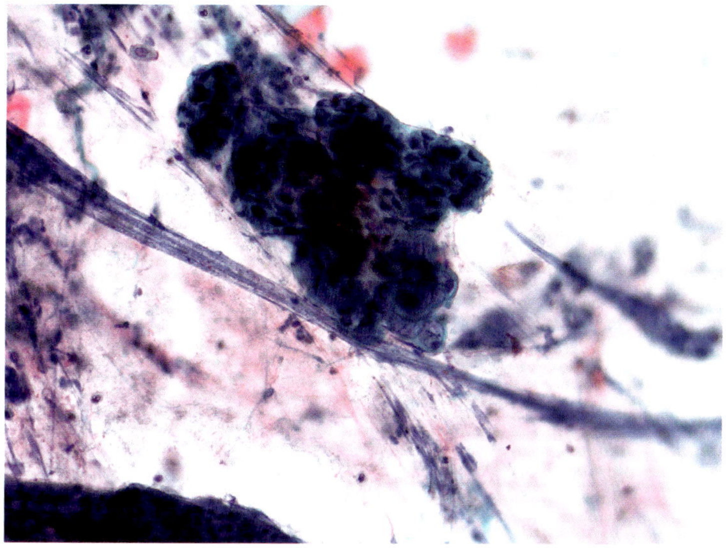

Figure 6.24a — Well-Differentiated Squamous Cell Carcinoma, Bronchial Brushing [Pap Stain; Medium Power]. The malignant cells are arranged in a tight, vaguely lobular pattern in the foreground. They can be recognized as malignant by the high nuclear:cytoplasmic ratio, nuclear membrane irregularity, hyperchromasia, and variable nuclear size (particularly prominent in the lower right of the lobule). The background contains several single exfoliated pink keratinized cells, suggesting a background of squamous metaplasia in this brush specimen. Neutrophils are noticeable within and around the cell cluster, which may be an additional feature of squamous carcinomas.

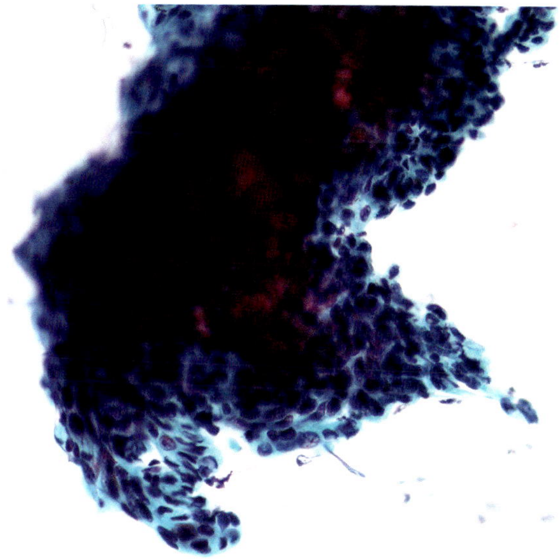

Figure 6.24b — Well-Differentiated Squamous Cell Carcinoma, Bronchial Brushing [Pap Stain; High Power]. Fragments of tissue such as this may be suggestive of malignancy due in part to the prominent hyperchromasia and pleomorphism. In areas, the cells have an almost "streaming" appearance and are tightly cohesive. Perhaps lacking is an immediate impression of squamous cell carcinoma, although the hard, "glassy," appearance of the cytoplasm points towards squamous differentiation, despite the lack of keratinized cells. Squamous cell carcinoma may be difficult to distinguish from dysplasia or even reactive metaplasia in well-differentiated cases, and caution is required during interpretation.

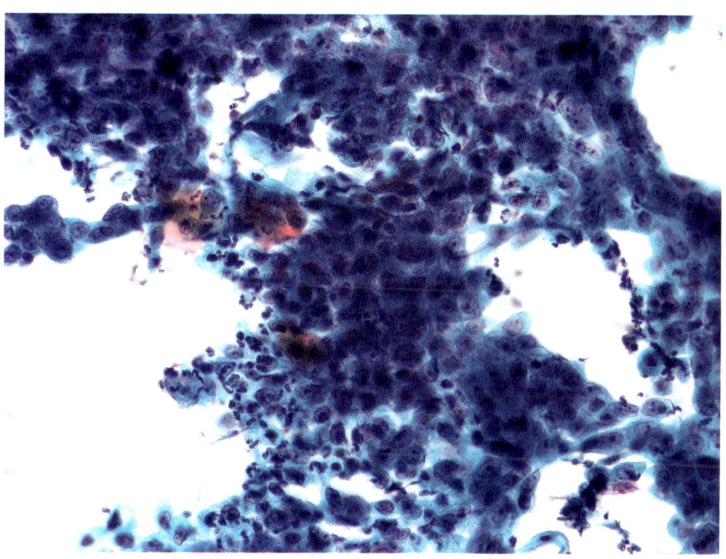

Figure 6.24c — Well-Differentiated Squamous Cell Carcinoma, Bronchial Washing [Diff-Quik Stain; High Power]. Sheets of cells appear to be pulled and stretched in many directions in this image. The cells all share nuclear enlargement with coarse chromatin and multiple nucleoli, in addition to the dense cytoplasm reaching in all directions due to strong cell-cell adhesions. Squamous cell carcinoma with extensive neutrophilic infiltration, as is prominent in this bronchial wash specimen, is occasionally seen. The differential diagnosis includes both infectious and reactive conditions.

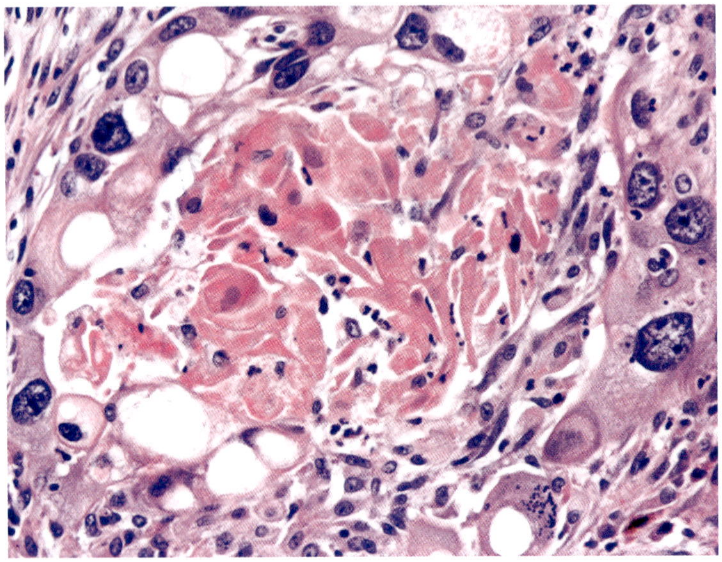

Figure 6.25 — Keratinizing Squamous Cell Carcinoma, Biopsy [H&E Stain; High Power]. This malignant squamous nest contains central dyskeratotic, partially necrotic cells surrounded by polygonal cells with dense pink cytoplasm and marked nuclear atypia. An atypical mitotic figure is present at the bottom right. A finding of keratinization, with or without keratin pearl formation and/or intercellular bridges, is sufficient for a diagnosis of squamous cell carcinoma in a resection specimen, if representative of the entire lesion. In small biopsies, the possibility of adenosquamous carcinoma cannot be confidently excluded. Studies show that adenosquamous tumors harbor adenocarcinoma-associated mutations at a rate similar to pure adenocarcinomas.

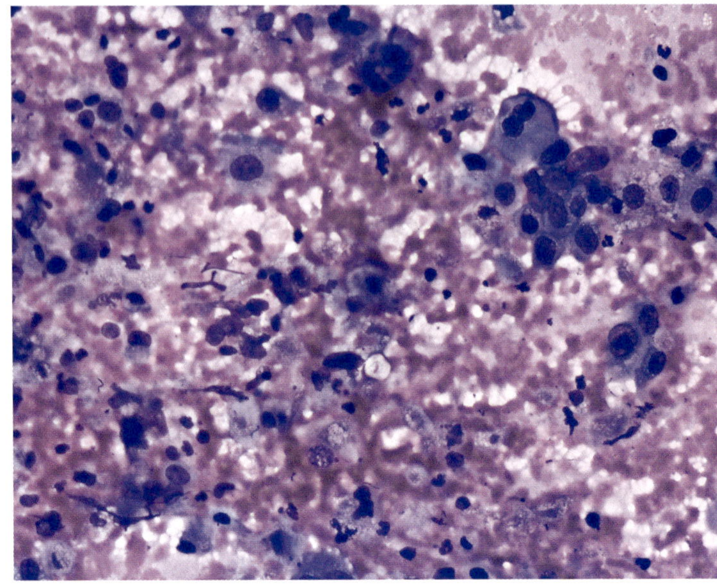

Figure 6.26a — Squamous Cell Carcinoma, Fine Needle Aspiration [Diff-Quik Stain; Medium Power]. This Diff-Quik stained aspirate specimen from a squamous cell carcinoma shows a loose population of malignant cells with large nuclei demonstrating irregular borders, occasional binucleated cells, moderate to abundant blue cytoplasm, and perinuclear fine vacuoles. The binucleation and cytoplasmic vacuoles are both features more often associated with malignant mesothelioma than squamous cell carcinoma but are not diagnostic of the former. These cells do not have the characteristic macronucleoli or two-toned cytoplasm of mesothelioma.

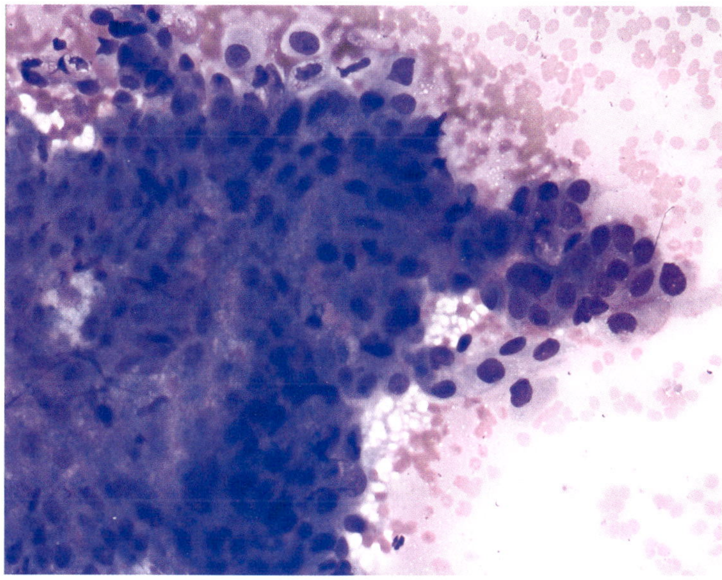

Figure 6.26b — Squamous Cell Carcinoma, Fine Needle Aspiration [Diff-Quik Stain; Medium Power]. Squamous cell carcinoma can mimic the morphology of other tumors, such as mesothelioma, as seen in this example. The tumor shown here appears more loosely cohesive around the edges, without apparent intercellular bridges at this magnification. Furthermore, the cells are vaguely rounded. No nucleoli are present, and there is a single cell with what appears to be a deep blue keratin cytoplasmic pearl to the right of the image center. The lack of obvious nucleoli also argues against mesothelioma.

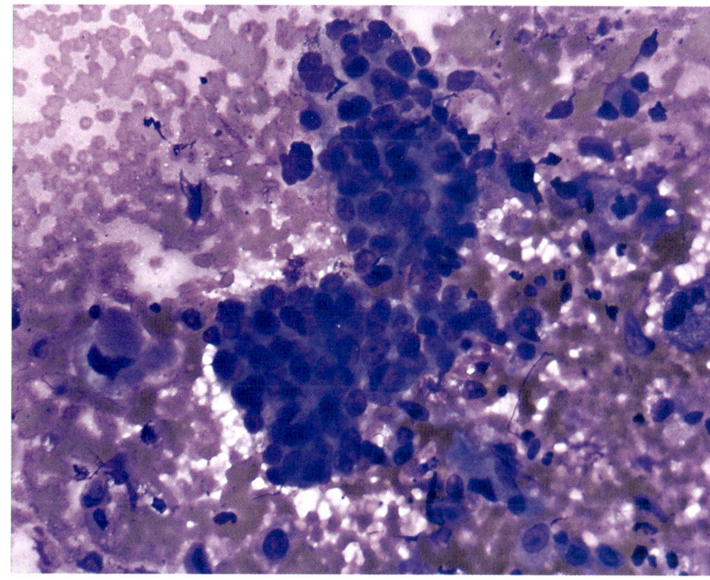

Figure 6.26c — Squamous Cell Carcinoma, Fine Needle Aspiration [Diff-Quik Stain; Medium Power]. This image of a pulmonary squamous cell carcinoma demonstrates some confusing features. These clusters of atypical cells display a prominent central nucleolus. Additionally, a multinucleated histiocyte at the right edge of the field could be mistaken for a multinucleated tumor cell. The cells do not show the "windows" or "ruffled border" characteristic of mesothelioma, but it would be difficult to definitively diagnose squamous cell carcinoma on this image alone.

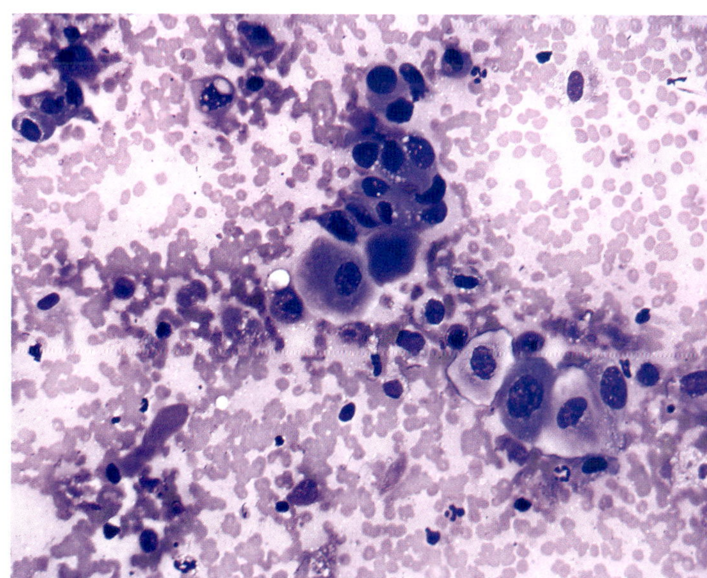

Figure 6.26d — Squamous Cell Carcinoma, Fine Needle Aspiration [Diff-Quik Stain; High Power]. This example of squamous cell carcinoma displays faint perinuclear vacuoles; a pale, ruffled cytoplasmic border; and the suggestion of "windows" between cells—all features of mesothelioma. The cytoplasm has more of the hard, glassy character of squamous lesions, and lacks any true "two-toned" ruffled edge; in addition, the nuclear features are not quite that of mesothelioma. Immunohistochemistry for WT-1 and calretinin would be negative in this case, arguing against mesothelial differentiation.

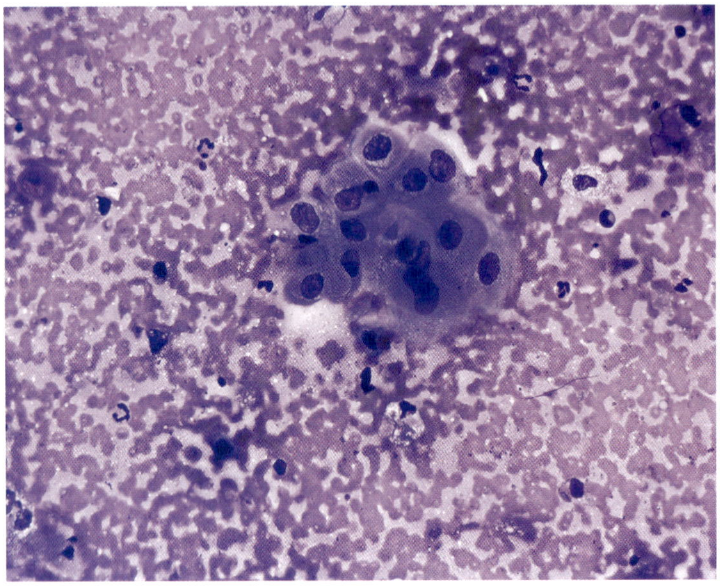

Figure 6.27a — Squamous Cell Carcinoma, Fine Needle Aspiration [Diff-Quik Stain; High Power]. The tumor cell aggregate has noticeable fine perinuclear vacuoles and distinct intercellular borders in this example, and some nuclei have easily visible nucleoli. The coloration and texture of the cytoplasm display the "hard" character often associated with squamous cell carcinoma, but without apparent intercellular bridges. A background without single atypical mesothelial cells, and with the presence of more "conventional" appearing atypical squamous cells, would favor the diagnosis of squamous cell carcinoma.

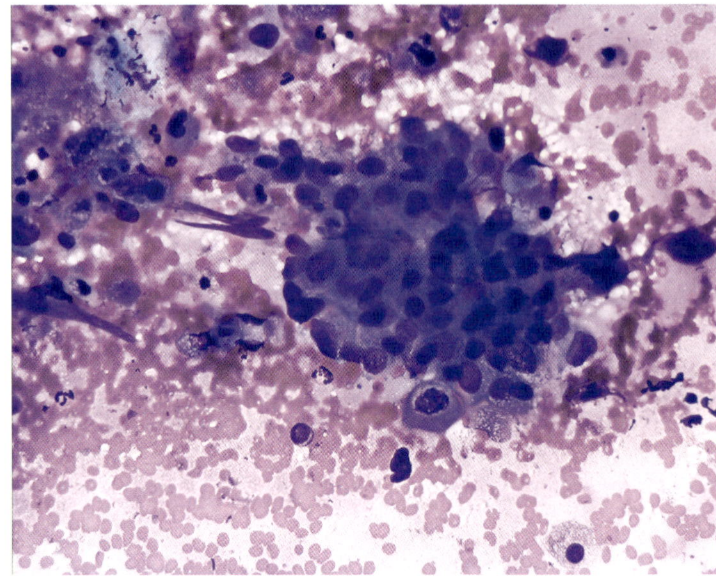

Figure 6.27b — Squamous Cell Carcinoma, Fine Needle Aspiration [Diff-Quik Stain; Medium Power]. Most of the tumor cells in this view are present in the central aggregate and display malignant features, but with no feature that proclaims a squamous origin. However, there is a cell to the left of the aggregate at 9:00 with a large, dense blue cytoplasmic inclusion highly suggestive of a keratin inclusion. Caution should be used with immunohistochemistry, as mesothelial cells and squamous cells both express CK5/6, although mesothelial cells are usually negative for p40. A broad panel with multiple markers of each lineage is generally most helpful.

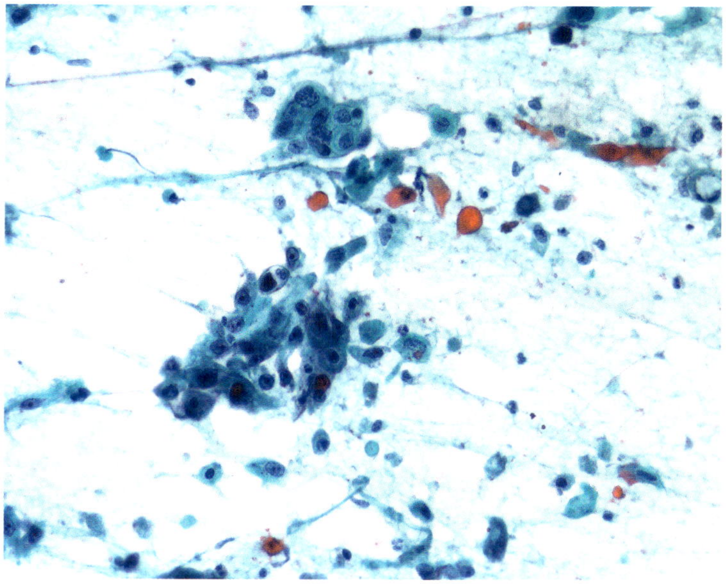

Figure 6.27c — Squamous Cell Carcinoma, Fine Needle Aspiration [Pap Stain; Medium Power]. The keratin pearls and irregularly shaped keratin fragments are a good clue to the squamous nature of this tumor; however, the groups of malignant cells in the center of the image do have prominent nucleoli, perinuclear clearing, and distinct cell borders, which should raise the consideration of mesothelioma. Squamous cell carcinoma is often a central lesion associated with a bronchus and is rarely present in pleural fluid, while mesothelioma is commonly diagnosed via thoracentesis and usually presents as a peripheral lesion "caking" the lung and with multiple pleural nodules.

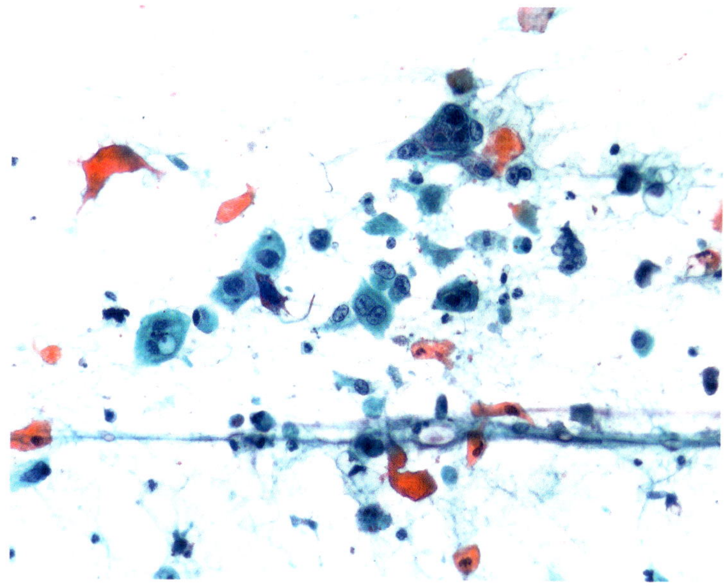

Figure 6.27d — Squamous Cell Carcinoma, Fine Needle Aspiration [Pap Stain; Medium Power]. The cells are mostly highly atypical and malignant, with some multinucleated cells and many cells with prominent nucleoli. The irregular fragments of orangeophilic keratin as well as the atypical keratinized cells are extremely helpful in making the diagnosis of squamous cell carcinoma. When the differential diagnosis includes mesothelioma and immunohistochemistry is necessary, recently BAP-1 loss has been demonstrated in mesothelioma.

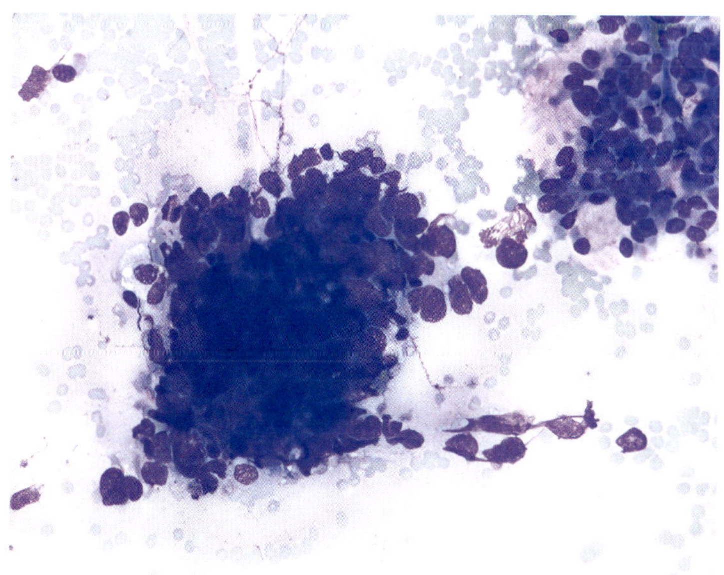

Figure 6.28a — Poorly Differentiated Squamous Cell Carcinoma, Bronchial Brushing [Diff-Quik Stain; High Power]. The array of cells in the center of the image demonstrate clear malignant features, such as irregular nuclear membranes, pleomorphism, overlapping, and elevated nuclear:cytoplasmic ratio, among others. The group of cells at the upper right provides a convenient internal comparison to benign cells with smooth nuclei, even chromatin, and ample cytoplasm. However, there is no clear indication of a line of differentiation of the malignant cells—only a poorly differentiated carcinoma. This case ultimately was a poorly differentiated squamous carcinoma. Determination of differentiation may require immunohistochemistry and expression of antigens such as p40 and CK5/6, which are suggestive of squamous differentiation.

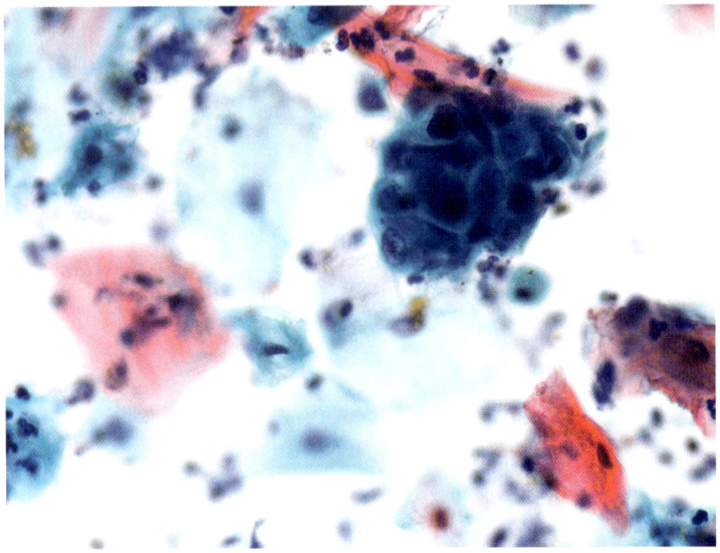

Figure 6.28b — Poorly Differentiated Squamous Cell Carcinoma, Sputum [Pap Stain; High Power]. A cluster of malignant cells is prominent in the upper right. The cells exhibit some molding and large, pleomorphic nuclei; some hyperchromatic while others have more open and pale chromatin and all exhibit irregular borders. Nucleoli are not prominent. The malignant cells tightly adhere to each other with little space between them, and in the far upper right seem to mold and curve around each other. The composition of the background is primarily superficial squamous cells, some of which are keratinized and others not and acute inflammation and granular, golden debris. The differential diagnosis at this point is broad for this poorly differentiated carcinoma. Patient history and possibly immunohistochemistry may be helpful. In this particular case, the final diagnosis was poorly differentiated squamous cell carcinoma.

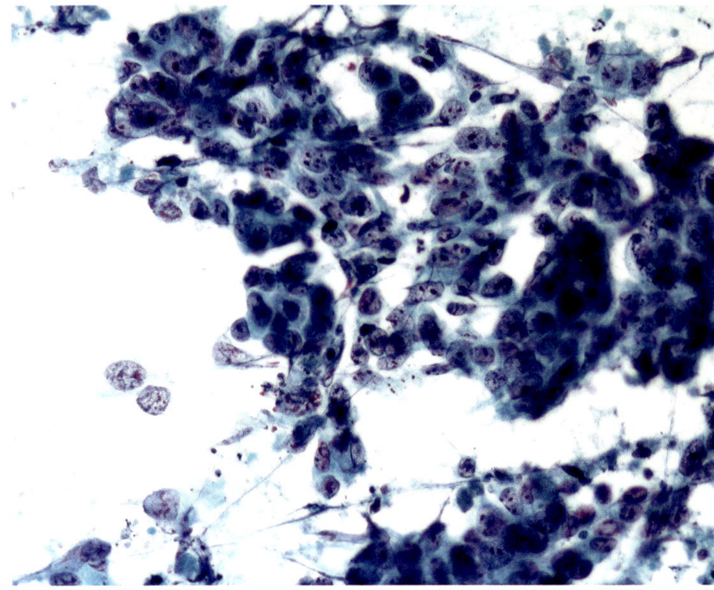

Figure 6.29a — Poorly Differentiated Squamous Cell Carcinoma, Fine Needle Aspiration [Pap Stain; High Power]. This image shows cells with large, irregular nuclei and multiple eccentric and variably sized nucleoli, with necrotic debris in the background. The presence of some areas with more distinct cell borders among small collections of cells hints at squamous differentiation. Identification of squamous cell carcinoma is important for treatment purposes; squamous carcinoma has been associated with sometimes fatal hemorrhages in patients who receive the monoclonal antibody bevacizumab as part of chemotherapy.

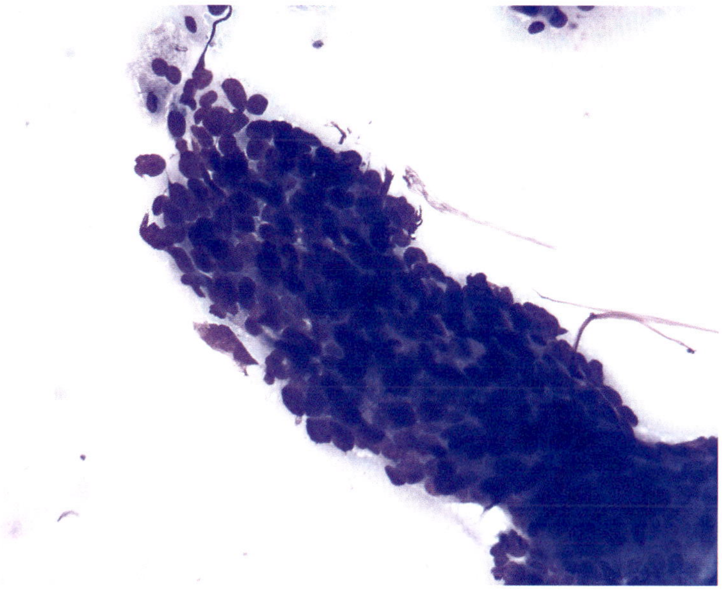

Figure 6.29b — Poorly Differentiated Squamous Cell Carcinoma, Fine Needle Aspiration [Diff-Quik Stain; High Power]. This aggregate of cells has high nuclear:cytoplasmic ratios and a sense of streaming but otherwise little indication of a line of differentiation. The nuclei have moderate pleomorphism and irregularity and there is dense cytoplasm. Squamous cell carcinomas may show such three-dimensional clusters on smear preparations, but it is not a diagnostic feature. A diagnosis of non–small cell carcinoma is appropriate if definitive evidence of squamous differentiation is absent.

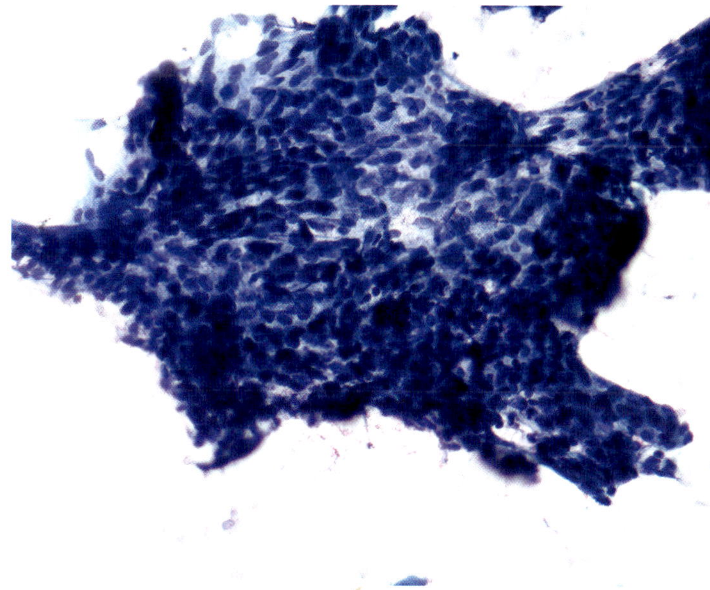

Figure 6.29c — Poorly Differentiated Squamous Cell Carcinoma, Fine Needle Aspiration [Pap Stain; High Power]. The specimen in this image nicely illustrates the sheeting that can be a component of squamous cell carcinomas. The tumor is poorly differentiated, and small cell carcinoma could enter the differential diagnosis, although there is more cytoplasm than would typically be seen in a small cell carcinoma, and less nuclear molding and fewer mitoses.

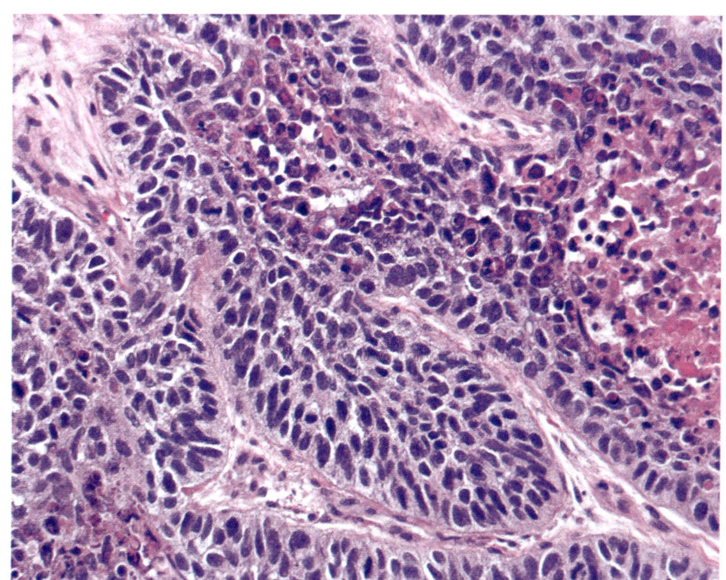

Figure 6.30a — Poorly Differentiated Squamous Cell Carcinoma, Lobectomy [H&E Stain; High Power]. This squamous cell carcinoma lacks unequivocal keratinization, and intercellular bridges are not demonstrable. Apoptotic zones are present centrally in some nests; the associated eosinophilia may be confused with keratin. This nested solid pattern occurs in both adenocarcinoma and squamous cell carcinoma; immunohistochemical stains are required for accurate classification. p40 is at present the most specific squamous marker; however, metastatic urothelial carcinoma also expresses p40 and may be morphologically similar. A positive GATA-3 stain is expected in most tumors of urothelial origin.

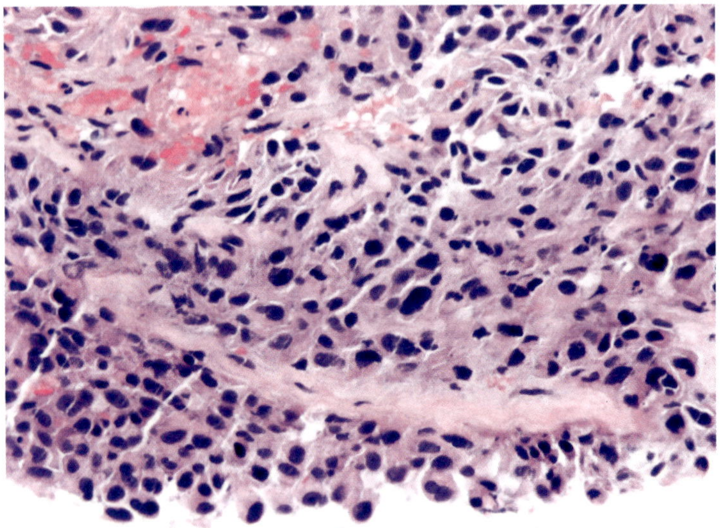

Figure 6.30b — Nonkeratinizing Squamous Cell Carcinoma, Biopsy [H&E Stain; High Power]. This biopsy sample of a poorly differentiated squamous cell carcinoma shows no cytoplasmic features of either squamous or glandular differentiation by hematoxylin and eosin staining. Differential considerations include solid-pattern adenocarcinoma (TTF-1 and/or napsin A+) and large cell carcinoma with null phenotype (non-small cell morphology, keratin+, negative for p40/p63, napsin A, and TTF-1). Urothelial carcinoma is also sometimes a mimic of squamous cell carcinoma, and can be addressed by patient history and immunohistochemical staining (GATA-3+, p40+, p63+, and often, CK7+ and CK20+).

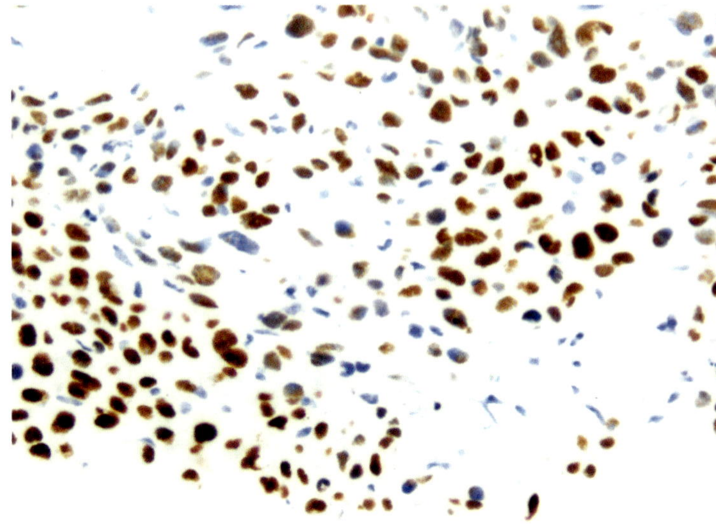

Figure 6.30c — Nonkeratinizing Squamous Cell Carcinoma, Biopsy [p40 Immunohistochemical Stain; High Power]. The tumor cells show strong and relatively uniform staining for p40. Stains for TTF-1 and napsin A were negative. This tumor was a single large hilar mass, consistent with primary pulmonary poorly differentiated nonkeratinizing squamous cell carcinoma.

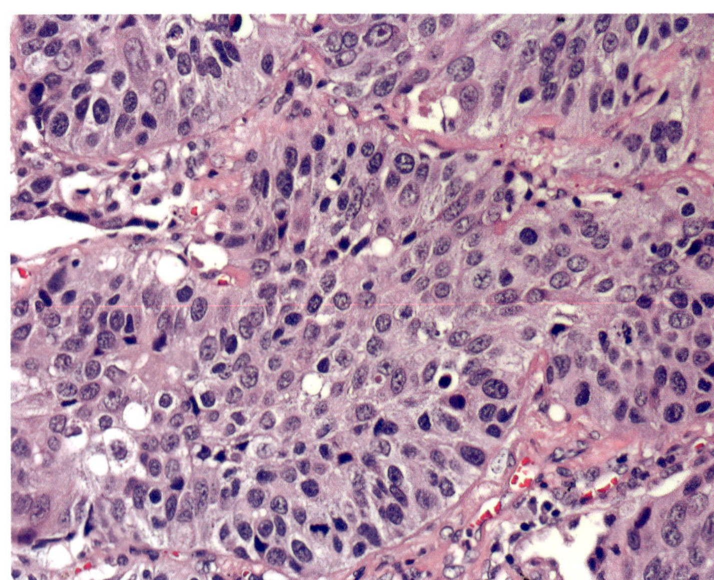

Figure 6.31 — Squamous Cell Carcinoma With Neuroendocrine Features, Lobectomy [H&E Stain; High Power]. This poorly differentiated nonkeratinizing squamous cell carcinoma shows a nested pattern with focal pseudopalisading (bottom center) and frequent mitoses, raising consideration for large cell neuroendocrine carcinoma. In the absence of unequivocal keratinization or intercellular bridges, immunostains are required to distinguish squamous cell carcinoma (p40+, p63+, CK5/6+, TTF-1-, synaptophysin-, CD56-) from large cell neuroendocrine carcinoma (synaptophysin+, CD56+, TTF-1 +/-, p40-, p63-) and from solid-pattern adenocarcinoma (napsin A+, TTF-1+, synaptophysin-, CD56-).

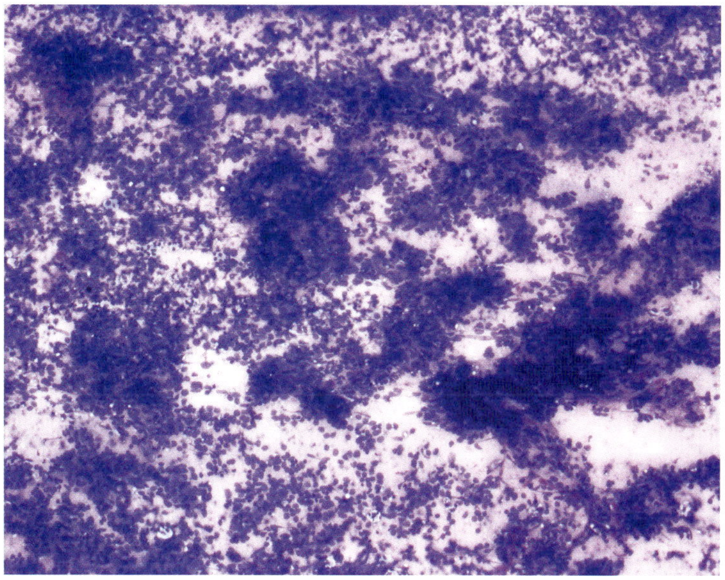

Figure 6.32a — Basaloid Squamous Cell Carcinoma, Fine Needle Aspiration [Diff-Quik Stain; Low Power]. The smear is strikingly cellular, as is often the case with basaloid squamous cell carcinoma, and the cells have enlarged, somewhat pleomorphic and irregular nuclei with scanty cytoplasm. The differential diagnosis in these cases includes small cell carcinoma and large cell carcinoma, among others.

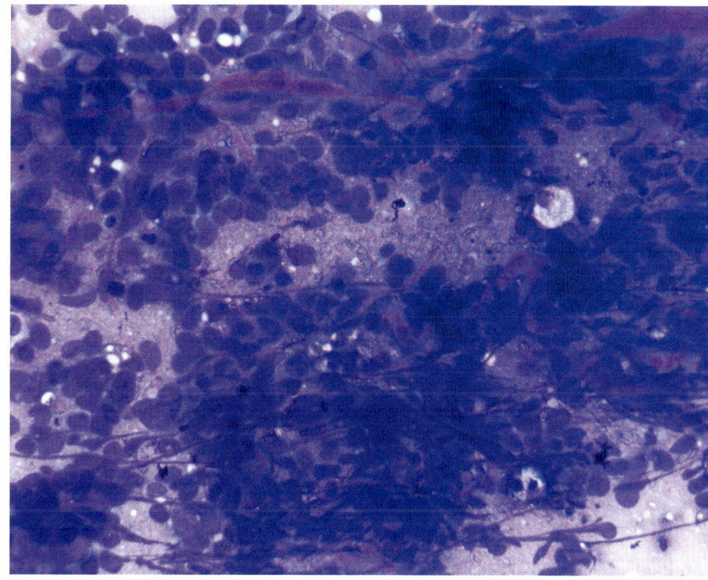

Figure 6.32b — Basaloid Squamous Cell Carcinoma, Fine Needle Aspiration [Diff-Quik Stain; Medium Power]. Basaloid squamous cell carcinomas may show extracellular matrix material, spectacularly displayed as sweeping, metachromatic ribbons across the upper part of this image, with scant clinging blue cytoplasm of the carcinoma cells forming a thin border. This matrix material may also be present in more spherical form, which can mimic adenoid cystic carcinoma, especially on H&E sections. However, basaloid squamous cell carcinoma has only one cell population and typically displays more atypia than adenoid cystic carcinoma. Immunohistochemistry or immunocytochemistry for markers such as p40 and S100 may be useful in difficult cases.

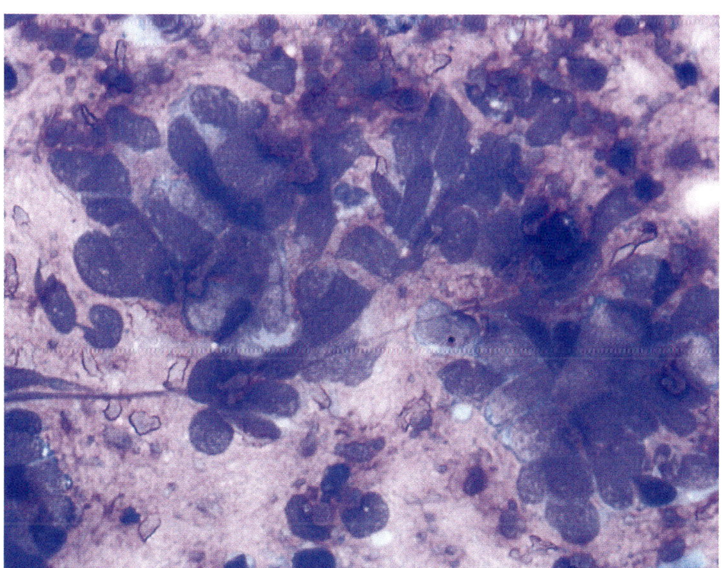

Figure 6.32c — Basaloid Squamous Cell Carcinoma, Fine Needle Aspiration [Diff-Quik Stain; High Power]. Sometimes basaloid squamous cell carcinomas show nuclear molding which simulates small cell carcinoma. Helpful features to distinguish the two include the presence of blue cytoplasm, increased pleomorphism, and lower mitotic rate seen in basaloid squamous carcinoma. All of these features are seen in this image. Basaloid squamous cell carcinomas should be negative for neuroendocrine markers and positive for more specific markers of squamous differentiation if uncertainty remains.

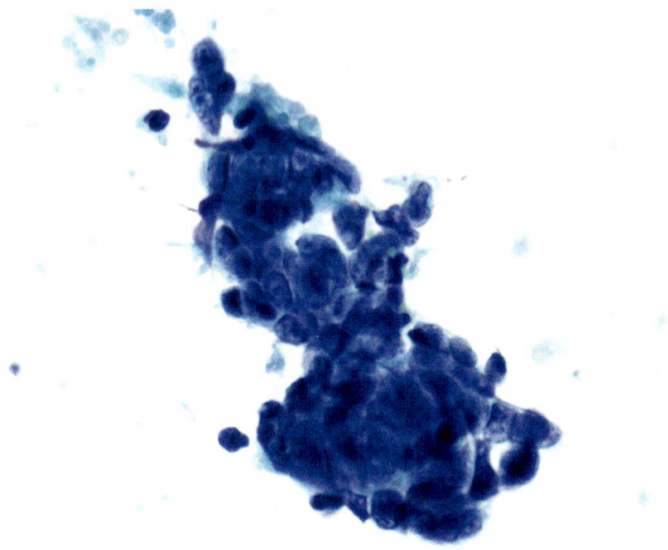

Figure 6.32d — Basaloid Squamous Cell Carcinoma, Fine Needle Aspiration [Pap Stain; High Power]. This Pap-stained high power image demonstrates again the nuclear molding of a basaloid squamous cell carcinoma and emphasizes that the differential diagnosis should include small cell carcinoma. This example shows very scant cytoplasm, although at the top of the image is a hint of blue, glassy cytoplasm around a few of the cells. There is also more nuclear pleomorphism than is typical for small cell carcinoma but expected in a squamous cell carcinoma. The chromatin is more coarse and irregular in this basaloid squamous cell carcinoma than is typical for small cell carcinomas.

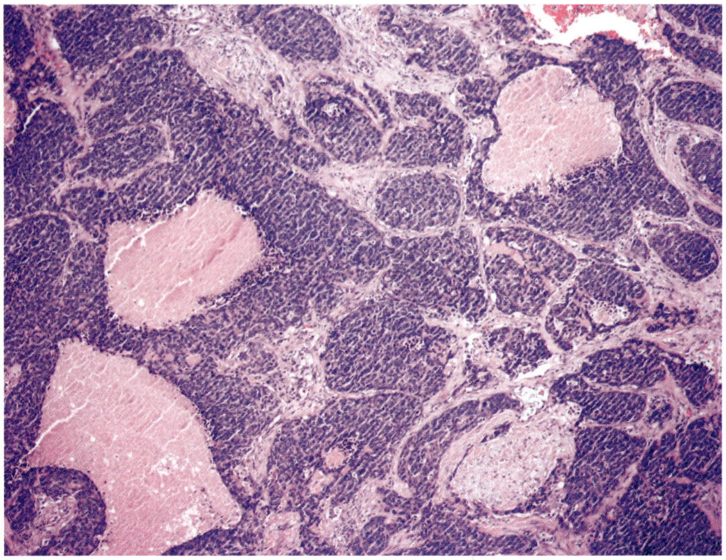

Figure 6.33a — Metastatic Tongue Base Cancer, Biopsy [H&E Stain; Low Power]. Nonkeratinizing squamous cell carcinoma of the oropharynx uncommonly metastasizes to the lung, where it may mimic primary basaloid squamous cell carcinoma or small cell carcinoma. This low-power view of a base-of-tongue metastasis has low power features suggestive of small cell carcinoma, including irregular nests of "blue cells" with zones of necrosis.

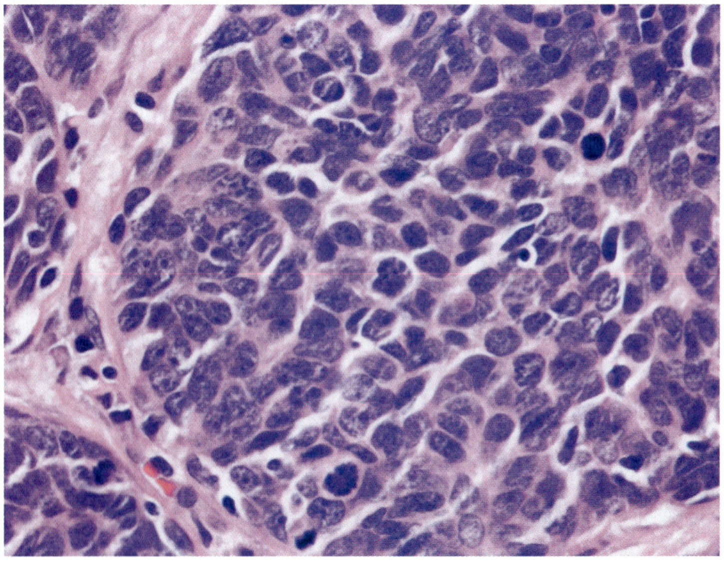

Figure 6.33b — Metastatic Tongue Base Cancer, Biopsy [H&E Stain; High Power]. At high power this metastasis lacks differentiation; it shows no keratinization or intercellular bridging. Several mitoses are present, and there is nuclear molding, suggestive of small cell carcinoma, although the presence of somewhat vesicular chromatin and readily identifiable nucleoli are not typical of small cell carcinoma.

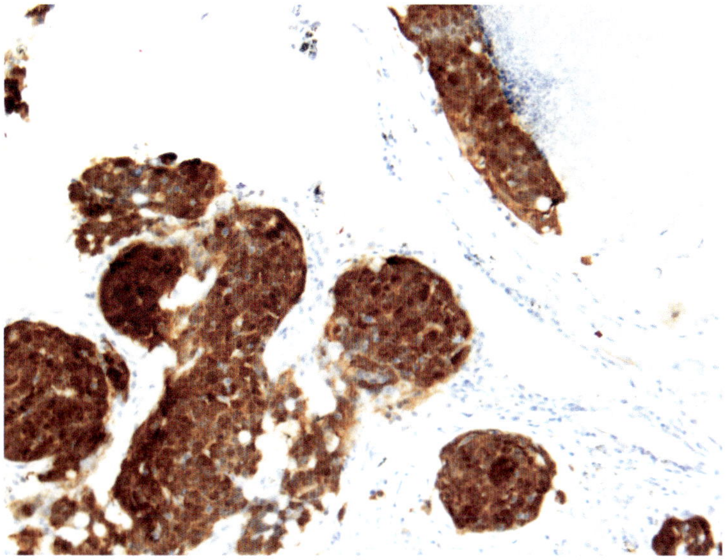

Figure 6.33c — Metastatic Tongue Base Cancer, Biopsy [p16 Immunohistochemical Stain; Low Power]. The tumor is diffusely positive for p16 (note absence of staining in necrotic zone at upper right). Tumor cells also expressed CK5/6 and nuclear p40, and were negative for synaptophysin, CD56, and TTF-1. Strong and uniform p16 expression is present in less than 5% of primary squamous cell carcinomas of the lung, and high-risk human papillomavirus DNA is virtually never detected.

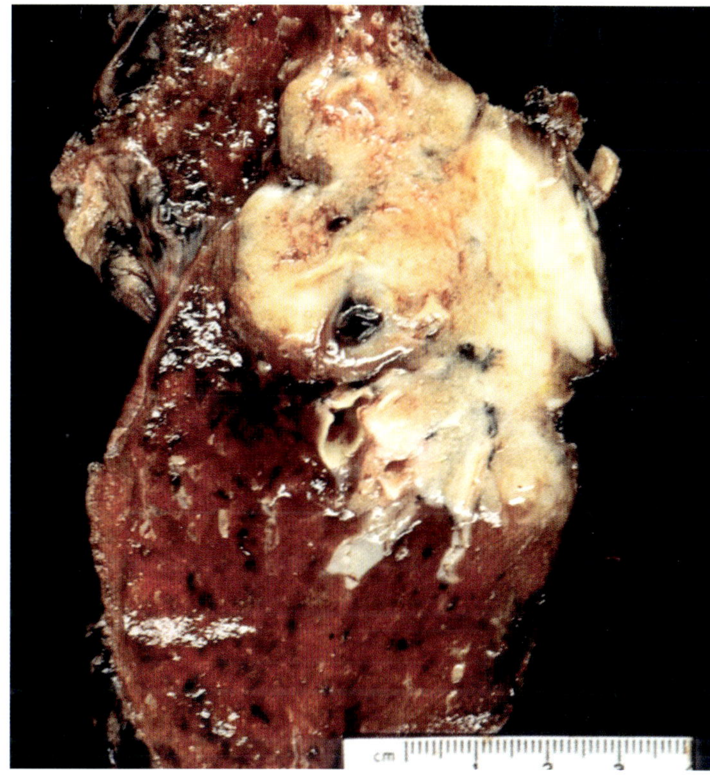

Figure 6.34 — Squamous Cell Carcinoma, Lobectomy [Gross Examination]. This pneumonectomy specimen demonstrates the characteristic gross features of squamous cell carcinoma, including large size, pushing borders, yellow-white color, and central location. Two small foci of cavitation with hemorrhage are present. Squamous tumors often cavitate, while adenocarcinomas rarely do.

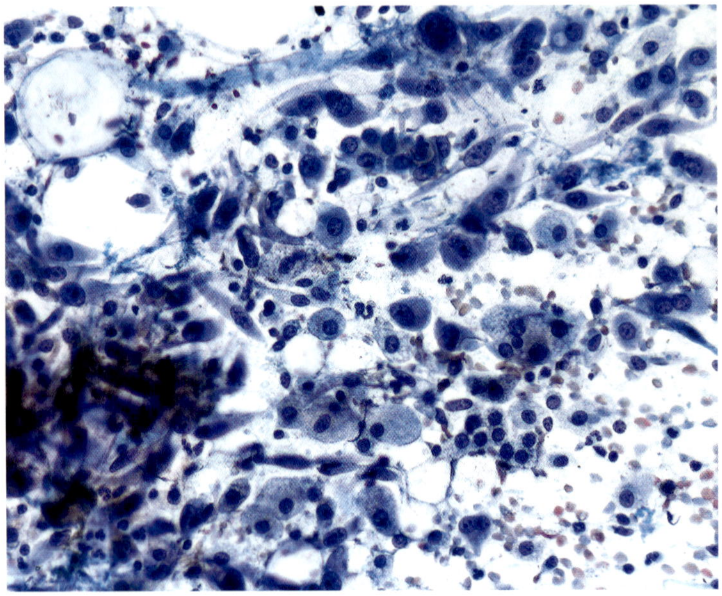

Figure 6.35a — Sarcomatoid Carcinoma, Fine Needle Aspiration [Pap Stain; Medium Power]. The current 2015 World Health Organization classification of lung tumors recognizes three histologic subtypes of carcinoma under the rubric of sarcomatoid carcinoma: pleomorphic, spindle cell, and giant cell carcinoma. In addition, it also categorizes carcinosarcoma and pulmonary blastoma as forms of sarcomatoid carcinoma. All are poorly differentiated malignancies composed of large cells defined histologically as having certain percentages of giant, pleomorphic, and spindle cell elements mixed with conventional non-small cell carcinoma and small cell carcinoma. As such, and per the World Health Organization classification, a definitive diagnosis of specific subtypes should only be attempted on resected lesions, not on core needle biopsy or cytology specimens. Pure forms of these various subtypes are extremely rare. Cytology smears are highly cellular and contain readily recognizable malignant cells. A randomly arranged mixture of malignant cells with epithelioid, pleomorphic, and spindle shapes is noticeable, along with a multinucleated cell that reflects the cellular heterogeneity encountered in sarcomatoid carcinoma.

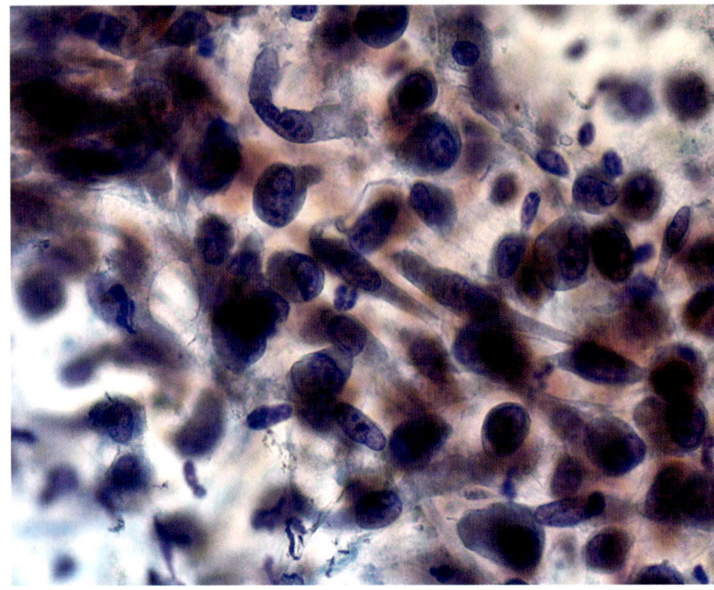

Figure 6.35b — Sarcomatoid Carcinoma, Fine Needle Aspiration [Pap Stain; High Power]. A high percentage (greater than 90%) of patients are smokers, and most are men; as these are clinically very aggressive neoplasms, patients have a poor prognosis. Since most sarcomatoid carcinomas arise in the peripheral lung, fine needle aspiration is the principal cytologic method used for diagnosis. This spindle cell-rich focus containing cells with markedly enlarged pleomorphic and vesicular nuclei, macronucleoli, and uni-/bipolar cytoplasmic processes imitates a mesenchymal malignancy. Although not illustrated, stromal components such as osteoid, chondroid, and myogenic differentiation may be seen. In such instances, the term *carcinosarcoma* has been used, which signifies a sarcomatoid carcinoma with heterologous differentiation. The differential diagnosis of these malignant spindle cell-rich smears includes high-grade sarcoma (e.g., leiomyosarcoma), metastatic sarcomatoid carcinoma, sarcomatoid mesothelioma, and malignant melanoma.

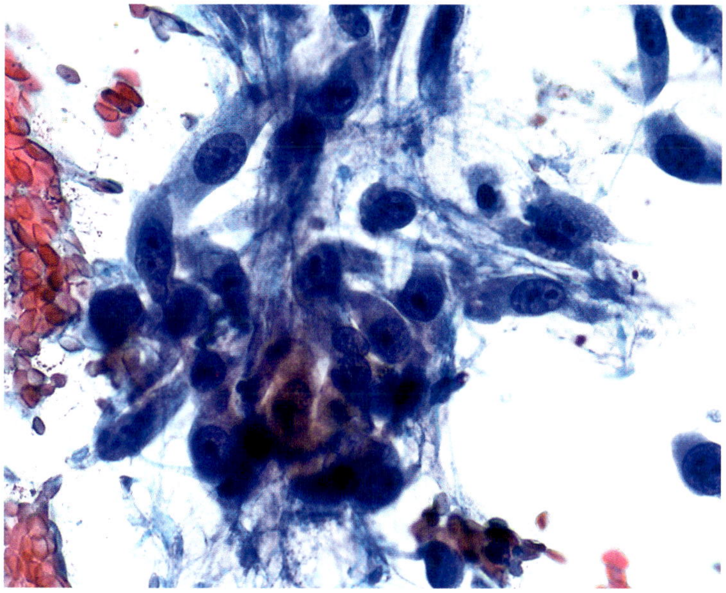

Figure 6.35c — Sarcomatoid Carcinoma, Fine Needle Aspiration [Pap Stain; High Power]. Polygonal and spindle cells show obvious nucleomegaly and some degree of pleomorphism. Immunohistochemistry shows variable results with epithelial and mesenchymal markers. Nearly all cells express vimentin, but cytokeratin expression—though present in differentiated epithelial cells such as adenocarcinoma and squamous carcinoma—may be absent to weakly positive in spindled and giant cells. Positive staining with TTF-1, p63, BerEp4, and p40, when present, are extremely helpful in distinguishing these spindle cells from a true sarcoma.

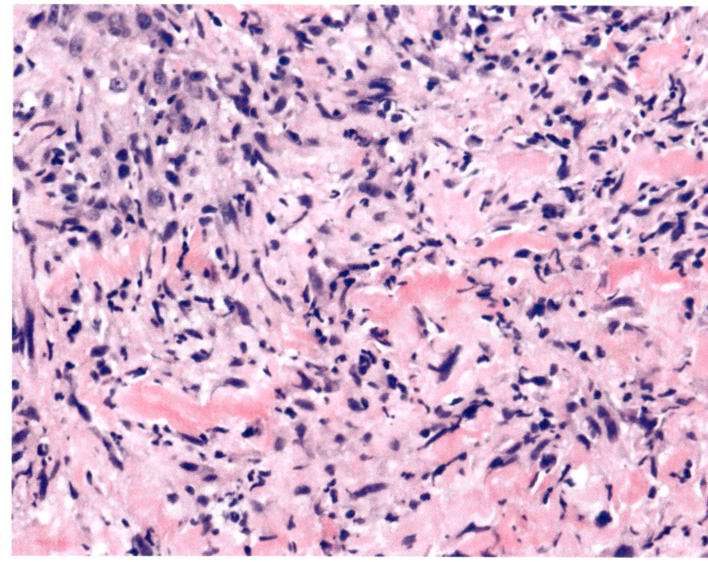

Figure 6.36a — Sarcomatoid Carcinoma, Spindle Cell Type, Bi-Lobectomy [H&E Stain; Low Power]. This spindle cell neoplasm is presented as a large mass with chest wall invasion. There is hypercellularity, including inflammation, with a few plumper cells at the upper left, but the predominant cell type is a bland spindle cell. No specific differentiation is apparent on hematoxylin and eosin stain; the histology suggests a fibroinflammatory process, sarcomatoid mesothelioma, or a sarcoma.

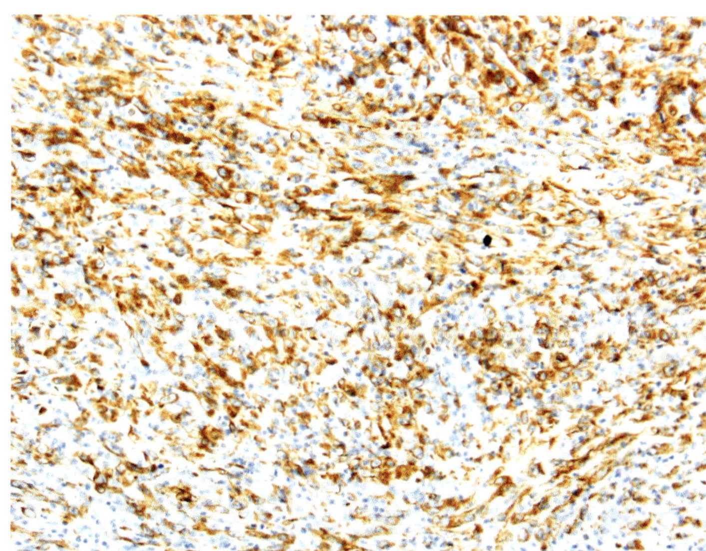

Figure 6.36b — Sarcomatoid Carcinoma, Spindle Cell Type, Bi-Lobectomy [CAM5.2 Immunohistochemical Stain; Low Power]. An immunostain for cytokeratin (CAM5.2) highlights a dense population of spindle cells with strong keratin expression. In addition to spindle cell carcinoma, differential considerations include reactive and neoplastic mesothelial proliferations. Mesothelial proliferations routinely express WT-1, calretinin, and D2-40 (podoplanin), and architectural cues are required to distinguish benign from malignant mesothelial lesions.

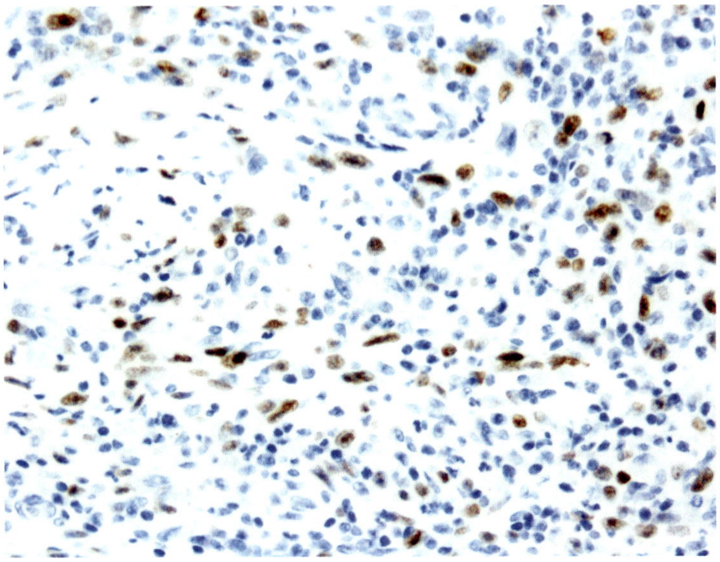

Figure 6.36c — Sarcomatoid Carcinoma, Spindle Cell Type, Bi-Lobectomy [TTF-1 Immunohistochemical Stain; Low Power]. An immunostain for TTF-1 shows moderate nuclear staining and strong evidence for spindle cell carcinoma, probably derived from a poorly differentiated adenocarcinoma. Mesothelial markers were negative.

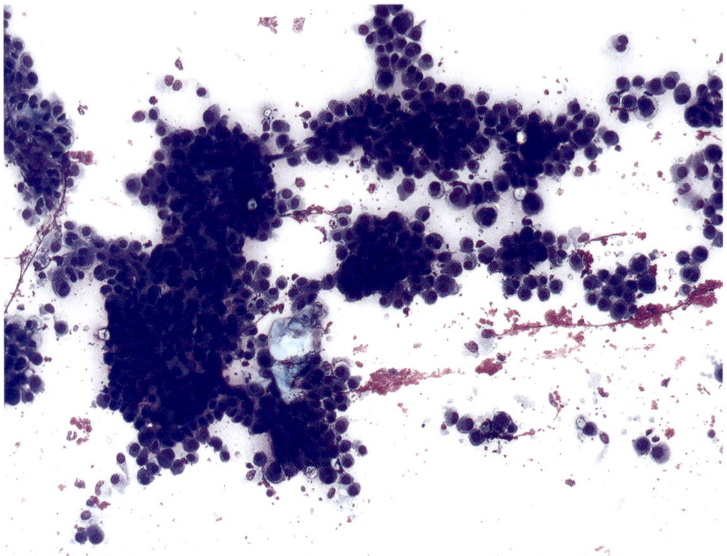

Figure 6.37a — Epithelioid Mesothelioma, Fine Needle Aspiration [Diff-Quik Stain; Low Power]. Mesothelioma is a malignant neoplasm of the pleura; thus, the majority of pulmonary cytologic specimens involve effusions although percutaneous aspiration biopsy of the pleura is also performed. The World Health Organization recognizes three histologic subtypes: sarcomatoid, biphasic, and epithelioid, with the latter being the most common. Mesothelioma is directly linked to asbestos overexposure with fewer cases due to therapeutic radiation. Diagnostically useful is the characteristic radiographic appearance of a diffuse rind-like circumferential pleural thickening. In some instances, multiple individual nodular plaques exist on the pleural surface; these eventually coalesce to form a single mass. Positive effusions almost always represent the epithelioid variant of mesothelioma, as the sarcomatoid variant rarely sheds cells into the pleural cavity. This image of a hypercellular slide shows cytologically bland mesothelial cells in clusters, flat sheets, and single forms. By itself, it is not diagnostic of mesothelioma.

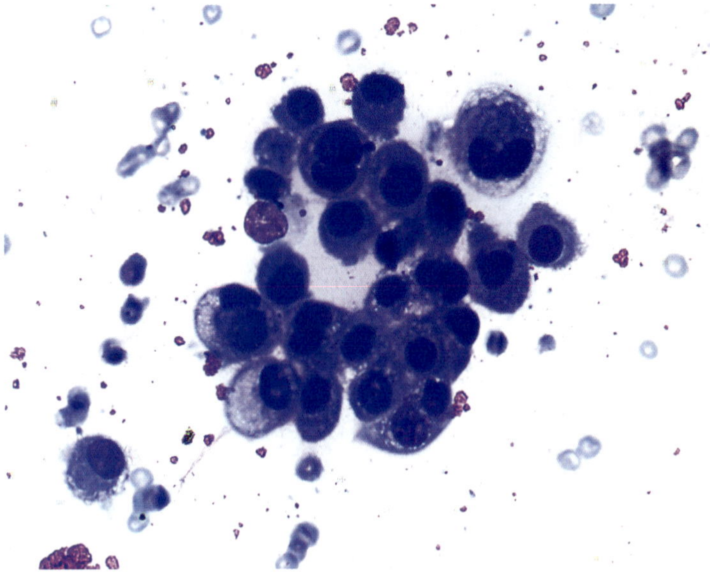

Figure 6.37b — Epithelioid Mesothelioma, Fine Needle Aspiration [Diff-Quik Stain; Medium Power]. The two major challenges in mesothelioma diagnosis are distinguishing it from reactive mesothelial cells and from adenocarcinoma. Tissue invasion, the hallmark of this malignancy, is not evaluable in cytologic preparations. Therefore, the sensitivity for a definitive diagnosis is low (20%–30% of cases).

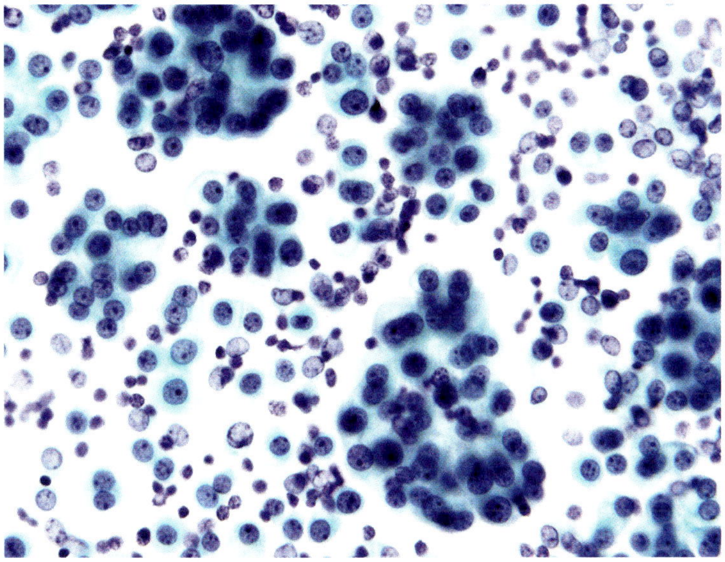

Figure 6.37c — Epithelioid Mesothelioma, Fine Needle Aspiration [Pap Stain; Medium Power]. The more common cytologic pattern in effusions is the morular pattern with either smooth, scalloped, or hobnail outer contours. Cells are more often arranged in flat sheets in fine needle aspiration smears. Individual cells are in loose clusters with slit-like spaces ("windows") separating them from one another. Cells possess large rounded nuclei with smooth outlines and a moderate amount of cytoplasm. Binucleation as seen here is not uncommon. Also common is the "two tone" dense endoplasm and pale peripheral ectoplasm seen in some of these cells. Single macronucleoli are typical.

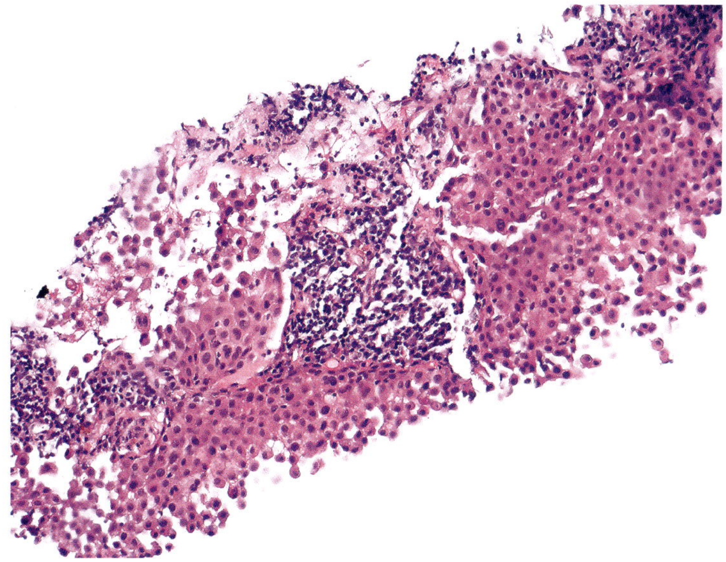

Figure 6.37d — Epithelioid Mesothelioma, Core Biopsy [H&E Stain; Medium Power]. This H&E-stained fragment contains a proliferation of cytologically bland and uniform mesothelial cells. Since ancillary testing is nearly always needed for a definitive diagnosis of mesothelioma, either a cell block or core needle biopsy become invaluable. These allow for performing a panel of immunohistochemical stains and genomic molecular study.

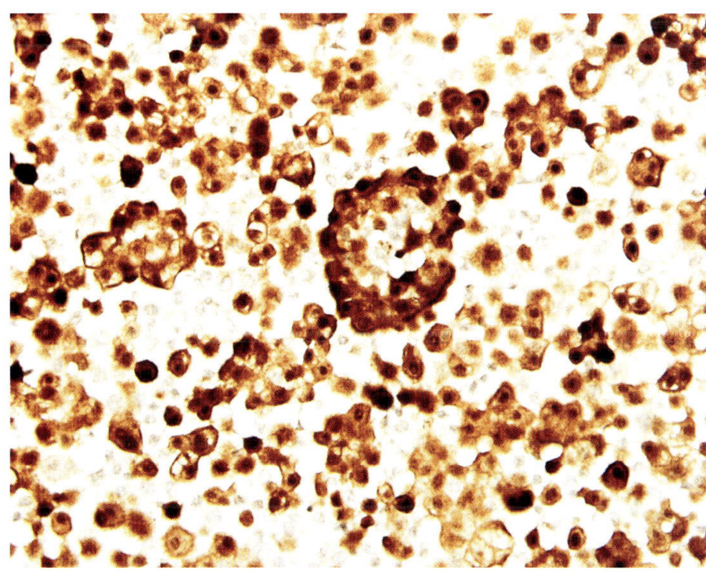

Figure 6.37e — Epithelioid Mesothelioma, Fine Needle Aspiration [Calretinin Immunohistochemical Stain; Medium Power]. Calretinin (shown here), CK5/6, D2-40, and WT1 expression can be used in cytospin preparations to support a diagnosis of mesothelioma or reactive mesothelial cells. However, BerEp4, MOC31, and TTF-1 expression, if present, would favor pulmonary adenocarcinoma. Since no immunohistochemical marker exists allowing for distinction between mesothelioma and a reactive, but benign mesothelial proliferation, fluorescence in situ hybridization testing for 9p21 deletion (present in the majority of mesotheliomas) is recommended. The International Mesothelioma Panel recommends use of the phrase "Atypical Mesothelial Proliferation" in equivocal cases of reactive mesothelial hyperplasia vs. malignant mesothelioma.

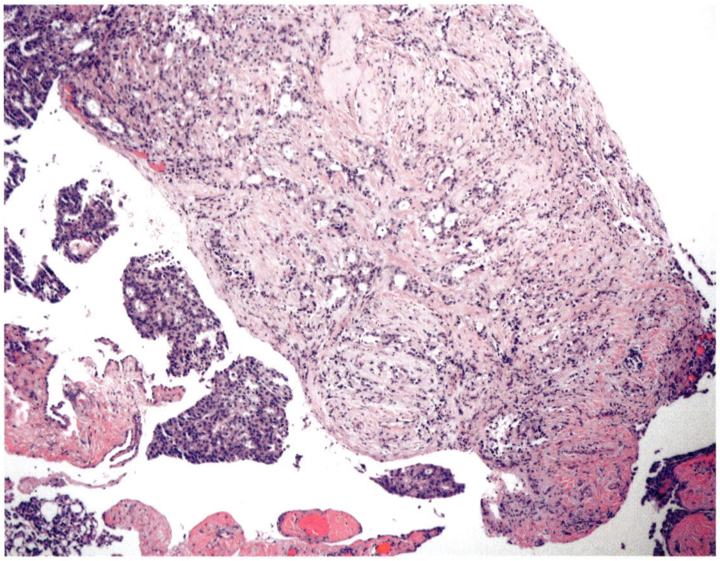

Figure 6.38a — Epithelioid Malignant Mesothelioma, Biopsy [H&E Stain; Low Power]. Within the dense rind of diffuse epithelioid malignant mesothelioma are embedded epithelioid tumor cells arranged in a polymorphous mix of patterns, here including tubulo-papillary with cribriform foci, and single-file strings of individual cells. Other examples may show solid, trabecular, and/or microcystic patterns; rare variants include deciduoid and small cell types. While inflammatory and reactive pleural injury may also be associated with fibrous thickening, malignant mesothelioma is distinguished by full-thickness infiltration of the dense collagenous pleura by neoplastic mesothelial cells in a haphazard, random distribution, in contrast to the layered organization of cells near the pleural surfaces observed in benign processes (including the chronic pleuritis observed in some patients with a history of asbestos exposure).

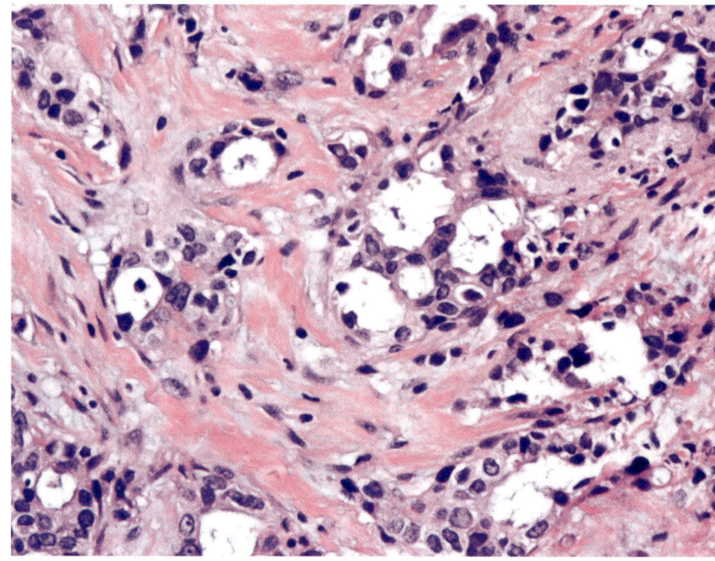

Figure 6.38b — Epithelioid Malignant Mesothelioma, Biopsy [H&E Stain; High Power]. While the individual cells of epithelioid malignant mesothelioma are most often relatively bland, this example shows moderate pleomorphism, with irregular vesicular nuclei and frequent nucleoli. In the setting of a new diagnosis, distinction from adenocarcinoma is not possible without a panel of immunohistochemical stains and detailed whole-body imaging studies. A few cases have high-grade or anaplastic cytology and require a panel of immunohistochemical stains to exclude sarcoma or anaplastic carcinoma. Any adenocarcinoma may involve the pleura, but the lung is the most frequent primary site for metastatic pleural disease, followed by the breast and stomach. Malignant vascular neoplasms may rarely involve the pleura and mimic mesothelioma; consideration of angiosarcoma and epithelioid hemangioendothelioma may be further evaluated with appropriate immunohistochemical stains (CD31, CD34, factor VIII, ERG).

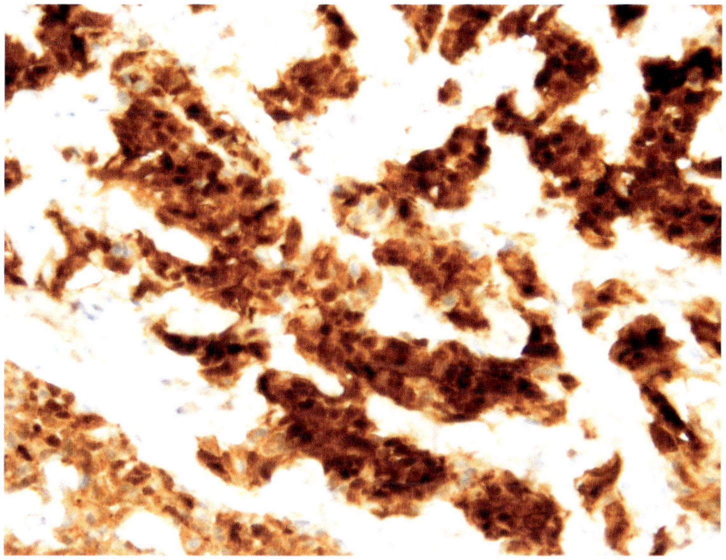

Figure 6.38c — Epithelioid Malignant Mesothelioma, Biopsy [Calretinin Immunohistochemical Stain; High Power]. Calretinin has greater than 90% sensitivity and specificity for epithelioid malignant mesothelioma, and is typically strong and uniform, as seen here. WT-1 somewhat less sensitive, but has close to 100% specificity. Other positive markers with a sufficient degree of sensitivity but somewhat less specificity include D2-40 (podoplanin) and CK5/6. MOC31 and BerEP4 are positive in most adenocarcinomas, and are routinely negative in mesothelioma. CEA, TTF-1, and CD15 (LeuM1) are somewhat less sensitive for adenocarcinoma, but, if positive, essentially exclude mesothelioma.

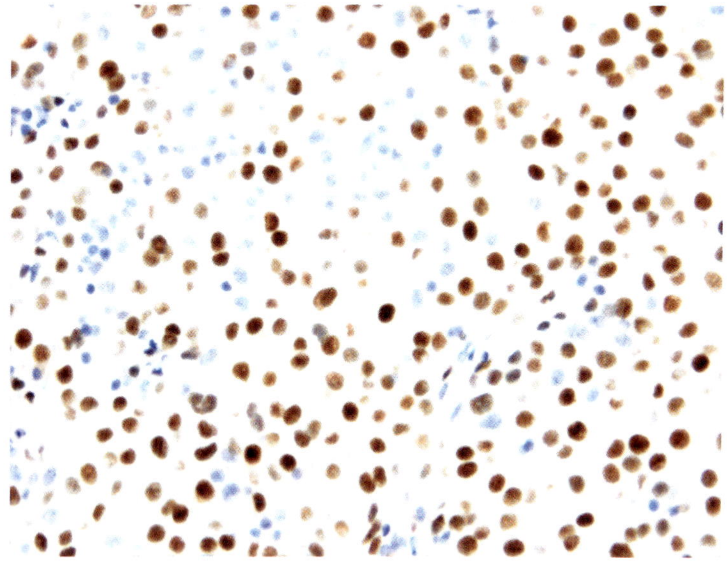

Figure 6.38d — Epithelioid Malignant Mesothelioma, Biopsy [WT-1 Immunohistochemical Stain; High Power]. WT-1 is a nuclear protein that is highly expressed in cells of the embryonic/fetal kidney and in the surface cells of the developing coelomic cavity. In mesotheliomas of all types, it is typically positive in more than 50% of cells, although intensity may vary. In epithelioid malignant mesothelioma, it is most often strong and uniform, as in this case. Normal resting mesothelium is usually negative, but reactive mesothelial cells may express this oncofetal antigen; a broad panel of immunostains and thorough assessment of atypia, imaging studies, and history are the best tools for excluding a reactive process.

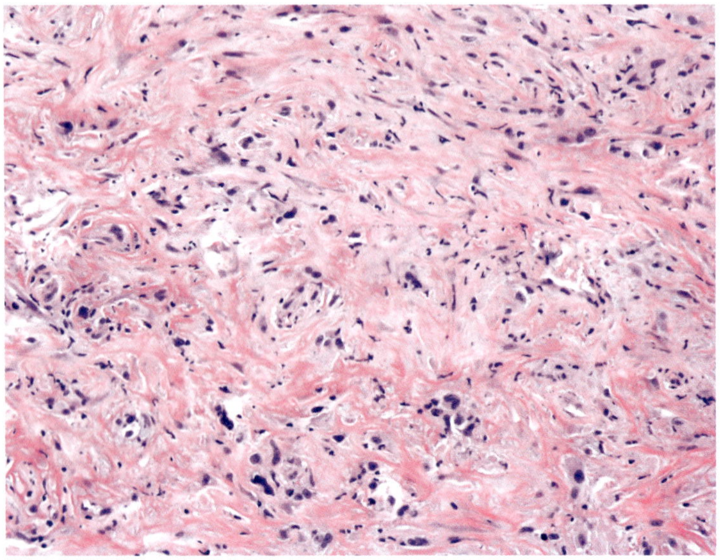

Figure 6.39 — Sarcomatoid Mesothelioma, Resection [H&E Stain; High Power]. Sarcomatoid variants have a gross appearance similar to that of the epithelioid type, but are characterized histologically by dense collagenous stroma and spindled neoplastic cells. "Biphasic" tumors have a mixed pattern, with at least 10% epithelioid and 10% spindled morphologies. "Desmoplastic" mesotheliomas are spindled, with a storiform or "patternless" growth pattern and dense stroma, reminiscent of desmoplastic melanomas in the skin. As in this example, atypia in sarcomatoid mesotheliomas may be minimal, or within the range of floridly reactive processes (e.g., chronic organizing empyema). Additional differential considerations include sarcoma and sarcomatoid carcinoma. Sarcomatoid mesothelioma typically retains expression of keratins and WT-1, at least focally; low power architecture, a broad panel of immunostains, and detailed imaging studies and history provide the key information required to establish an accurate diagnosis.

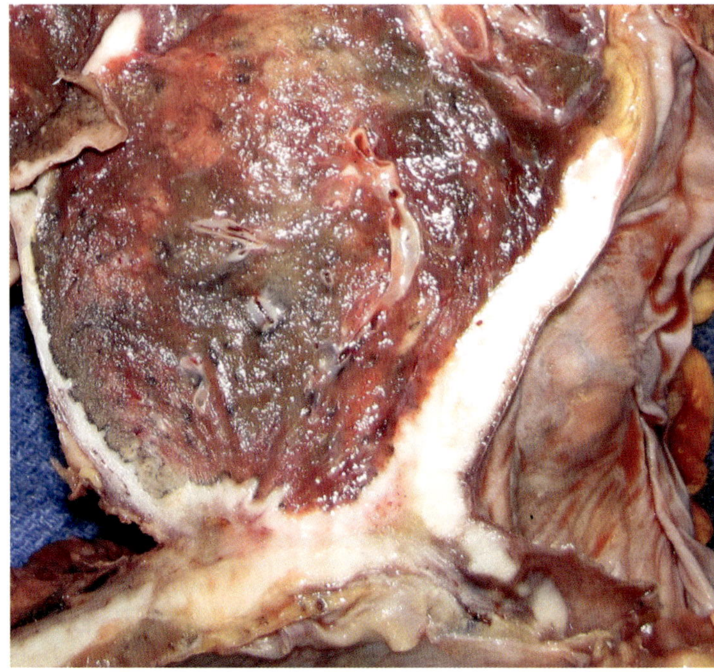

Figure 6.40 — Mesothelioma, Resection [Gross Examination]. This pleural neoplasm involves the lung base, infiltrating the diaphragm and adjacent lung parenchyma, and extending superiorly along the pleural surfaces. Fusion of the visceral and parietal pleurae by a rind several centimeters thick is the usual result; in nonfused areas, large pleural effusions often accumulate. A focus of bronchopneumonia, a frequent complication, is present at the upper left. Restrictive physiology develops when a tumor is extensive.

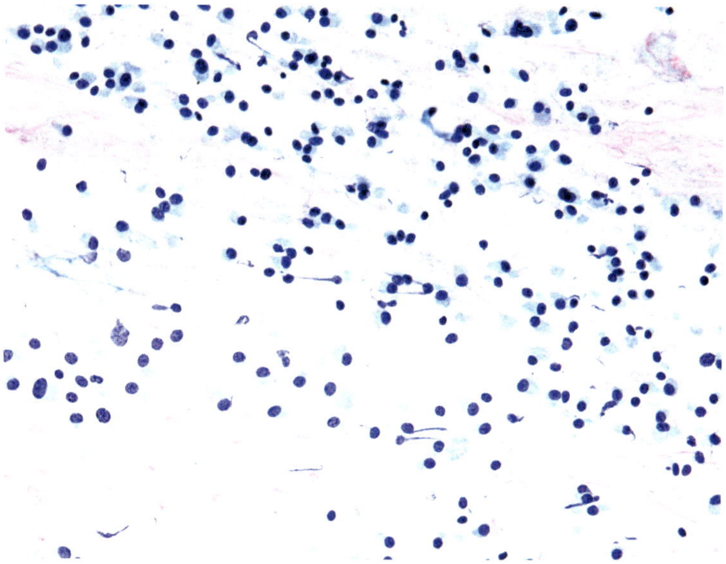

Figure 6.41a — Carcinoid Tumor, Fine Needle Aspiration [Pap Stain; Low Power]. Typical carcinoid tumor is a solitary neoplasm that arises in the central airways just below the surface of the bronchial mucosa; a small percentage arise in the peripheral airways. Because of this central submucosal location, carcinoid tumor is amenable to cytologic diagnosis using bronchial brushings and washings (if superficially ulcerated) as well as fine needle aspiration biopsy, but rarely sputum cytology. Most patients present in the fifth decade of life, which is younger than individuals with other forms of pulmonary neuroendocrine neoplasia. The cellularity of carcinoid tumor in bronchial brushings is variable. Most are moderately cellular as in this image and contain monomorphic cells arranged singly and in short chains. Other patterns on occasion include acinar and 3-dimensional clusters. A clean smear background as seen here is typical, and is diagnostically useful in separating this subtype of neuroendocrine neoplasia from more aggressive variants.

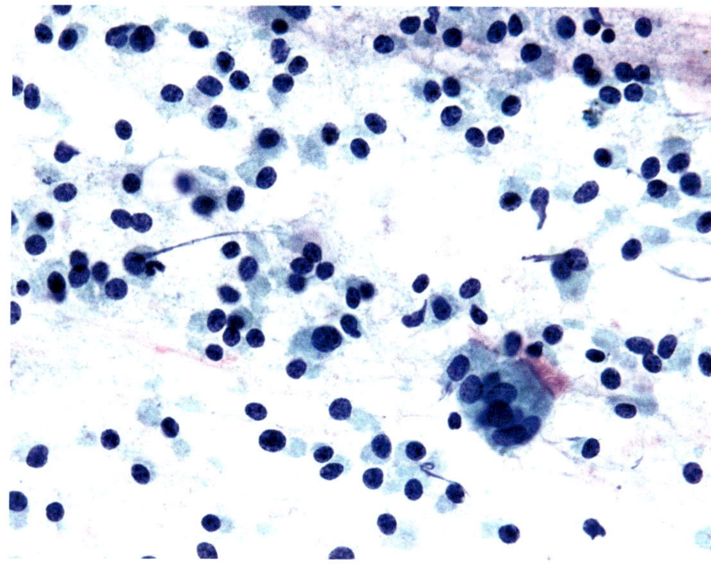

Figure 6.41b — Carcinoid Tumor, Fine Needle Aspiration [Pap Stain; High Power]. As the least aggressive subtype of neuroendocrine carcinoma, carcinoid tumor has a 5-year survival rate of over 90%, yet it still has a metastatic potential of 10% to 15% to regional lymph nodes, and approximately 5% to extrapulmonary sites. Closer examination of bronchial brushing preparations highlights the nuclear monotony and eccentric nuclear positioning within cells. Note that the size and shape of carcinoid tumor nuclei closely mirror those of the bronchial cells present in this single cluster. Unlike bronchial cells, however, carcinoid tumor cells are less cohesive and of course lack a terminal bar and cilia.

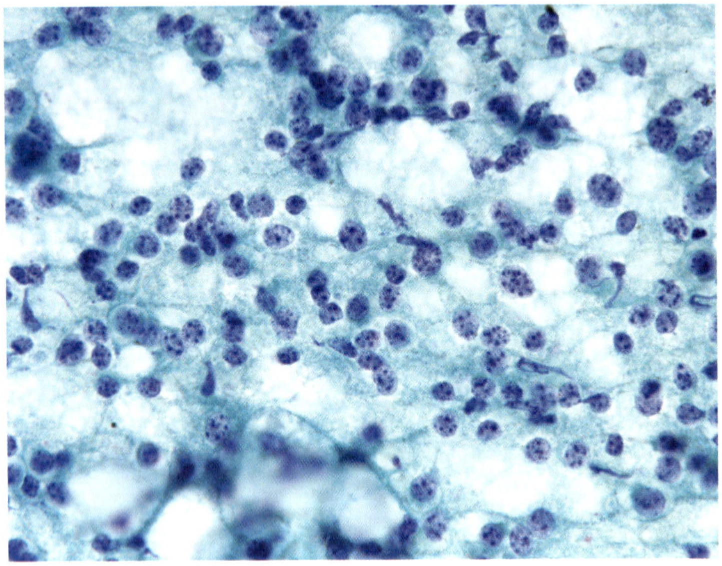

Figure 6.41c — Carcinoid Tumor, Fine Needle Aspiration [Pap Stain; High Power]. As noted in several of these images of carcinoid tumor, the granularity of nuclear chromatin can vary from fine and evenly dispersed to a more coarse and uneven distribution within the nucleus. In this example, coarse granularity creates the so-called classic "salt and pepper" chromatin pattern that is highly suggestive of neuroendocrine cells. Since cell cytoplasm is often less apparent in alcohol-fixed preparations than in air-dried smears, carcinoid tumor cells more easily mimic lymphocytes/lymphoma and non-lymphoid malignant small round cell tumors. Nonetheless, the cell monotony and classic nuclear features, plus an absence of mitotic figures, individual cell necrosis, and background tumor diathesis, are strong morphologic criteria for recognizing this image as carcinoid tumor.

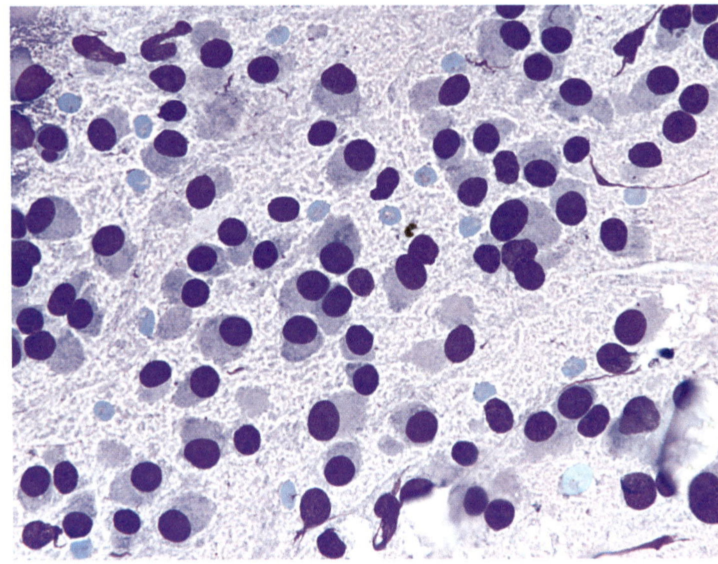

Figure 6.41d — Carcinoid Tumor, Oncocytic, Fine Needle Aspiration [Diff-Quik Stain; High Power]. In contrast to the prior image, the oncocytic variant of carcinoid tumor contains a greater amount of cytoplasm, which is finely granular. Cell nuclei appear smudged and lack the granularity seen in prior images in part due to the cell preparation. Fine cytologic detail such as chromatin granularity and nuclear chromatin arrangement, as well as nuclear contour, are often less apparent in air-dried smears. The dissociated cell pattern and eccentric placement of cell nuclei produce a "plasmacytoid" appearance to these oncocytic cells, thus evoking several diagnostic possibilities including plasma cell myeloma, lobular breast carcinoma, metastatic pheochromocytoma, metastatic thyroid carcinoma, and malignant melanoma. An unusual feature of carcinoid tumor in this case is the presence of strands of cytoplasm creating a so-called tigroid pattern in the smear background.

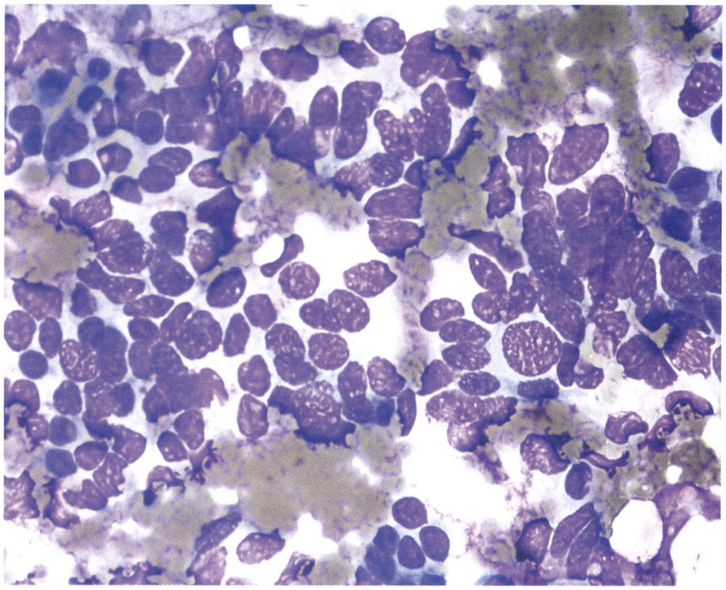

Figure 6.42a — Carcinoid Tumor, Fine Needle Aspiration [Diff-Quik Stain; High Power]. On occasion, cells of carcinoid tumor show crush artifact with extreme cell clustering and "molding" of nuclei against one another, thereby mimicking the cytomorphology of small cell carcinoma. Helpful features to avoid a mistaken diagnosis of small cell carcinoma include the absence of mitoses, individually necrotic/apoptotic cells, and a necrotic cellular background as seen in this field. Ki-67 staining serves a valuable role in separating carcinoid tumor from small cell carcinoma. In contrast to small cell carcinoma or large cell neuroendocrine carcinoma, the Ki-67 staining index of carcinoid tumor is less than 10% to 20%, whereas it is always greater than 50% and often as high as 90% in small cell carcinoma.

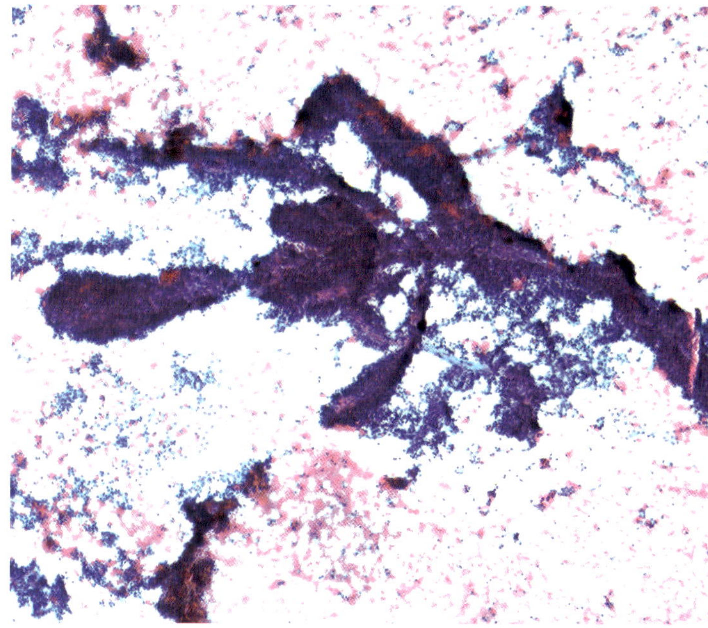

Figure 6.42b — Carcinoid Tumor, Fine Needle Aspiration [Pap Stain; Low Power]. Due to its extensive vascular network, some aspirates of carcinoid tumor capture large vascularized tissue fragments, creating a papillary appearance. In addition to the branching thick 3-dimensional papillary fragments, single cells, bare nuclei, and loose cell clusters are scattered about. Nuclear features are identical to those seen in prior images.

Figure 6.42c — Carcinoid Tumor, Fine Needle Aspiration [Synaptophysin Immunohistochemical Stain; Low Power]. The diagnosis of all subtypes of neuroendocrine neoplasia is aided substantially by the application of immunohistochemical markers. Synaptophysin (as illustrated here) is the single most reliable neuroendocrine marker, but it is not entirely specific, being aberrantly expressed in melanoma and parathyroid adenoma, for example. Synaptophysin is often used in conjunction with chromogranin A, and sometimes CD56 and TTF-1 (the latter is positive in about a third of cases). Neuron-specific enolase is much too nonspecific a marker to be of practical value. In addition to pan-keratin staining, carcinoid tumor can also show punctate staining with vimentin, and rarely S100. It should be remembered that the intensity of many immunohistochemical stains are reduced in alcohol-fixed smears.

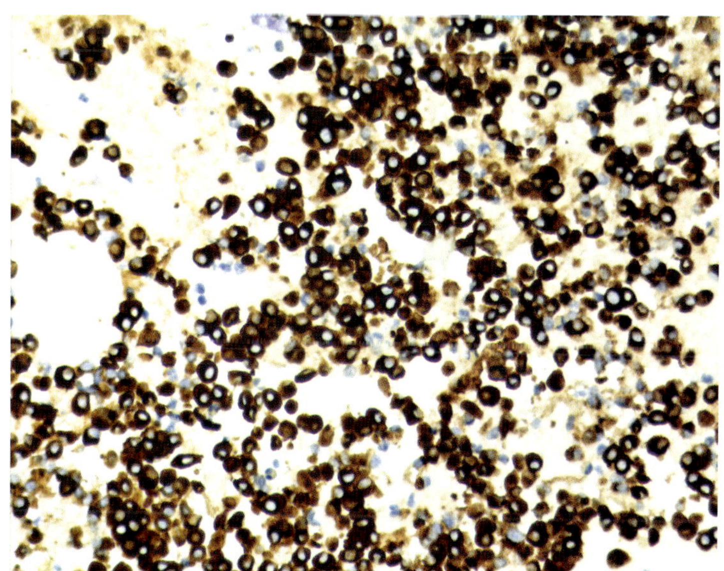

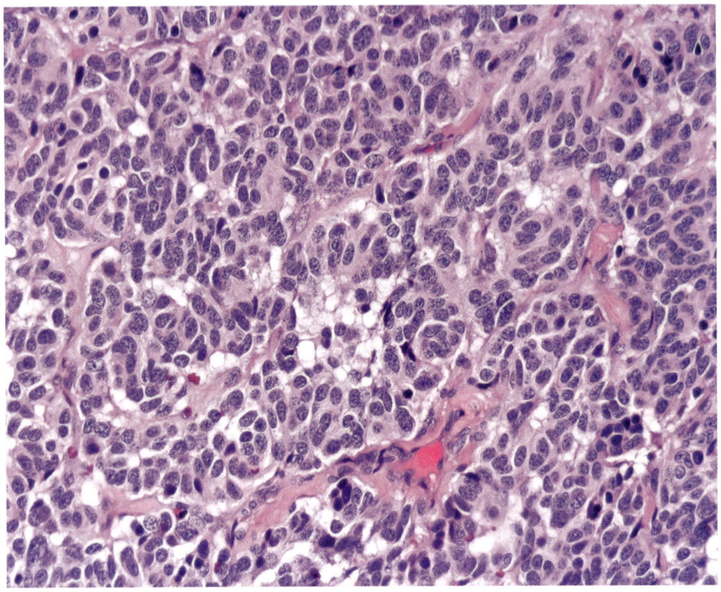

Figure 6.43a — Typical Carcinoid, Lobectomy [H&E Stain; High Power]. This example of a typical carcinoid tumor demonstrates an organoid nested pattern, without necrosis or demonstrable mitotic figures. The tumor cells are polygonal, with finely granular chromatin and relatively abundant eosinophilic cytoplasm; nucleoli are inconspicuous. Some cases will have pronounced pleomorphism and/or large nucleoli. Peripheral lesions often have a more spindled cytology. Note the extensive fibrous septation, which contains this tumor's rich vasculature. With adequate tissue sample size, typical carcinoid can be distinguished from atypical carcinoid tumor, which is similar, but has notable mitotic activity (2 to 10 per 2 mm^2, assessed on H and E) and/or punctate or zonal necrosis.

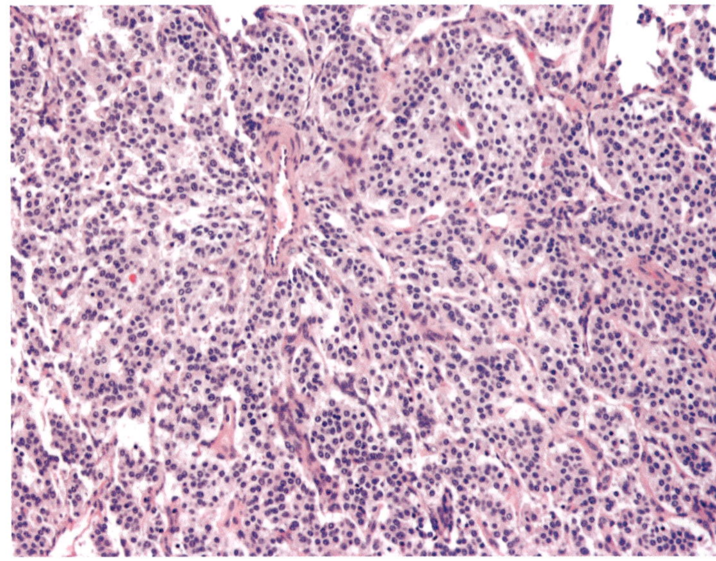

Figure 6.43b — Typical Carcinoid, Lobectomy [H&E Stain; Low Power]. This Example Shows the Characteristic "Zellballen" Nested Pattern (Right), with a More Trabecular Pattern at Far Left. Rosettes or papillae may also be seen. The dividing septa are richly vascular; small biopsies of these tumors may be associated with significant bleeding. Most carcinoid tumors arise centrally and are endobronchial, but about 20% to 30% are peripheral, with a more spindled cytology.

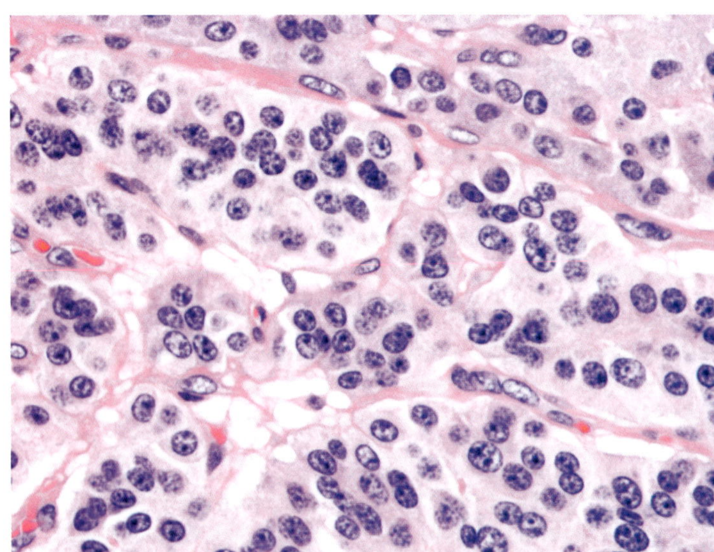

Figure 6.43c — Typical Carcinoid, Lobectomy [H&E Stain; High Power]. The cells of this nested tumor are round to polygonal with abundant eosinophilic cytoplasm. The nuclei have stippled, granular, open chromatin ("salt-and-pepper" type). In small biopsies with any degree of crush artifact, immunostains may be helpful in excluding non–small cell carcinoma; carcinoid tumors express cytokeratin, chromogranin, synaptophysin, and CD56, and are negative for TTF-1 and p40. Atypical carcinoid tumors are histologically similar, but are defined by a mitotic rate of 2 to 10/2 mm^2, and/or the presence of necrosis, which is typically punctate rather than zonal. Peripheral tumors are more likely to meet criteria for atypical carcinoid. Confident exclusion of atypical carcinoid is often not possible on a small biopsy.

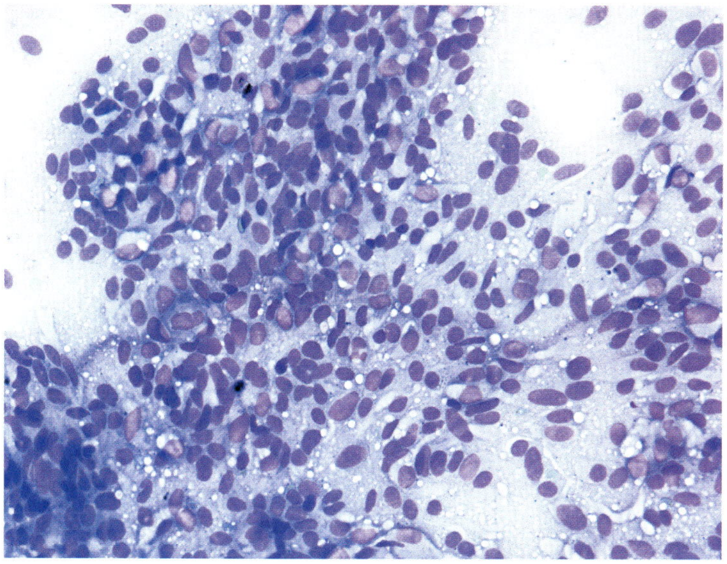

Figure 6.44a — Carcinoid Tumor, Spindle Cell, Fine Needle Aspiration [Diff-Quik Stain; Medium Power]. Spindle cell carcinoid tumor is more commonly encountered in the peripheral lung. These are typically single, well-circumscribed nodules rarely greater than 3 cm. Aspirate smears are mainly hypercellular and dominated by a spindle cell population in loose clusters with little anisocytosis. Elongated cytoplasmic processes produce a spindled appearance to cell nuclei, which can be ovoid, elongated, and infrequently rounded. Nuclear chromatin is similar to that described for typical carcinoid tumor except that nuclear molding is possible, but only focally, raising the possibility of small cell carcinoma. Mitoses are rarely if ever encountered and the lack of necrosis favors carcinoid tumor.

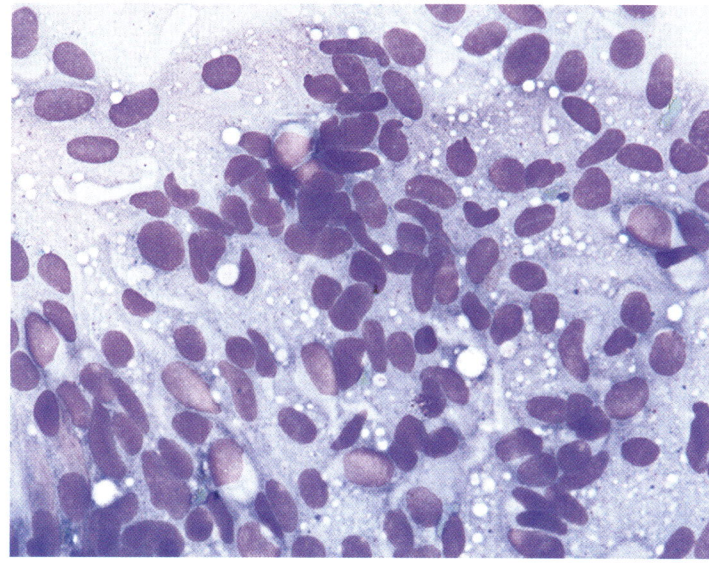

Figure 6.44b — Carcinoid Tumor, Spindle Cell, Fine Needle Aspiration [Diff-Quik Stain; High Power]. This syncytial cellular cluster of spindle cells contains hypochromic nuclei. The air-dried nature of this preparation precludes one from appreciating the fine granularity of nucleoplasm that is characteristic of carcinoid tumor. Nonetheless, the absence of enlarged nucleoli, mitoses, necrotic debris, and extensive nuclear molding helps eliminate a diagnosis of large cell neuroendocrine carcinoma. Note that some of these elongated nuclei exhibit slight indentations mimicking the nuclear shape of epithelioid histiocytes. Ancillary immunostaining is helpful in distinguishing this neoplasm from other spindle cell neoplasms primary and metastatic to the lung including spindle cell melanoma, spindle cell squamous carcinoma, and a host of mesenchymal neoplasms including solitary fibrous tumor, synovial sarcoma, leiomyosarcoma, and malignant peripheral nerve sheath tumor.

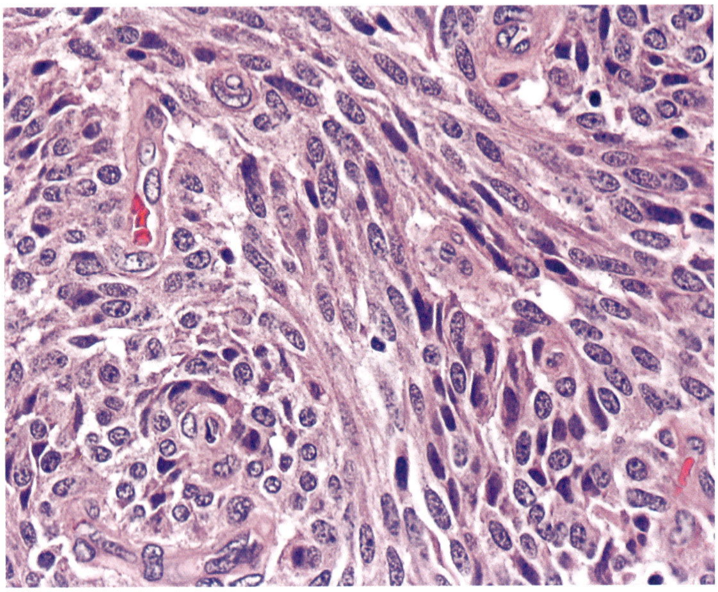

Figure 6.44c — Carcinoid Tumor, Spindle Cell, Lobectomy [H&E Stain; High Power]. Spindle cell cytology is more common in peripheral carcinoid tumors, but the typical nested pattern and vascularized septa are still present, and the tumor cells express the characteristic carcinoid markers (chromogranin, synaptophysin, CD56). Given the peripheral location and spindled cytology, solitary fibrous tumor may enter the differential diagnosis. The cells of solitary fibrous tumor have denser chromatin and are separated individually by thin bands of collagen fibers, and express CD34, bcl-2, and STAT6.

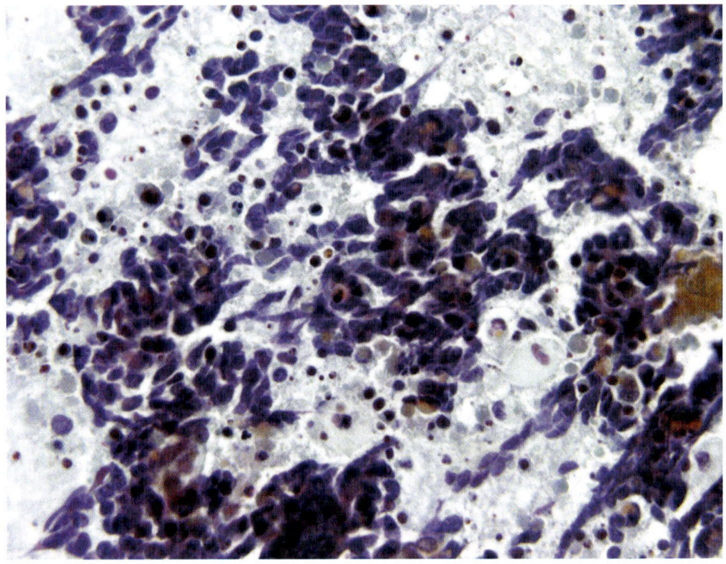

Figure 6.44d — Atypical Carcinoid, Fine Needle Aspiration [Pap Stain; High Power]. In the classification spectrum of pulmonary neuroendocrine tumors, atypical carcinoid conceptually occupies a mid-point between the relatively indolent carcinoid tumor and highly aggressive small cell carcinomas and large cell neuroendocrine carcinomas. For this reason, many pathologists consider this a "moderately differentiated" subtype of neuroendocrine carcinoma. Atypical carcinoid is strictly defined by the World Health Organization as a neoplasm that shares the morphologic growth patterns and immunohistochemical profile of carcinoid tumor, but contains two additional diagnostic criteria: the presence of necrosis and mitoses. Necrosis is typically comedo-like group necrosis as well as punctate individual cell necrosis, and mitotic activity is defined as 2 to 10 mitoses per 2 mm^2. Because of this latter histologic definition, the cytologic diagnosis of atypical carcinoid can only be suggested. Because necrosis is so common in atypical carcinoid, most fine-needle aspirates mimic the smears of high-grade neuroendocrine carcinomas. Cells are dispersed singly as well as in loose and tightly clustered groups with occasional 3-dimensional stacking of cells upon one another. Slides often exhibit nuclear molding of cells, coarsely granular nuclear chromatin, crush artifact, nuclear smearing, and minimal visible cytoplasm. A tumor diathesis of necrotic cellular debris is common. The image illustrated here is easily misinterpreted as small cell carcinoma, yet upon surgical removal the mass proved to be an atypical carcinoid.

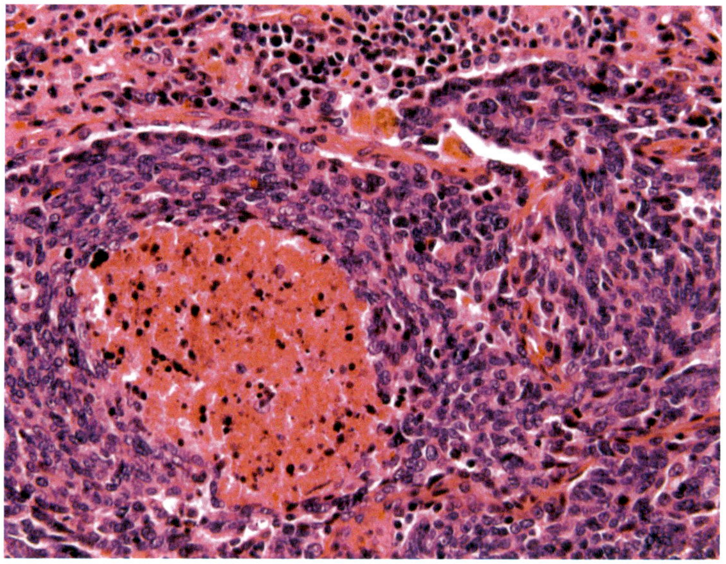

Figure 6.44e — Atypical Carcinoid, Lobectomy [H&E Stain; High Power]. Unlike carcinoid tumor, which has no association with cigarette smoking, a weak association exists with atypical carcinoid. Also, regional lymph node metastases are seen in 40% to 50% of atypical carcinoid patients, in contrast to 15% or less with carcinoid tumor. Atypical carcinoid is usually peripherally situated in the lung. This organoid cluster of slightly swirling malignant cells shows a circumscribed border and an obvious focus of comedo-type necrosis. Mitotic figures are readily noticeable. Tumor cell nuclei are about 3 times the size of adjacent lymphocytes seen at the top of this image. They display coarsely granular chromatin without discernable nucleoli, and contain only a meager amount of cytoplasm. Ki-67 staining has been used in cytology cell blocks to assist with distinguishing small cell carcinoma from atypical carcinoid with the latter typically having a Ki-67 index of 25% or less while small cell carcinoma is generally greater than 50%.

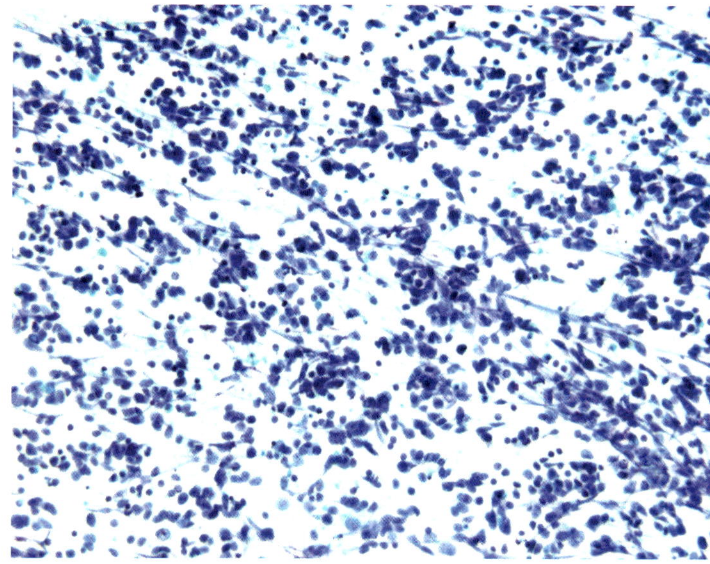

Figure 6.45a — Small Cell Carcinoma, Fine Needle Aspiration [Pap Stain; Low Power]. Small cell carcinoma is one of the more common forms of lung cancer. Virtually all patients provide a history of prolonged and heavy cigarette smoking. As small cell carcinoma arises in the central endobronchial portion of the lung (about 5% arise in the lung periphery), it is highly amenable to cytologic diagnosis using bronchial washings, bronchial brushings, and occasionally sputum. Transbronchial and endobronchial ultrasound--guided fine needle aspiration are used to sample parenchymal masses and mediastinal lymph nodes–the latter for clinical staging purposes. Metastases are common at the time of presentation. Paraneoplastic syndromes associated with small cell carcinoma include Cushing syndrome, inappropriate antidiuretic hormone syndrome, and Lambert-Eaton myasthenic syndrome. Cytopathology is diagnostically sensitive and specific for small cell carcinoma. Smears are extremely cellular due to a lack of stromal fibrosis within the cancer. At low power, a dual population of seemingly larger and smaller cells is noticed due to the individually necrotic/apoptotic nature of the latter as a consequence of rapid cell turnover.

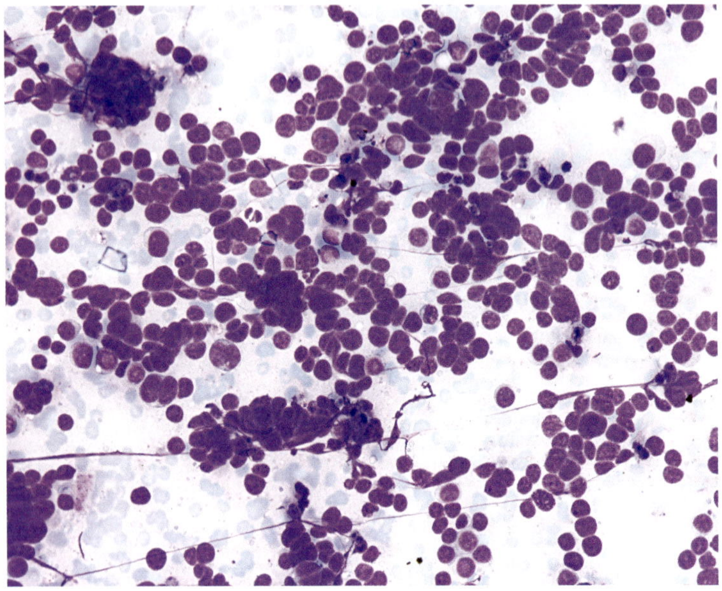

Figure 6.45b — Small Cell Carcinoma, Fine Needle Aspiration [Diff-Quik Stain; Medium Power]. Smears typically show cells arranged in aggregates and singly dispersed. These cell clusters may be irregularly formed, or show nuclei in tandem with short cords of cells and in an occasional rosette formation. In air-dried smears, cell nuclei appear larger and rounded such that they imitate large lymphocytes or a non–small cell carcinoma. Angulation of nuclei—so-called "molding"—is commonplace as they crowd together. Although not specific for small cell carcinoma, nuclear molding is one of the more consistent and reliable morphologic criteria used to recognize this neoplasm. Note the "clean" background in this image in contrast to the "tumor diathesis" of the prior image.

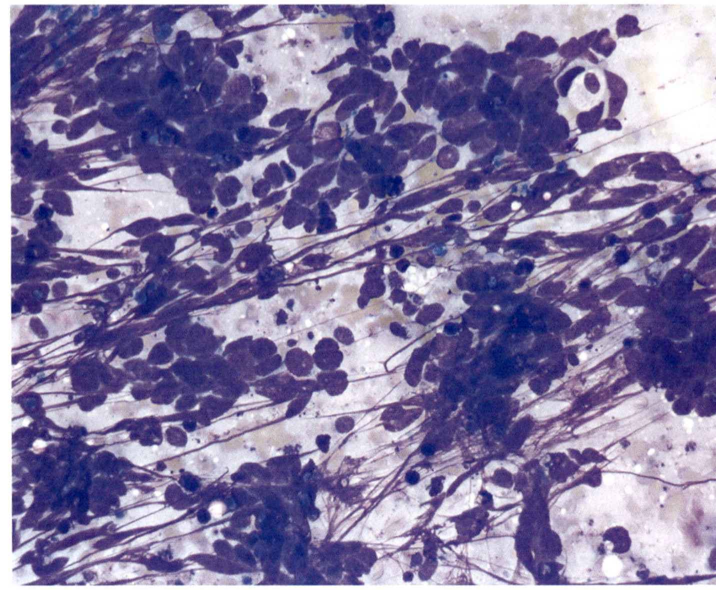

Figure 6.45c — Small Cell Carcinoma, Fine Needle Aspiration [Diff-Quik Stain; Medium Power]. Due to their fragility, nuclei of small cell carcinoma are easily disrupted. Therefore, smearing or streaking of nuclear chromatin along with bare nuclei is routinely seen in cytologic slides. You will notice tiny intensely blue globules having a "glassy" appearance in this image. These so-called "blue bodies" appear to represent cytoplasmic fragments. Along with nuclear molding and nuclear streaking, they are characteristic of small cell carcinoma. Also, misshapen fragments of nuclear debris are seen in the background.

Figure 6.45d — Small Cell Carcinoma, Fine Needle Aspiration [Diff-Quik Stain; High Power]. This image illustrates the "plasticity" of small cell carcinoma nuclei as some of them are rounded, some are fusiform, some have a V-shaped indentation allowing for a glimpse of meager cytoplasm, and some use extreme molding to form into angulated (triangular) shapes or thin wafer-like structures, or are elongated and indented into "banana" configurations (upper right). Mitoses are often found in almost every high-power field. The center of this image shows nuclei organized into short chains. A potential mimicker of small cell carcinoma, reserve cell hyperplasia of the lung also consists of small cells with smudged nuclei and minimal cytoplasm that can demonstrate nuclear molding and be distributed into short chains. However, the cells of reserve cell hyperplasia are even smaller than those encountered in small cell carcinoma, and lack the mitoses and cellular necrosis that are virtually constant in small cell carcinoma.

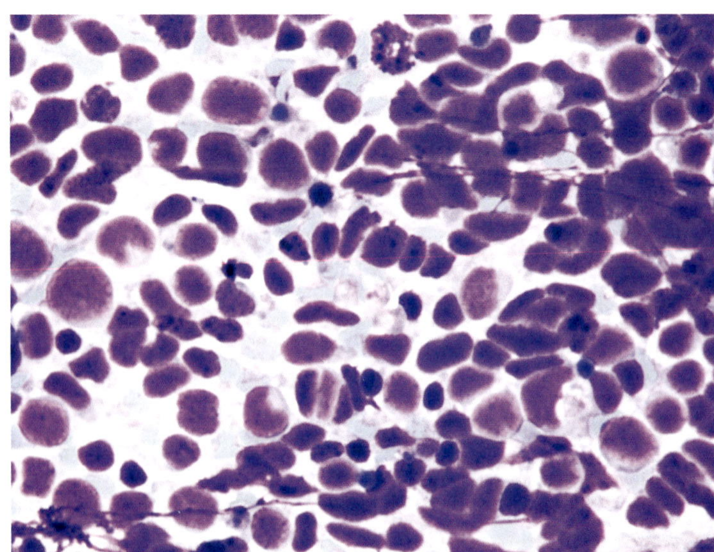

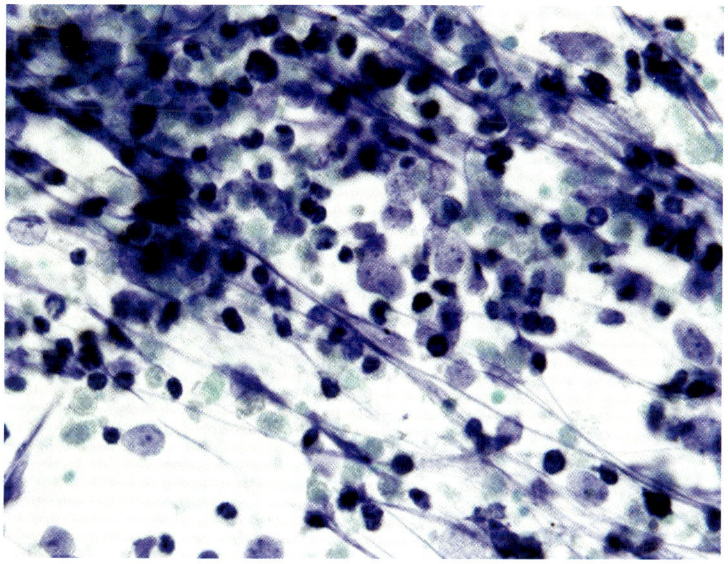

Figure 6.46a — Small Cell Carcinoma, Fine Needle Aspiration [Pap Stain; High Power]. In contrast to the numerous apoptotic cells that appear as small intensely hyperchromatic globules, intact malignant cells display a characteristic delicate, finely textured, and evenly dispersed granularity of nuclear chromatin minus nucleoli. Cell cytoplasm of these intact cells is so meager, it is virtually impossible to identify. Potentially confusing aspects of this image include the spherical hyperchromatic globules that have been mistaken as small lymphocytes and the background cyanophilic fragments ("ghost cells") that may be mistaken as lymphoglandular bodies, leading to an erroneous diagnosis of malignant lymphoma. Though not present in this slide, tingible-body macrophages are not uncommon in aspirates of small cell carcinoma and may be a further confounding factor.

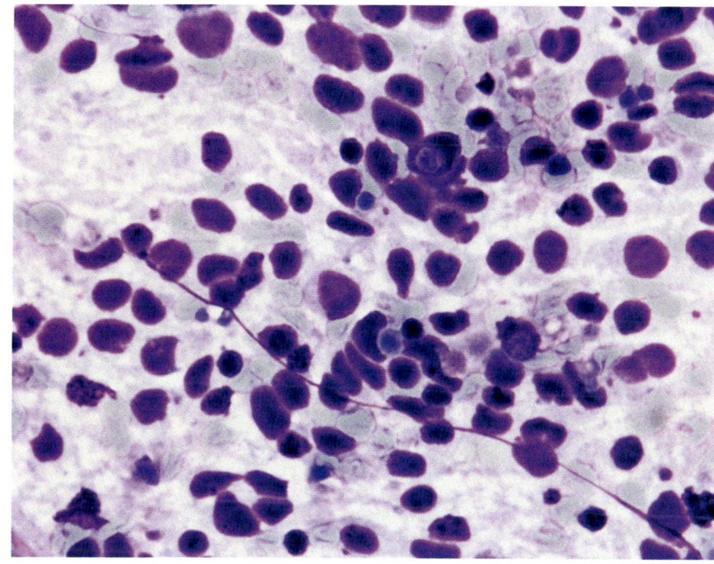

Figure 6.46b — Small Cell Carcinoma, Fine Needle Aspiration [Diff-Quik Stain; High Power]. A paranuclear "blue body" partially indenting the cell nucleus is situated near the center of this image, and another lies almost directly above it. The deep blue and "glassy" quality of this structure varies in quantity from case to case. Cytoplasmic mucinous vacuoles, unlike "blue bodies," are typically clear or pale in both air-dried and alcohol-fixed smears. "Blue bodies" presumably represent the remnant of necrotic cells, and are more difficult to identify in Papanicolaou-stained slides due to their paleness. Although characteristic of small cell carcinoma, they are by no means pathognomonic. The basaloid variant of squamous cell carcinoma that superficially resembles small cell carcinoma typically lacks its cellular fragility and rapid cell turnover such that the nuclear streaking, crush artifact, mitotic activity, and cellular diathesis help distinguish it from small cell carcinoma. Additionally, individually keratinized squamous cells can often be found in basaloid squamous carcinoma if diligently searched for.

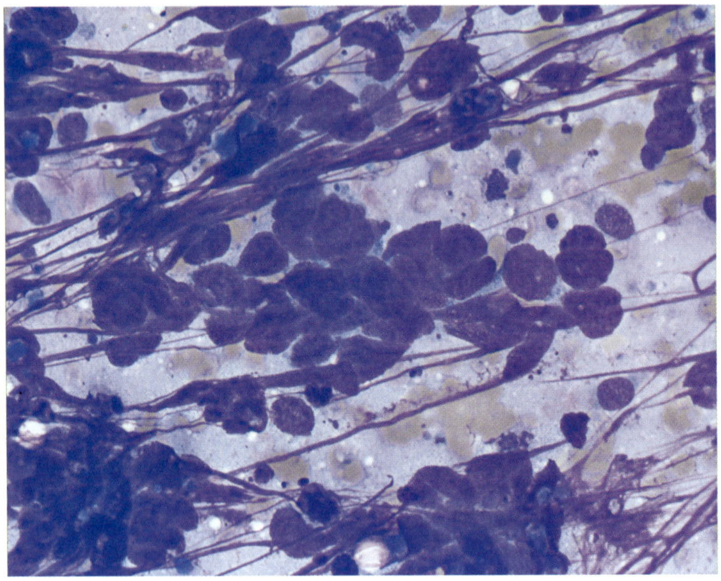

Figure 6.46c — Small Cell Carcinoma, Fine Needle Aspiration [Diff-Quik Stain; High Power]. The nuclei of small cell carcinoma are about 2 to 3 times larger than the diameter of resting lymphocytes; thus, "small" is a relative term. In air-dried smears, they can occasionally assume a larger diameter and be mistaken for large cell neuroendocrine carcinoma. The degree of nuclear disruption (chromatin streaking) with long strands of nucleoplasm being stretched across this image is not unusual in small cell carcinoma. Since intact vessels are rarely encountered in cytologic preparations, the nuclear encrustation sometimes seen in tissue sections (Azzopardi phenomenon) cannot be appreciated cytologically.

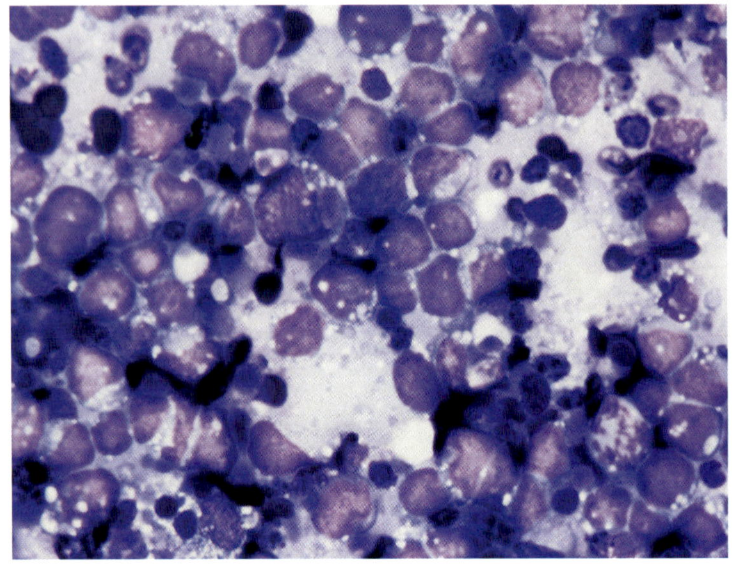

Figure 6.46d — Small Cell Carcinoma, Fine Needle Aspiration [Diff-Quik Stain; High Power]. A diagnostically challenging form of small cell carcinoma is this unusual example that harbors cytoplasmic vacuoles. In addition to the lymphoid appearance of these cells, this aspirate from a hilar lymph node in a histologically and immunohistochemically proven example of pulmonary small cell carcinoma contained cytoplasmic fragments reminiscent of lymphoglandular bodies. Although some nuclear molding, individual cell necrosis, and a mitotic figure are seen, this focus is easily mistaken for a large cell lymphoma. Other areas of the smear showed more typical features of small cell carcinoma.

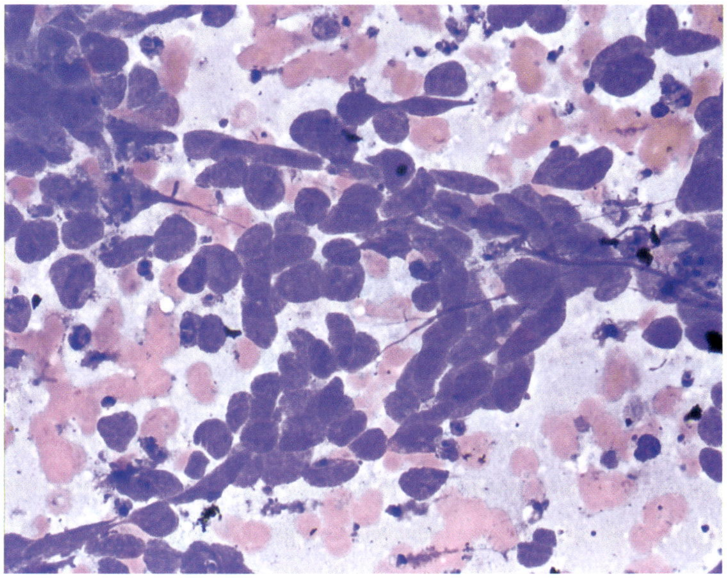

Figure 6.47a — Small Cell Carcinoma, Fine Needle Aspiration [Diff-Quik Stain; High Power]. Abundant nuclear debris and apoptotic bodies are scattered throughout the field with occasional smearing artifacts. The viable cells have a very high nuclear:cytoplasmic ratio, appearing almost as "naked nuclei," and demonstrate nuclear molding. Small cell carcinoma is an aggressive disease, usually disseminated beyond the point of surgical resection at the time of diagnosis. Despite combination chemotherapy and radiation, the 5-year survival rate remains poor.

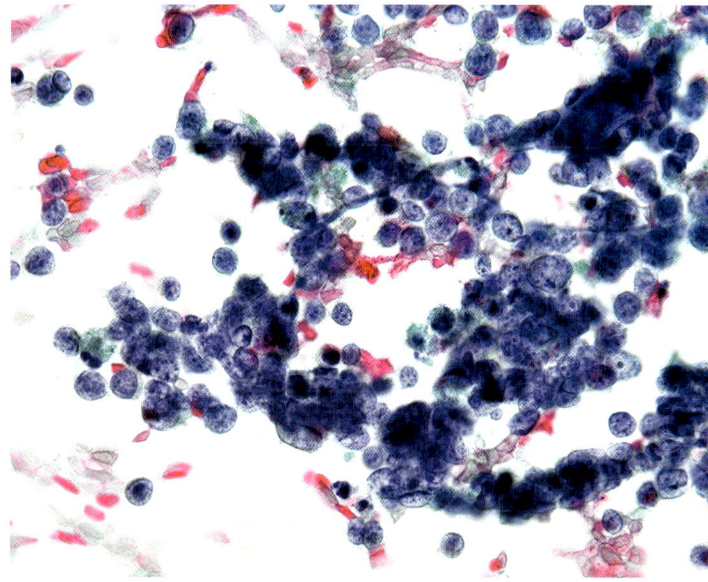

Figure 6.47b — Small Cell Carcinoma, Fine Needle Aspiration [Pap Stain; High Power]. The cells are relatively uniform in size and small (approximately 1.5 to 2x size of a lymphocyte) with a thin rim of pale cytoplasm. The chromatin is granular and hyperchromatic, and nucleoli are inconspicuous or absent. Nuclear molding is evident in the lower right and apoptotic cells are prominent. Although not seen in this field, necrosis and a background tumor diathesis are common features. A subset of patients manifest symptoms due to tumor secretion of ectopic hormones (typically antidiuretic hormone or adrenocorticotropic hormone).

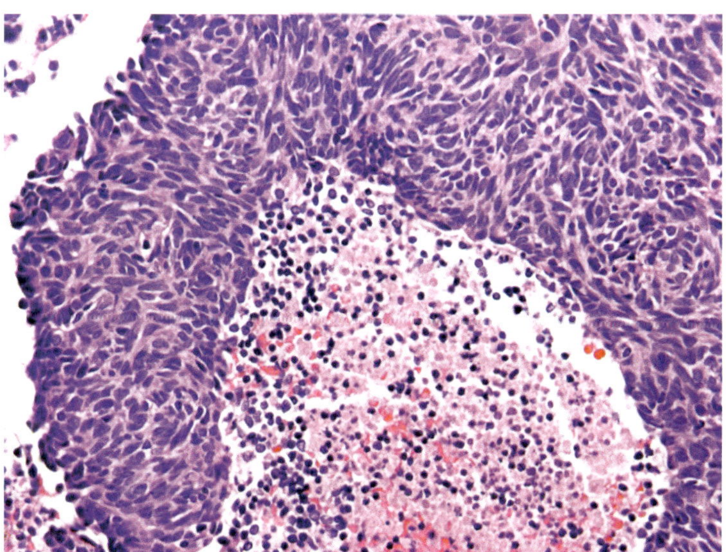

Figure 6.47c — Small Cell Carcinoma, Fine Needle Aspiration [H&E Stain; Medium Power]. Cell blocks are extremely useful and practical for documenting neuroendocrine differentiation in small cell carcinoma. This cell block illustrates not only the necrosis and nuclear molding typical of small cell carcinoma, but highlights the overwhelming fusiform nuclear shape seen in a high percentage of small cell carcinoma cases. Immunostains should include expression with a pan-cytokeratin antibody such as AE1/AE3 or CAM 5.2 displaying dot-like paranuclear or diffuse cytoplasmic staining, as well as staining with synaptophysin, TTF-1, chromogranin, and CD56. The latter is the least specific, but a highly sensitive marker. Ki-67 staining can be used in problematic instances as small cell carcinoma has a proliferative index of greater than 50%.

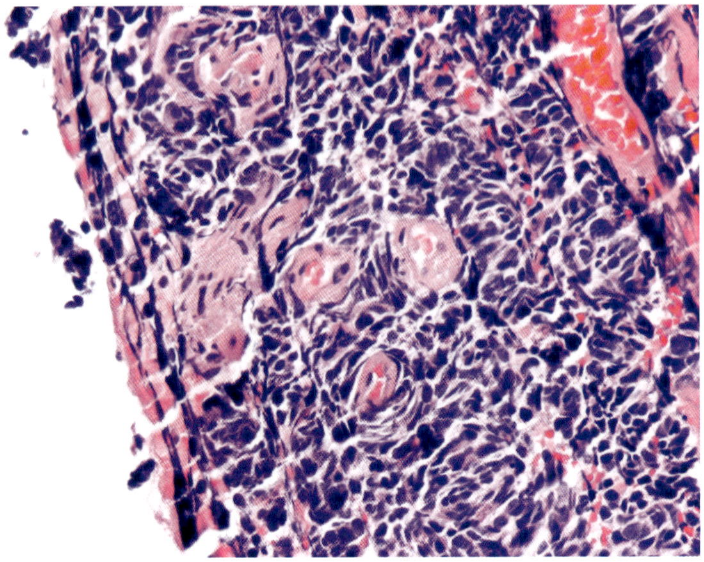

Figure 6.47d — Small Cell Carcinoma, Biopsy [H&E Stain; Low Power]. The absence of significant stroma and the minimal cytoplasm of individual tumor cells confer the typical "sheet of nuclei" appearance associated with extreme fragility of tumor tissue in biopsy specimens. The resulting crush and "chatter" artifacts often obscure the cell features, but are in themselves diagnostic clues. Note also the rich vascularity. Nesting and organoid growth are uncommon; disorganized sheets of dyshesive cells are the rule. The major differential diagnostic consideration is malignant lymphoma; a wide variety of other small blue cell tumors may enter into consideration, and appropriate immunohistochemical evaluation is routinely required. Large cell neuroendocrine carcinoma must be excluded on morphologic grounds (more cytoplasm; prominent nucleoli; organoid pattern).

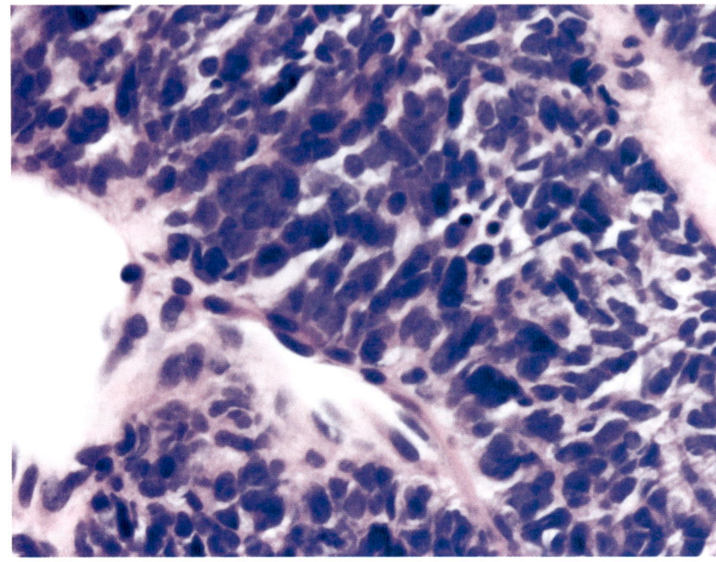

Figure 6.47e — Small Cell Carcinoma, Biopsy [H&E Stain; High Power]. The tumor cells are crowded and overlapping, with frequent nuclear molding. Hyperchromasia without identifiable nucleoli is characteristic. A focus of apoptosis is at the right of center. Zones of coagulative necrosis are characteristic but often not demonstrable in small tissue biopsies, although this feature is often present in fine needle aspiration samples as granular necrotic debris. Proliferative rates as assessed by Ki-67 staining typically exceed 80%.

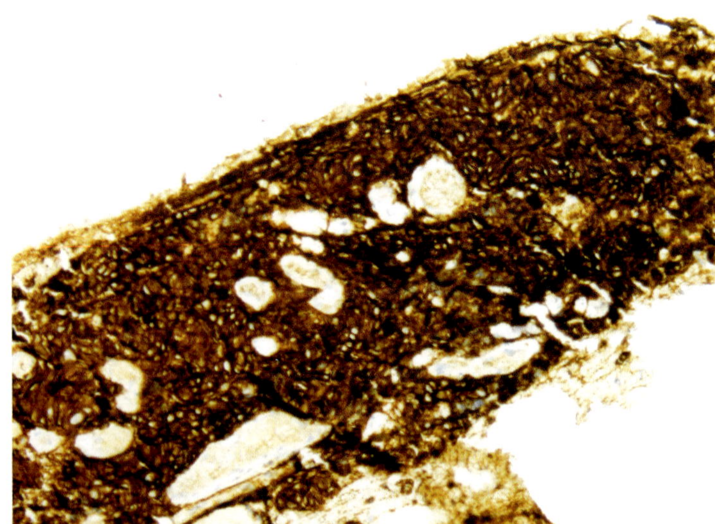

Figure 6.47f — Small Cell Carcinoma, Biopsy [CD56 Immunohistochemical Stain; Low Power]. This tumor is strongly and diffusely positive for CD56 NCAM, a highly sensitive neuroendocrine marker with relatively low specificity. Synaptophysin and chromogranin are also typically positive. Not uncommonly, a small cell carcinoma will drop a neuroendocrine marker, most often chromogranin; a panel of neuroendocrine stains is therefore optimal. If neuroendocrine stains are negative in the setting of positive keratins, basaloid squamous cell carcinoma (p40+, p63+) should be considered.

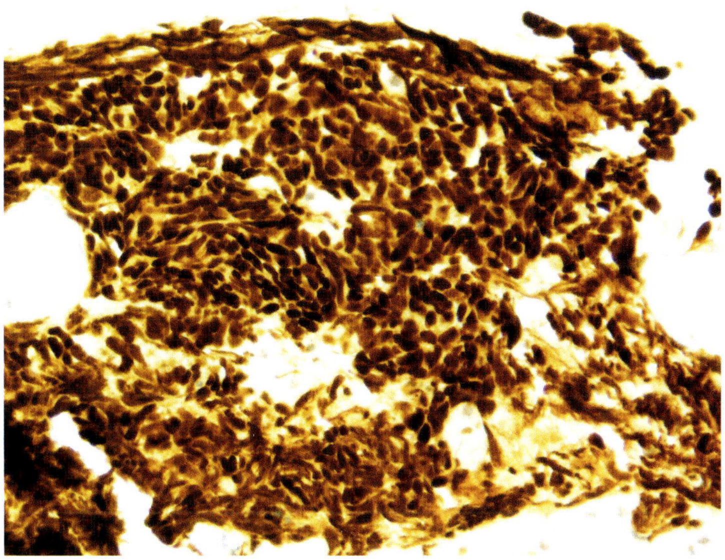

Figure 6.47g — Small Cell Carcinoma, Biopsy [TTF-1 Immunohistochemical Stain; Low Power]. This tumor shows strong and uniform nuclear expression of TTF-1. Depending on the clone used, greater than 90% of small cell carcinomas express TTF-1. If TTF-1 is negative, consideration should be given to basaloid squamous cell carcinoma (p40+, p63+, TTF-1-) or large cell neuroendocrine carcinoma, which is more often TTF-1-negative (50%) than is small cell carcinoma. Metastatic neuroendocrine carcinoma from other sites may enter into consideration in some cases; GI neuroendocrine tumors often express CDX2, and are TTF-1-negative.

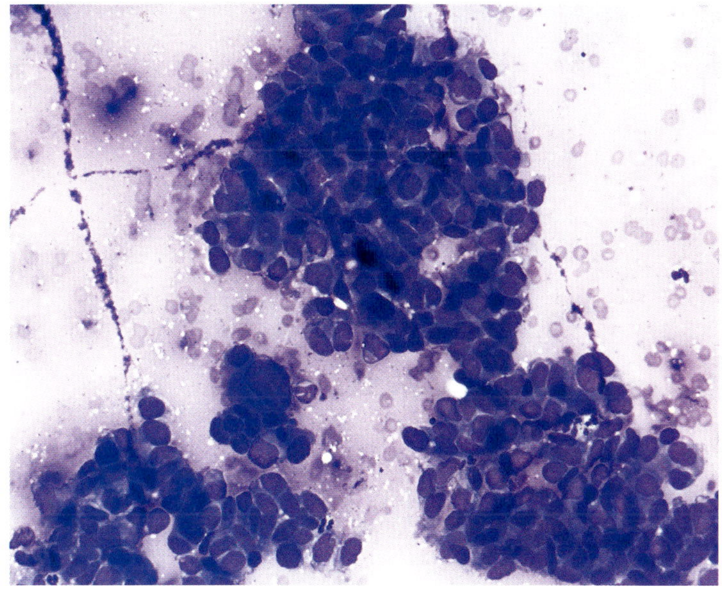

Figure 6.48a — Large Cell Neuroendocrine Carcinoma, Fine Needle Aspiration [Diff-Quik Stain; High Power]. Large cell neuroendocrine carcinoma is a large cell malignancy that exhibits neuroendocrine features such as trabecular and nested growth patterns with rosette formation that are best displayed in tissue sections, but often very difficult to appreciate in cytologic preparations. Like small cell carcinoma, it most often develops in heavy smokers over the age of 50 years. Sometimes, large cell neuroendocrine carcinoma is combined with components of squamous carcinoma, adenocarcinoma, or spindle cell carcinoma, which can present a confusing cytomorphologic picture. Slides are hypercellular and show cells dispersed singly, in small clusters with nuclear molding, and in large 3-dimensional aggregates as seen in this image. On occasion, these aggregates may show peripheral palisading. In contrast to small cell carcinoma, cells are much larger (usually 2 to 3 times larger than those of small cell carcinoma), have a modest amount of visible cytoplasm, have a greater degree of anisonucleosis, and importantly have discrete nucleoli in a high percentage of cases. Nonetheless, some morphologic overlap with small cell carcinoma and poorly differentiated non–small cell carcinoma exists. If a distinction between small cell carcinoma and large cell neuroendocrine carcinoma is not possible cytologically, it is best to diagnose these as high-grade neuroendocrine carcinomas.

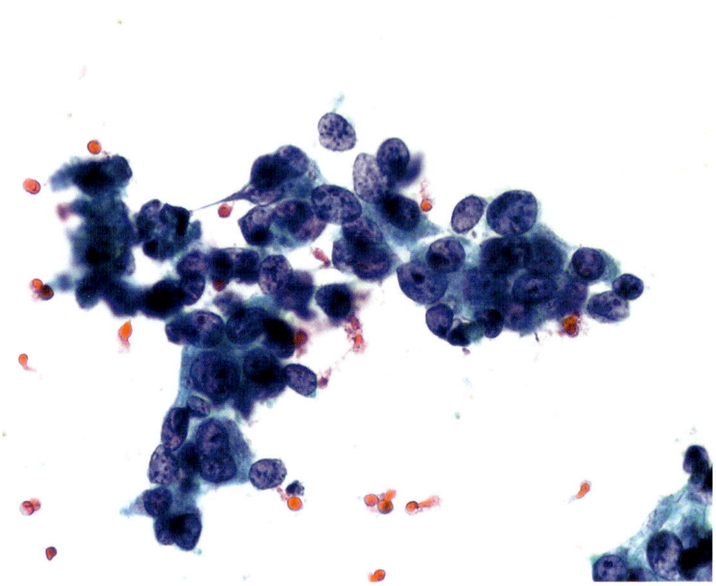

Figure 6.48b — Large Cell Neuroendocrine Carcinoma, Fine Needle Aspiration [Pap Stain; High Power]. Although most examples arise in the peripheral lung, and intermittently invading the pleura and chest wall, when located centrally large cell neuroendocrine carcinoma shows endobronchial invasion and can be recognized using bronchial brushings or washings. This particular loose syncytial aggregate of malignant large cells shows fine to coarsely granular nuclear chromatin and a small but definite amount of cyanophilic cytoplasm. Distinctive nucleoli are present in some but not all nuclei. Since nuclear borders are smooth without evidence of nuclear molding in this cluster, it is easily mistaken for a non–small cell carcinoma such as adenocarcinoma. Most examples of large cell neuroendocrine carcinoma contain a background tumor diathesis with crushed cells, many individually apoptotic nuclei, cellular debris, and mitotic figures (absent in this image). Mitotic counts per 10 high power fields as measured in tissue sections are not applicable to cytologic smears.

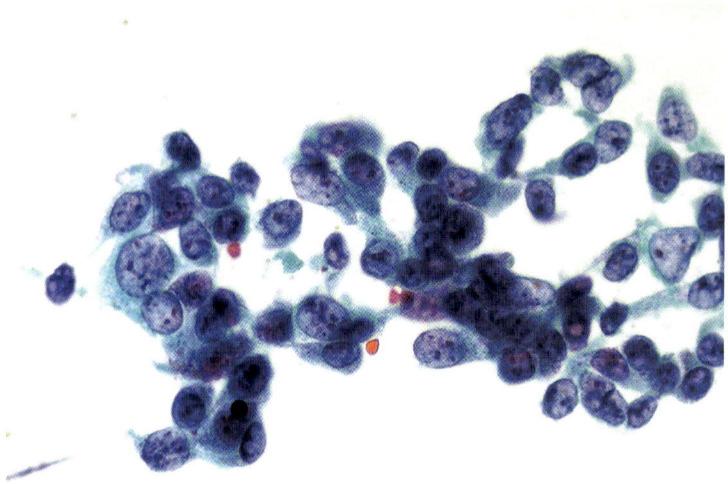

Figure 6.48c — Large Cell Neuroendocrine Carcinoma, Fine Needle Aspiration [Pap Stain; High Power]. This image of large cell neuroendocrine carcinoma would require immunohistochemical staining to recognize it as such; in particular, to distinguish it from a poorly differentiated adenocarcinoma or possibly squamous carcinoma. Some studies have shown that precise classification of neuroendocrine neoplasms is correct in less than half of cases. In addition to synaptophysin, both chromogranin A and CD56 are helpful in documenting the neuroendocrine nature of these malignant cells.

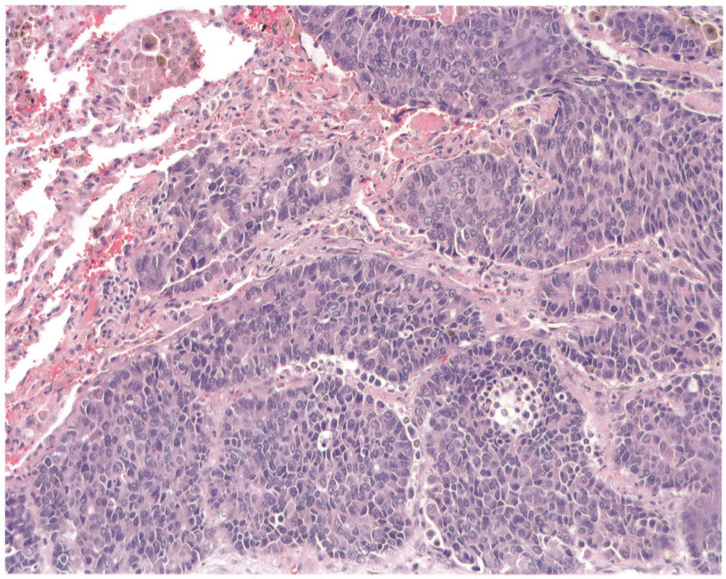

Figure 6.49a — Large Cell Neuroendocrine Carcinoma, Lobectomy [H&E Stain; Low Power]. Large cell neuroendocrine carcinoma is characterized in part by histologic features of neuroendocrine differentiation, particularly organoid nesting, rosettes, and peripheral palisading, all demonstrated here. Some examples have multiple rosettes within a single nest, conferring a cribriform pattern. Zonal or punctate necrosis is the rule. The tumor's interface with adjacent lung tissue is relatively circumscribed, one feature that distinguishes large cell neuroendocrine carcinoma from small cell carcinoma.

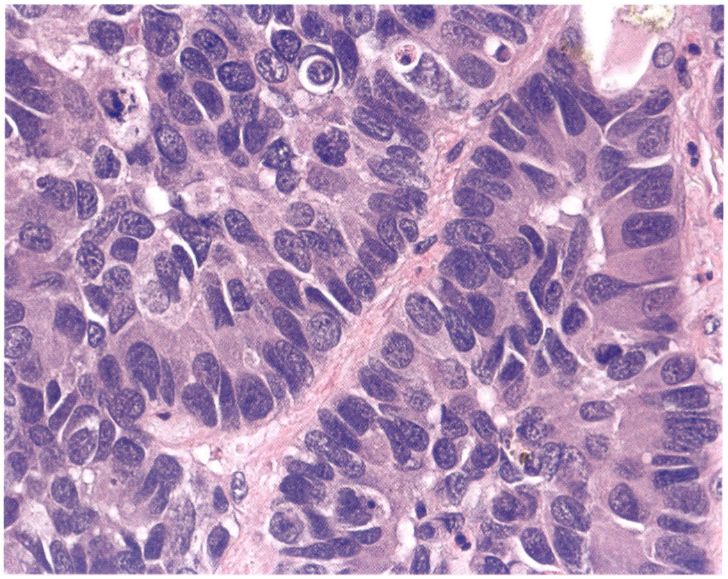

Figure 6.49b — Large Cell Neuroendocrine Carcinoma, Lobectomy [H&E Stain; High Power]. The finely granular "salt and pepper" chromatin and nuclear overlap and molding are seen here, characteristic features of neuroendocrine neoplasms. Additionally, the cells of large cell neuroendocrine carcinoma are large, with moderate to abundant cytoplasm and frequent nucleoli, features that distinguish large cell neuroendocrine carcinoma from small cell carcinoma. A mitosis is present at the upper left; large cell neuroendocrine carcinoma has greater than10 mitoses/2 mm^2, with a reported average of 75. Some large cell neuroendocrine carcinomas have lesser degrees of atypia and may resemble atypical carcinoid tumors, but can be recognized by a significantly elevated mitotic rate: large cell neuroendocrine carcinomas rarely have fewer than 30/2 mm^2. Additionally, definitive diagnosis of large cell neuroendocrine carcinoma requires immunohistochemical confirmation of neuroendocrine differentiation (synaptophysin, chromogranin, and/or CD56); at least one neuroendocrine marker should be unequivocally positive in 10% or more of tumor cells. Small biopsies may lack one or more features of large cell neuroendocrine carcinoma, and a diagnosis of "non-small cell carcinoma, favor large cell neuroendocrine carcinoma" may be indicated in such cases.

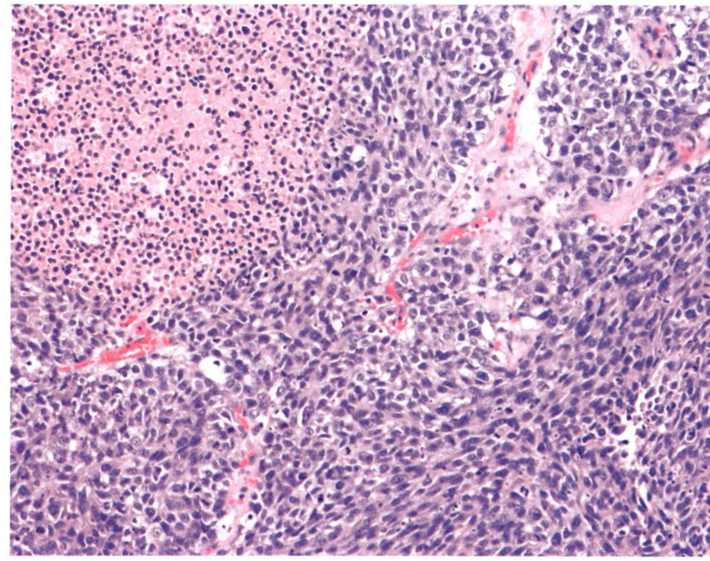

Figure 6.49c — Large Cell Neuroendocrine Carcinoma, Biopsy [H&E Stain; Low Power]. This example of large cell neuroendocrine carcinoma shows an irregular nested pattern, with surrounding vasculature. A confluent zone of necrosis is at the upper left. Some cases have a punctate, rather than zonal, pattern of necrosis. Frequent apoptotic nuclei are present in the nonnecrotic nests. At low power, the nonnecrotic areas could also represent solid-pattern adenocarcinoma or poorly differentiated nonkeratinizing squamous cell carcinoma.

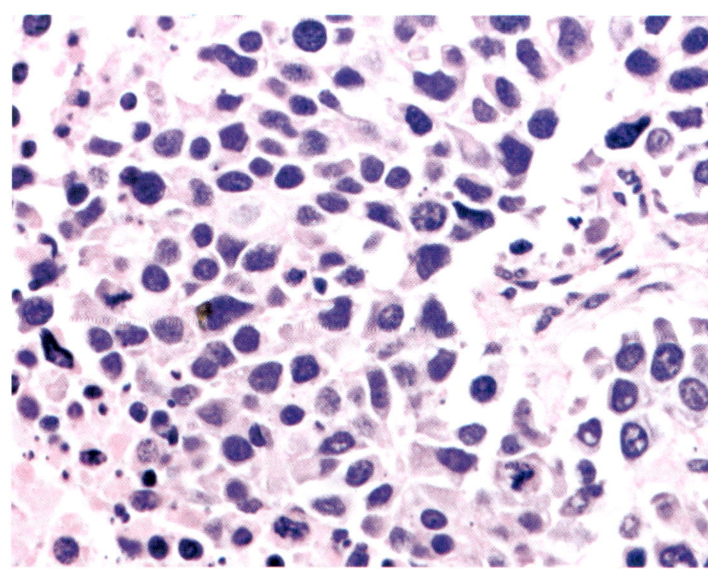

Figure 6.49d — Large Cell Neuroendocrine Carcinoma, Biopsy [H&E Stain; High Power]. On high power, the cells are dyshesive, and have a moderate amount of eosinophilic cytoplasm; some cells have an eccentrically placed nucleus, conferring a plasmacytoid appearance. The nuclei show stippled "salt-and-pepper" chromatin, and there are occasional nucleoli. Several mitoses are present, and a zone of necrosis is at the lower left. Large cell neuroendocrine carcinoma is defined in part by a mitotic rate of greater than10/2 mm^2, with a median of 70/2 mm^2.

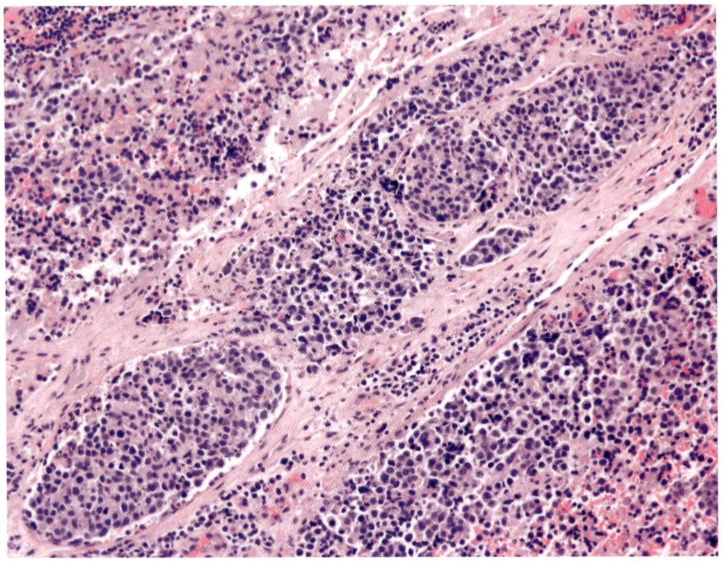

Figure 6.50a — Metastatic Large Cell Neuroendocrine Carcinoma, Biopsy [H&E Stain; Low Power]. Large cell neuroendocrine carcinoma has aggressive biology, similar to that of small cell carcinoma. This image shows nests of tumor cells within intracapsular afferent lymphatic channels. A subcapsular nodal metastasis is at the lower right. Due to dyshesion and cytologic similarities to large lymphocytes, large cell neuroendocrine carcinoma can be difficult to visualize in lymph nodes, and keratin staining may be a helpful adjunct in accurate staging.

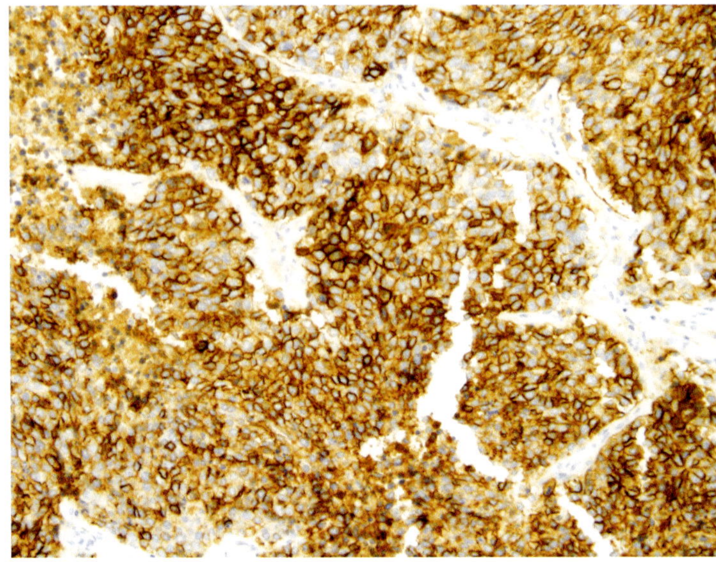

Figure 6.50b — Large Cell Neuroendocrine Carcinoma, Biopsy [CD56 Immunohistochemical Stain; Low Power]. This tumor is strongly and uniformly positive for CD56, which marks greater than 90% of all large cell neuroendocrine carcinoma. While the specificity of CD56 for neuroendocrine differentiation is lower than ideal, its high sensitivity in the setting of neuroendocrine morphology makes it a useful marker for diagnosis of large cell neuroendocrine carcinoma. The sensitivity of both synaptophysin and chromogranin is about 80%. Not infrequently, one or more neuroendocrine markers may be negative; one marker is enough if it is unequivocally positive. TTF-1 is expressed in large cell neuroendocrine carcinoma only 50% of the time.

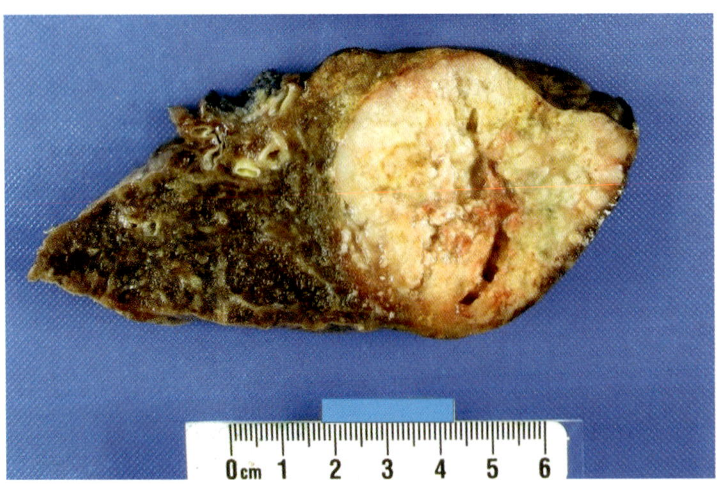

Figure 6.51 — Large Cell Neuroendocrine Carcinoma, Lobectomy [Gross Examination]. This upper lobe large cell neuroendocrine carcinoma is characteristically large, relatively circumscribed, friable, and peripheral, with extensive necrosis. Chest wall invasion by large cell neuroendocrine carcinoma is not uncommon, and rib resection may be required to achieve a negative margin. Frank cavitation, a common feature of squamous cell carcinoma, is rare in large cell neuroendocrine carcinoma.

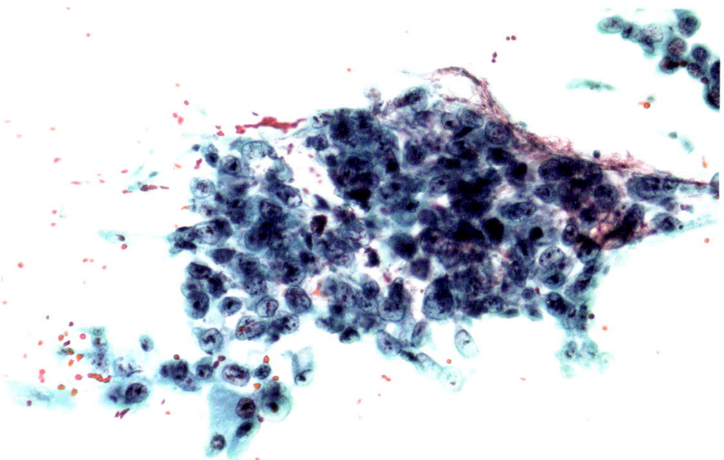

Figure 6.52a — Large Cell (Undifferentiated) Carcinoma, Fine Needle Aspiration [Pap Stain; Medium Power]. Large cell (undifferentiated) carcinoma is a non-small cell carcinoma lacking any morphologic or immunohistochemical features of squamous carcinoma, adenocarcinoma, or neuroendocrine carcinoma. The 2015 World Health Organization classification of lung tumors states that this diagnosis is one of exclusion, and therefore unreliable using either core needle biopsy or cytologic specimens. With the recent advent of immunohistochemical markers such as TTF-1, p63, napsin-A, CK5/6, and p40, the incidence of large cell (undifferentiated) carcinoma has decreased as pathologists have been able to more specifically categorize these neoplasms into specific tumor subtypes. As pictured here, this loosely clustered arrangement of epithelioid cells lacking gland formation, and any specific cytoplasmic features of differentiation such as keratinization, cytoplasmic vacuolization, secretory granules, or mucinous change, precludes a specific diagnosis other than non–small cell carcinoma unless immunohistochemical staining provides expression of a specific positive marker.

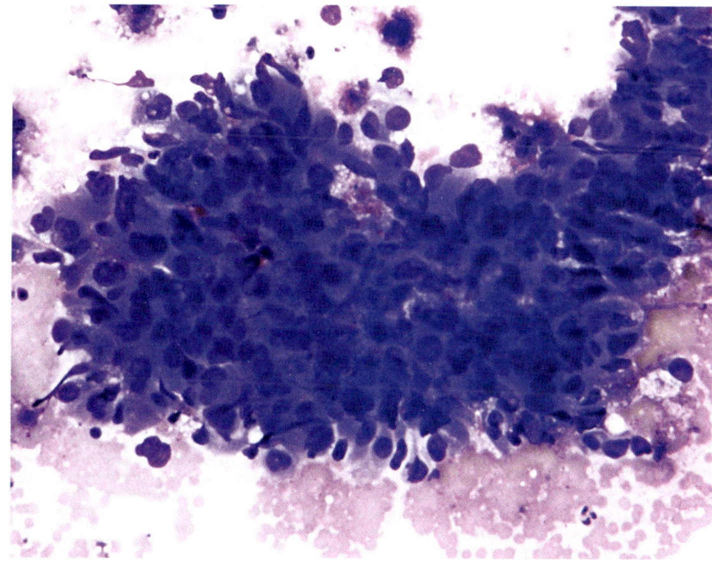

Figure 6.52b — Large Cell (Undifferentiated) Carcinoma, Fine Needle Aspiration [Diff-Quik Stain; Medium Power]. Cytologic slides are hypercellular in most instances with cells dispersed in a dissociated single-cell pattern, and in variably sized (often large) clusters. Due to their large size, high nuclear/cytoplasmic ratio, abnormal chromatin distribution, and enlarged nucleoli (better seen with Papanicolaou-stained slides), cells are invariably recognized as malignant, and as epithelial due in part to their polygonal shape and tendency to aggregate in tight clusters. Unlike better differentiated examples of adenocarcinoma, these aggregates lack a smooth so-called "community border." Just above this particular aggregate, large fragments of necrotic cellular material were seen on this slide—a common feature of large cell (undifferentiated) carcinoma.

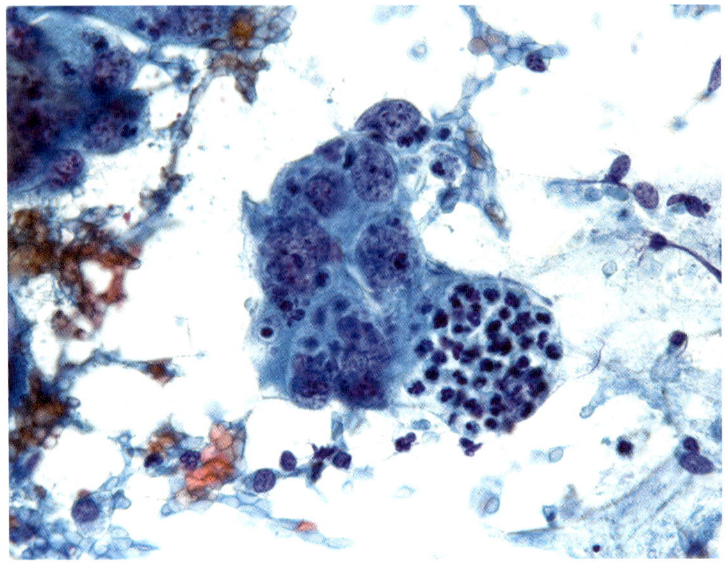

Figure 6.52c — Large Cell (Undifferentiated) Carcinoma, Fine Needle Aspiration [Pap Stain; High Power]. This group of unequivocally malignant cells is emblematic of large cell (undifferentiated) carcinoma having tremendously enlarged nuclei, minimal cytoplasm, and no evidence of glandular, squamous, or neuroendocrine differentiation. Neutrophilic emperipolesis, as seen here, is not uncommon, but it is nonspecific for large cell (undifferentiated) carcinoma being commonplace in sarcomatoid carcinoma, as well as other poorly differentiated malignancies. As clinicians have added newer therapeutic agents to their armamentarium based on molecular results (e.g., epidermal growth factor receptor status), an attempt to garner cells for immunostaining from a cell-block preparation to more specifically subtype this carcinoma, and potentially perform fluorescence in situ hybridization testing, is critical in these cases of non–small cell carcinoma.

7

Unusual and Metastatic Lesions

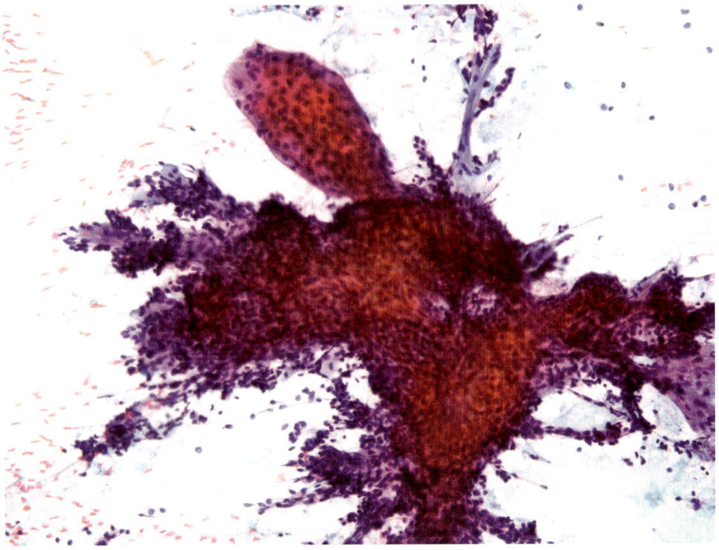

Figure 7.1a — Fetal Adenocarcinoma, Fine Needle Aspiration [Pap Stain; Low Power]. Fetal adenocarcinoma is a peripherally based lung adenocarcinoma composed of tubular and cribriform structures often in a complex back-to-back arrangement histologically mimicking the appearance of fetal lung between 10 and 16 weeks gestation. Both low-grade and high-grade variants exist, with the former arising in the fourth to fifth decade of life, and the latter about 2 decades later. Interposed between glandular structures are small solid so-called "morular" nests of cytologically bland cells as seen jutting from the top and in the center of this microfragment. Cellular smears contain densely clustered aggregates that show thin papillary strands projecting from the fragment edge.

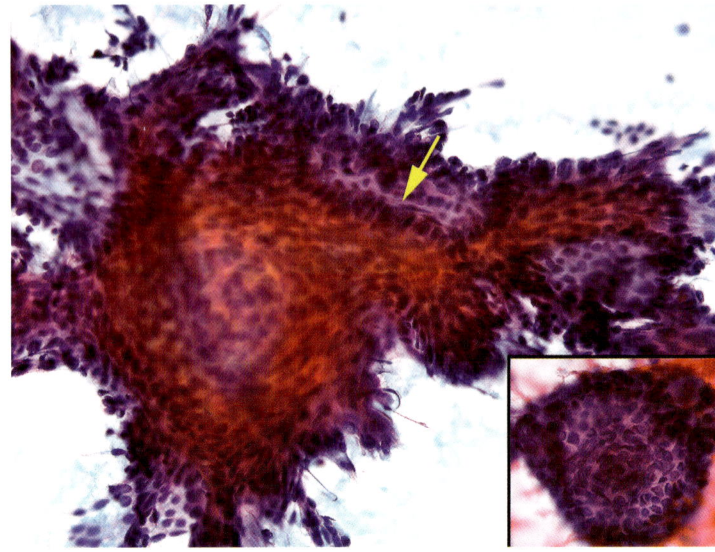

Figure 7.1b — Fetal Adenocarcinoma, Fine Needle Aspiration [Pap Stain; Medium Power]. Three-dimensional microfragments may show peripheral palisading (arrow). The glands in both low and high-grade subtypes contain glycogen-rich cells with cytoplasmic vacuoles imitating secretory endometrium. Although subnuclear or supranuclear vacuoles may be seen in Romanowsky-stained slides, they are rarely visible in alcohol-fixed preparations. A well-formed squamous "morule" composed of cytologically uniform cells with banal nuclei is seen in the inset. There is no specific immunohistochemical profile for fetal adenocarcinoma; however, these neoplasms show diffuse TTF-1 staining as well as aberrant nuclear staining with β-catenin, which can be diagnostically helpful. Since a high percentage express synaptophysin and chromogranin A, these aspirates may be mistaken for carcinoid tumor. Other entities in the differential diagnosis include endometriosis, well-differentiated adenocarcinoma not otherwise specified, and pulmonary blastoma.

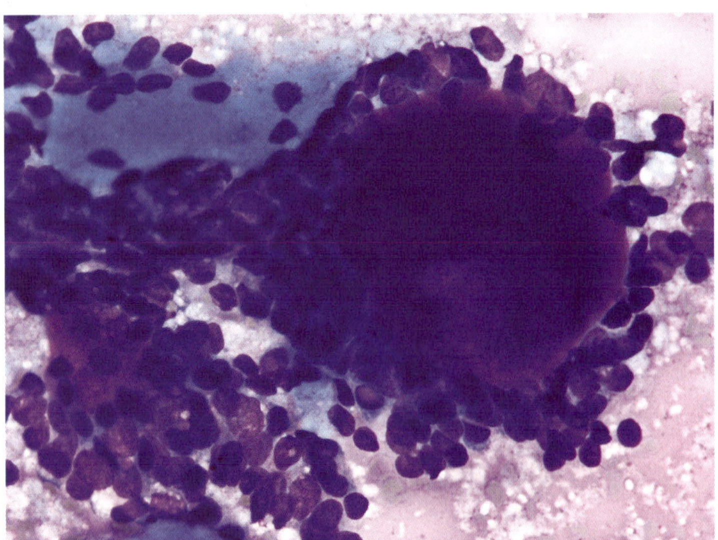

Figure 7.1c — Fetal Adenocarcinoma, Fine Needle Aspiration [Diff-Quik Stain; High Power]. One of the more striking features of fetal adenocarcinoma is the presence of dense hyaline globules with sharp, smooth borders somewhat evocative of adenoid cystic carcinoma. These globules are pale in Papanicolaou-stained slides, and densely metachromatic as illustrated in this Romanowsky-stained smear. Surrounding these globules, cells have a basaloid appearance with overlapping nuclei and nuclear molding. Smear background is typically clean in fetal adenocarcinoma lacking the tumor diathesis so regularly encountered in small cell neuroendocrine carcinoma. A "tigroid" background characterized by linear strips of detached cytoplasmic material has been reported in some instances of fetal adenocarcinoma. However, a "tigroid" background (initially promulgated as characteristic of seminoma) is not unusual in any neoplasm with high cytoplasmic glycogen content.

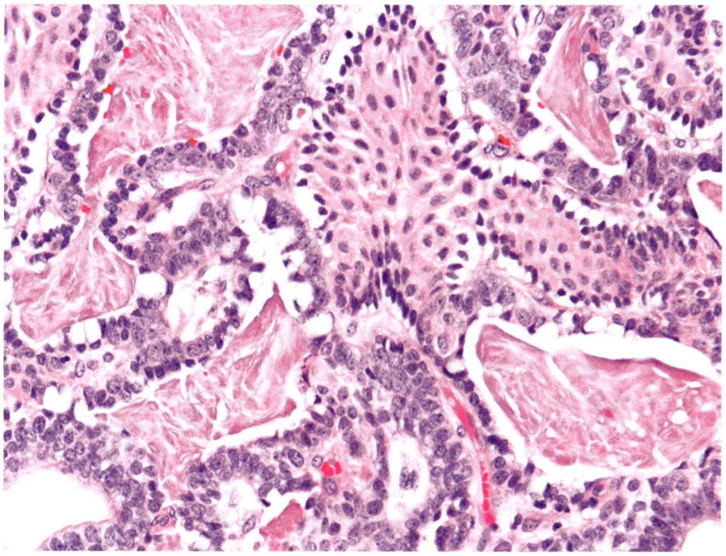

Figure 7.1d — Fetal Adenocarcinoma, Lobectomy [H&E Stain; High Power]. This low-grade fetal adenocarcinoma resembles the pseudoglandular phase of fetal lung development, with sub- and supranuclear glycogen-rich (i.e., Periodic acid-Schiff-positive, diastase-sensitive) vacuoles within uniform tall columnar nonciliated cells, with small, uniform, low-grade nuclei. TTF-1 will routinely be positive. This example contains prominent squamoid morules. Low-grade tumors have pure fetal morphology and typically affect young smokers, while high-grade variants are more often found in elderly male smokers. High-grade tumors have at least 50% fetal morphology, but also contain more common adenocarcinoma patterns, often with foci of necrosis, and lack morules. Unlike their low-grade counterparts, high-grade lesions may express AFP, glypican-3, and SALL4.

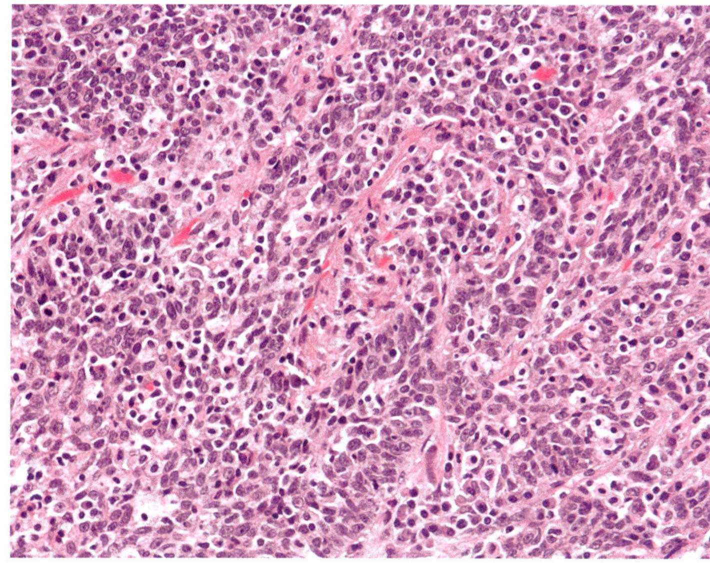

Figure 7.2 — Lymphoepithelioma-Like Carcinoma, Lobectomy [H&E Stain; High Power]. This tumor is composed of anastomosing syncytia of undifferentiated malignant epithelial cells, extensively infiltrated and often obscured by a dense reactive lymphoid infiltrate (CD3/CD8+ and CD20+). The neoplastic cells are large, with round to oval vesicular nuclei with irregular nuclear membranes and prominent eosinophilic nucleoli. In some cases, the tumor cells are more spindled. Immunohistochemical stains usually show expression of CK5/6, p40, and p63, suggesting squamous differentiation. Evaluation for the presence of Epstein–Barr virus by immunohistochemistry or in situ hybridization is routinely positive in the neoplastic cells. Differential diagnostic considerations include metastatic nasopharyngeal carcinoma (distinction requires history and/or imaging) and lymphocyte-rich thymoma (Epstein–Barr virus-negative; characteristic imaging). Granulomatous inflammation can be excluded with immunohistochemical staining for keratins and CD68.

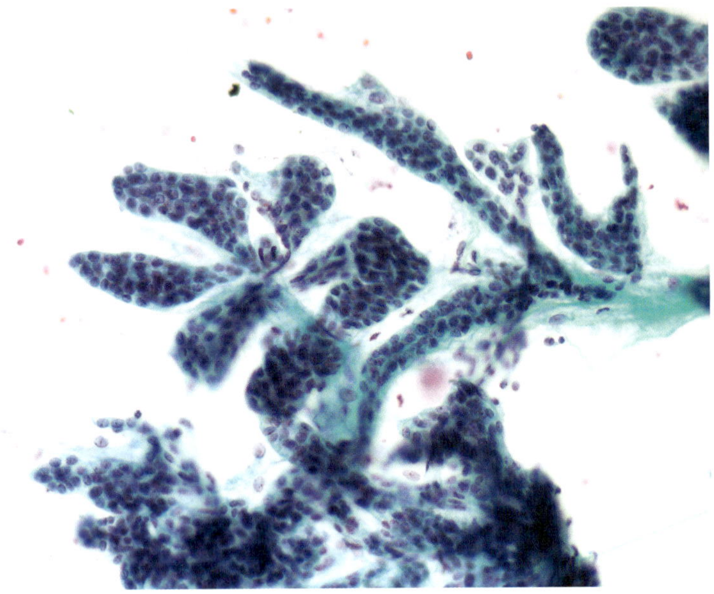

Figure 7.3a — Adenoid Cystic Carcinoma, Fine Needle Aspiration [Pap Stain; Medium Power]. Multiple finger-like bulbous papillae project from a scant amount of basal lamina producing a “fir tree” configuration in this image. Because adenoid cystic carcinoma of the lung commonly involves large airways, an endobronchial component resulting in a papillary architecture is not unusual, and can be potentially mistaken for squamous papilloma. Cell nuclei are typically small, isomorphic, and basaloid with much less cytoplasm than seen in the exfoliated squames from squamous papilloma. Within the tracheobronchial tree, adenoid cystic carcinoma is the most common salivary gland-type neoplasm, accounting for 70% to 80% of cases.

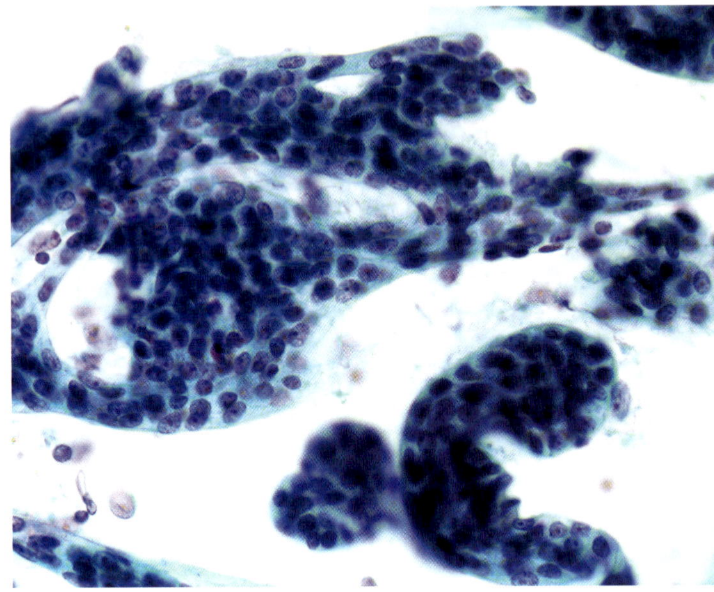

Figure 7.3b — Adenoid Cystic Carcinoma, Fine Needle Aspiration [Pap Stain; High Power]. Smoothly contoured papillary fronds and microacini contain a monotonous basaloid population with indistinct cell borders and a meager amount of cytoplasm. Nuclear chromatin is evenly dispersed, and unlike many small cell/basaloid neoplasms of the lung, nuclear molding is largely absent. The classic cribriform/“Swiss-cheese” architecture containing translucent globules is not always present. Unlike squamous papilloma or small cell carcinoma, single cells are largely absent in adenoid cystic carcinoma smears.

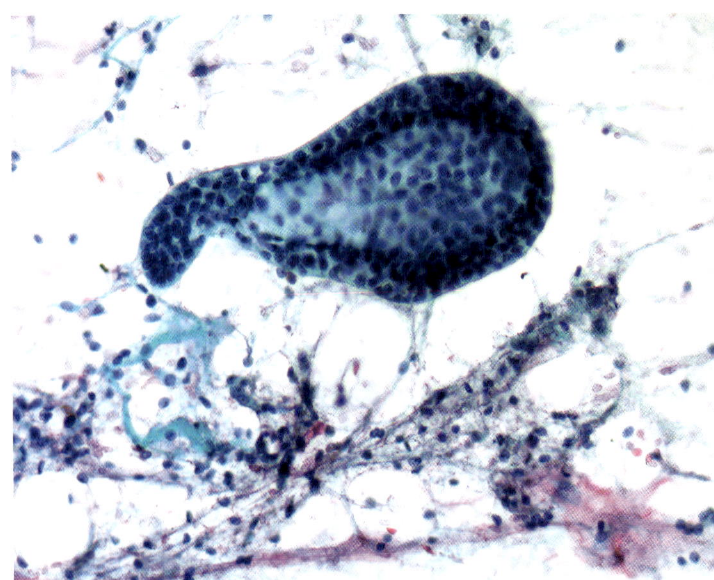

Figure 7.3c — Adenoid Cystic Carcinoma, Fine Needle Aspiration [Pap Stain; Medium Power]. A sharp smooth-edged “double-contour” configuration results from the 3-dimensional nature of this single microacinar fragment. Fine focusing on this cluster is required to appreciate any cells or stroma that may be in the center of this microacinus. The clean smear background lacking a tumor diathesis helps distinguish this basaloid neoplasm from more common entities such as small cell carcinoma. Immunostains from a cell block show positive myoepithelial marker (e.g., p63, smooth muscle actin, calponin, S100, and SOX-10) that help to distinguish adenoid cystic carcinoma from other basaloid malignancies.

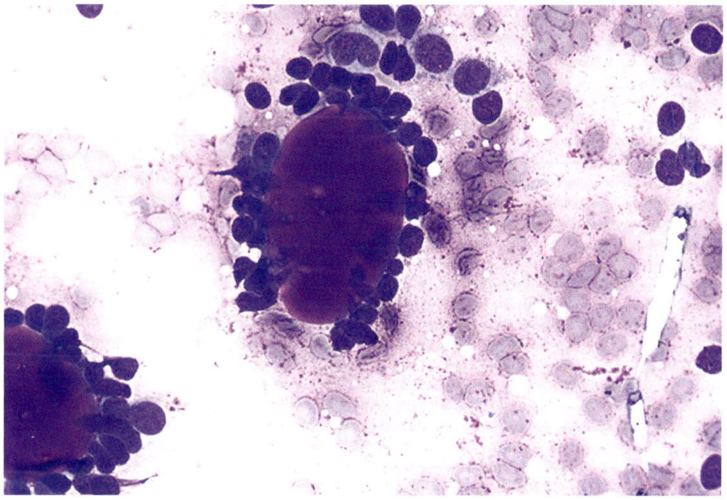

Figure 7.4a — Adenoid Cystic Carcinoma, Fine Needle Aspiration [Diff-Quik Stain; High Power]. This field provides an example of the classic appearance of adenoid cystic carcinoma–note the oval, magenta-colored globules with smooth borders ringed by basaloid cells. This is a contrast to the "inside out" pattern of pleomorphic adenoma, in which cells are imbedded in magenta-colored stroma that engulfs the neoplastic cells. While adenoid cystic carcinoma may be primary to the lung, which contains salivary tissue, there have been reported instances in which adenoid cystic carcinoma invades from a distant site along a nerve.

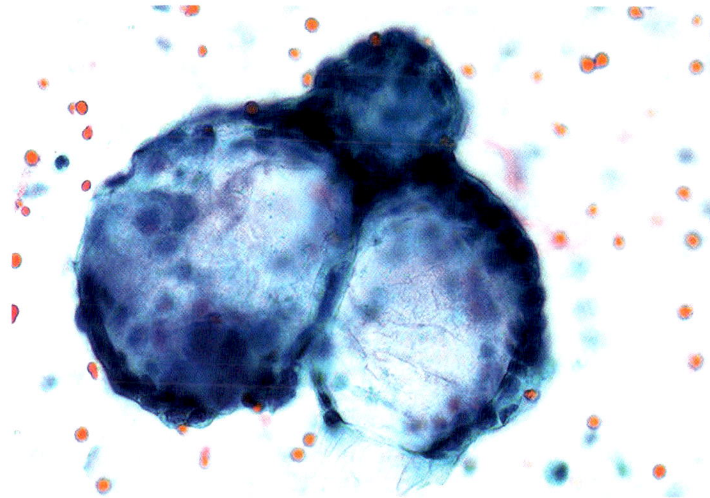

Figure 7.4b — Adenoid Cystic Carcinoma, Fine Needle Aspiration [Pap Stain; High Power]. On the Pap stain, the globular material of adenoid cystic carcinoma is not as obvious but still detectable. The neoplastic cells appear smaller, but are more visible throughout the surface of the globules rather than simply at the edges. Because the structures are symmetrical, they may be initially ignored on a Pap stain preparation if not present in great numbers.

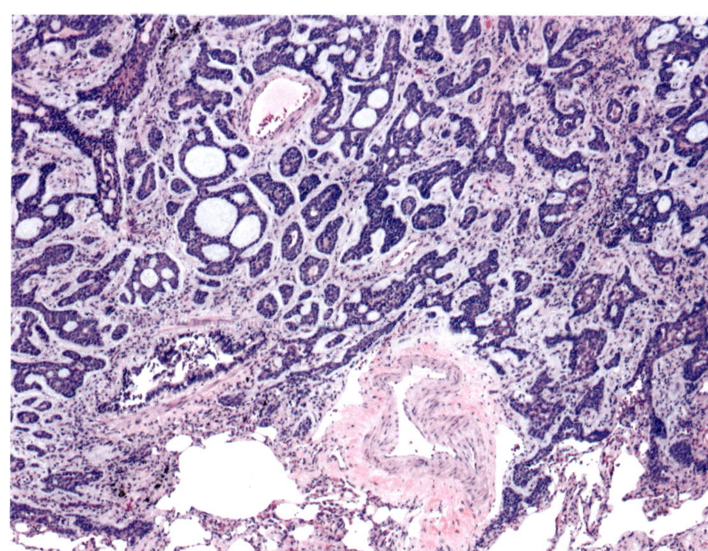

Figure 7.4c — Metastatic Adenoid Cystic Carcinoma, Biopsy [H&E Stain; Low Power]. This metastatic lesion shows the classic low power pattern of adenoid cystic carcinoma, with irregular cribriform, tubular, and solid nests of tumor cells, embedded in a myxohyaline stroma. The tumor infiltrates adjacent normal lung parenchyma, including a bronchovascular bundle, at the bottom of the image. Primary adenoid cystic carcinomas are histologically indistinguishable from metastatic lesions, but arise centrally from the seromucinous glands of the bronchi; the peripheral intraparenchymal location of this lesion is characteristic of a metastasis. This patient had a documented history of adenoid cystic carcinoma of the parotid gland.

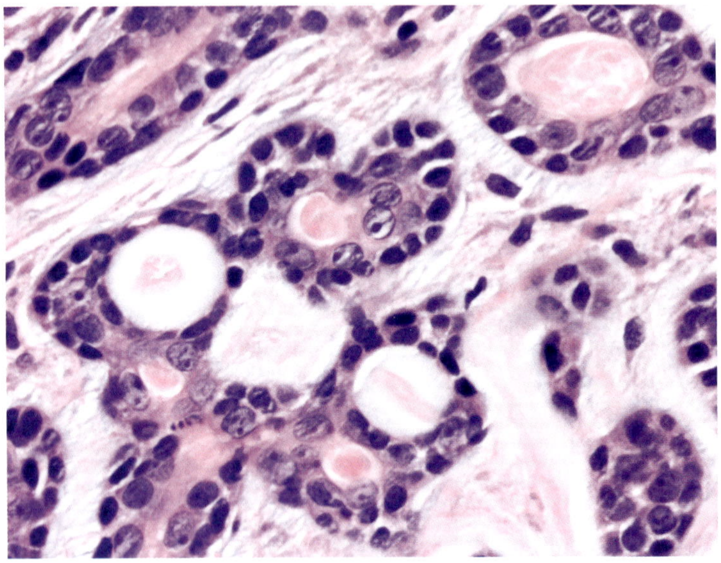

Figure 7.4d — Metastatic Adenoid Cystic Carcinoma, Biopsy [H&E Stain; High Power]. The glands of adenoid cystic carcinoma are lined by a dual layer of cells: a luminal cuboidal surface cell and a spindled, myoepithelial-type cell peripherally. The lumens contain a core of myxoid or hyalinized matrix.

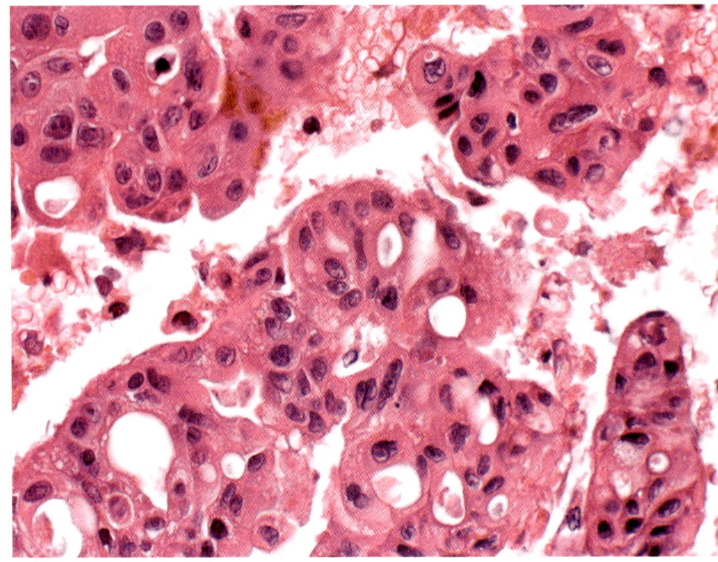

Figure 7.5a — Mucoepidermoid Carcinoma, Fine Needle Aspiration [H&E Stain; High Power]. If cell block material is created, a mucicarmine stain can be used to verify the presence of mucin with gland-like spaces. Mucoepidermoid carcinoma typically affects young patients and is found within large airway spaces. If patients have the tumor surgically resected, the prognosis is excellent. While immunohistochemical studies performed on tissue biopsies may help exclude a classic lung adenocarcinoma or squamous cell carcinoma, the interpretation is substantially more difficult on cell block material.

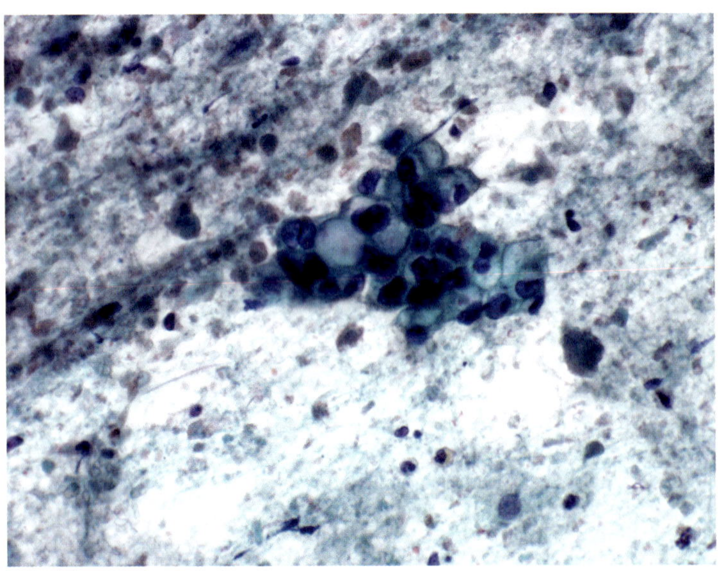

Figure 7.5b — Mucoepidermoid Carcinoma, Fine Needle Aspiration [Pap Stain; High Power]. These cells contain mucinous vacuoles, form a glandular space, and have hyperchromatic nuclei with irregular nuclear borders and distinct nucleoli. The intracytoplasmic vacuoles have the bubbly appearance suggestive of mucinous contents. A squamous component is not readily apparent. The background contains granular debris, which may be necrotic material or degenerated mucin. While mucoepidermoid carcinomas can be low or high grade, the majority are low-grade carcinomas. However, grading of mucoepidermoid carcinoma on cytologic material is not usually possible.

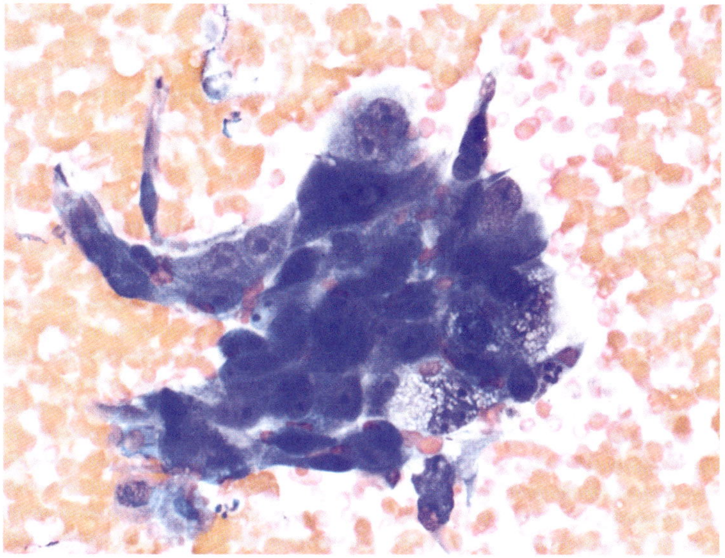

Figure 7.5c — Mucoepidermoid Carcinoma, Fine Needle Aspiration [Diff-Quik Stain; High Power]. This fragment contains a mixture of cell types, including squamoid cells with prominent nucleoli and spindled morphology, as well as vacuolated histiocytic-like, clear mucinous cells. The cells seen here are overtly malignant, with greatly enlarged nuclei, anisonucleosis, and a disorganized arrangement within the fragment.

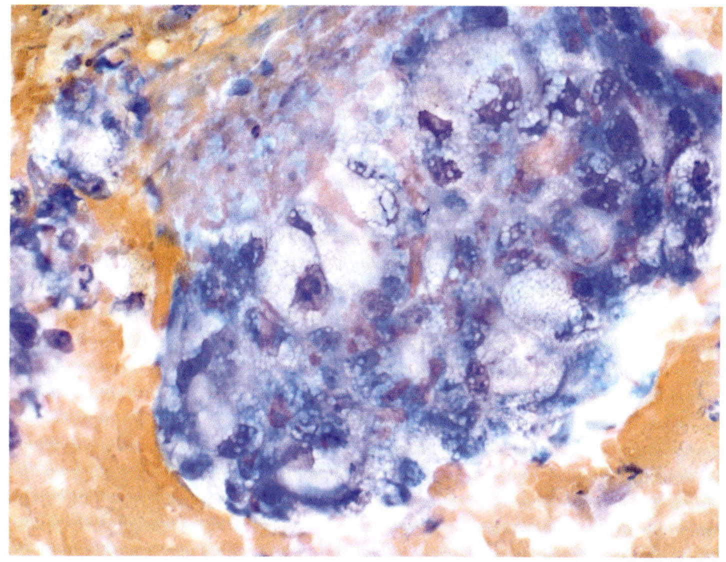

Figure 7.5d — Mucoepidermoid Carcinoma, Fine Needle Aspiration [Diff-Quik Stain; High Power]. Mucoepidermoid carcinoma may develop in the lung salivary tissue. Mucoepidermoid carcinoma is a diagnostic challenge because it contains both malignant squamoid and glandular elements. If only one element is sampled, such as the glandular component seen here, it may raise concern for either an adenocarcinoma or a squamous cell carcinoma. If both glandular and squamous components are seen, the differential includes an adenosquamous carcinoma of the lung.

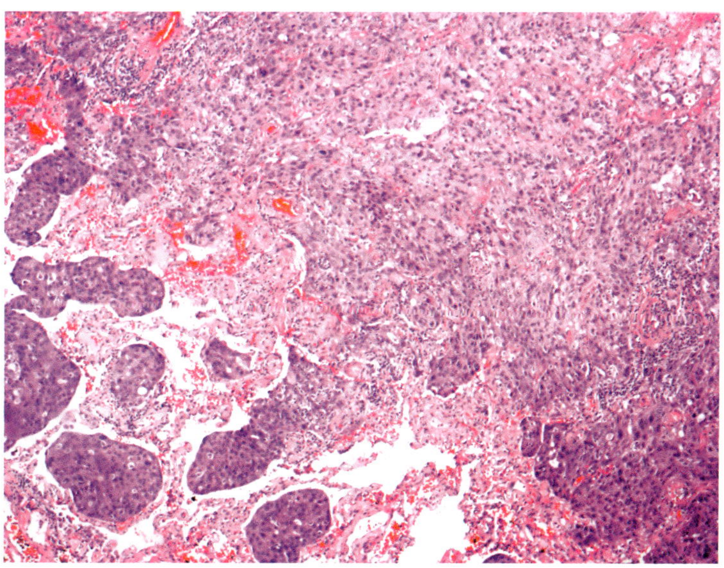

Figure 7.6a — Metastatic Mucoepidermoid Carcinoma, Biopsy [H&E Stain; Low Power]. At low power, nests of malignant squamous ("epidermoid") tumor cells are seen spreading through air spaces at the periphery of this metastasis. Non-small cell carcinoma is a consideration, and history is of critical importance in establishing the correct diagnosis. This patient had a documented history of mucoepidermoid carcinoma of the parotid gland.

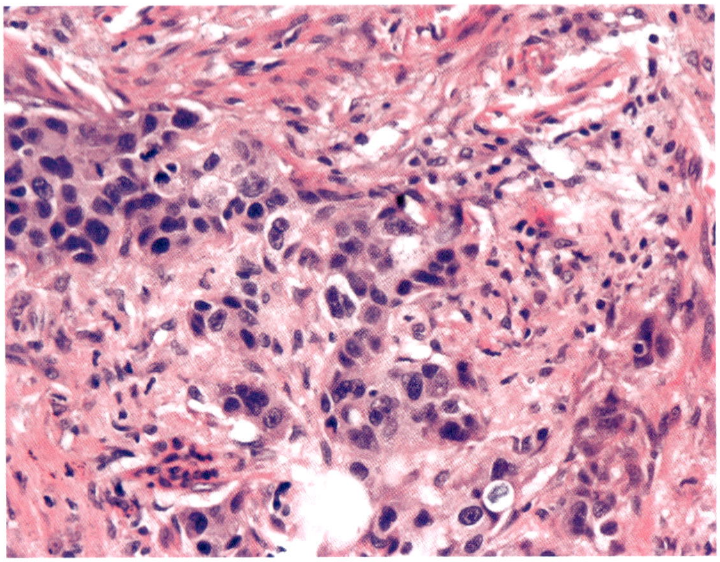

Figure 7.6b — Metastatic Mucoepidermoid Carcinoma, Biopsy [H&E Stain; High Power]. At high power, both components of this neoplasm can be appreciated. The squamous component dominates, and is at the upper left, while a mucin vacuole is present at the bottom, right of center. Mucicarmine staining and/or immunostaining for CK7 or EMA can be used to highlight the glandular component, which may be subtle on hematoxylin and eosin stain. The squamous nests express p40/p63 as well as CK5/6. Primary adenosquamous carcinoma of the lung may be difficult to exclude with certainty, especially in the absence of a clear history of a prior salivary lesion.

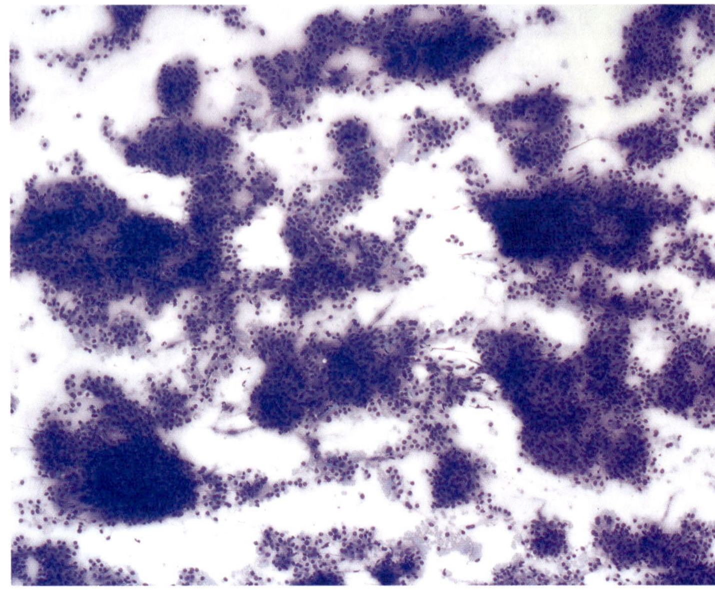

Figure 7.7a — Meningioma, Fine Needle Aspiration [Diff-Quik Stain; Low Power]. Primary pulmonary meningiomas are exceptionally rare. Metastatic deposits to the lung from intracranial neoplasms are also very uncommon. Meningiomas presumably derive from pluripotent cells, ectopic embryonic arachnoid cells, or from meningothelial nodules. A wide age range has been reported with most patients being of middle age. Most examples are single, incidentally encountered, well-demarcated nodules in the lung periphery. Aspirates are highly cellular, composed primarily of syncytial aggregates with few single forms. The smear background is clean.

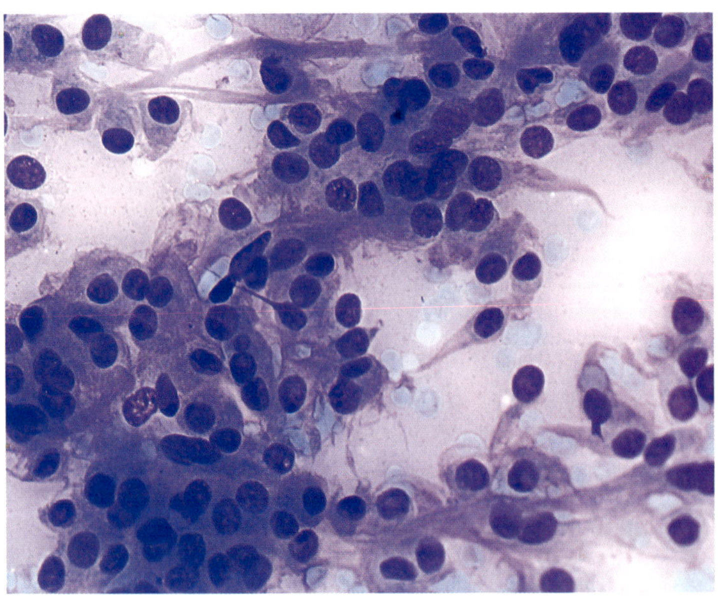

Figure 7.7b — Meningioma, Fine Needle Aspiration [Diff-Quik Stain; High Power]. Upon closer inspection, cells within these loose syncytial aggregates appear identical to one another with rounded to oval smoothly contoured nuclei, indistinct nucleoli, occasional nuclear grooves, and intranuclear cytoplasmic invaginations (absent here). Some cells have eccentrically placed nuclei, giving them a plasmacytoid "look." The moderate to abundant wispy cytoplasm interconnects among cells without sharp cell borders. Cell cytoplasm projects from single cells in long tapering strands. In contrast to this meningothelial variant, cells in the fibrous variant are also cytologically bland, but spindle shaped and mimic a mesenchymal neoplasm.

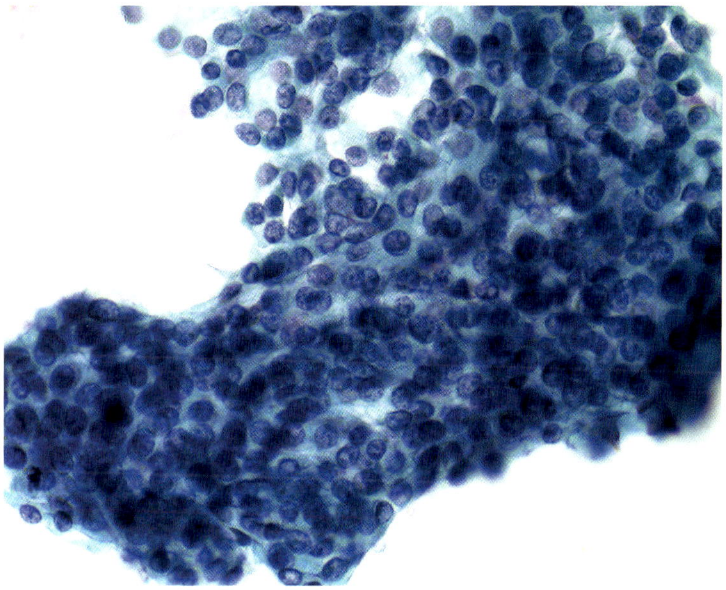

Figure 7.7c — Meningioma, Fine Needle Aspiration [Pap Stain; High Power]. Cells of meningioma may be arranged in well-formed whorled nests, particularly in the meningothelial variant. In many instances, however, this concentric cellular arrangement is incomplete, and instead cells form a smooth bulbous contour but lack well-developed circumferential streaming (lower left). Depending on the histologic subtype, psammoma bodies may be encountered in aspirate smears, but are usually infrequent. Note the absence of mitotic figures and individual cell necrosis in these images of meningioma.

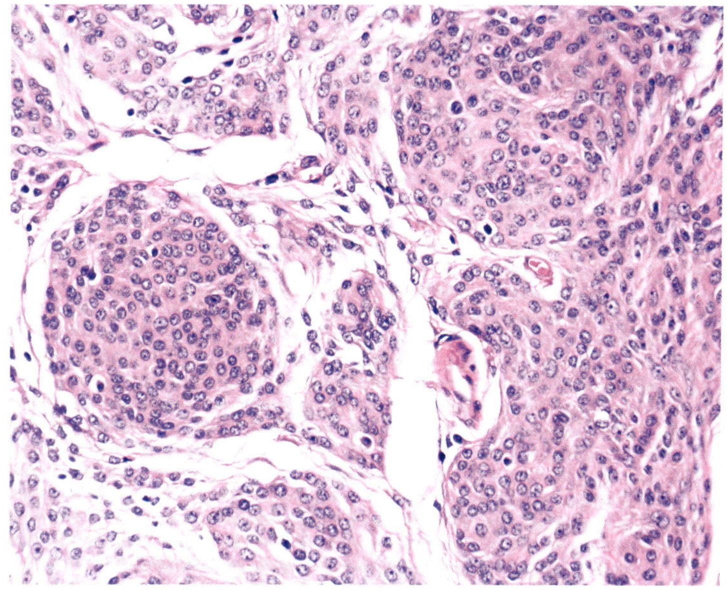

Figure 7.7d — Meningioma, Core Needle Biopsy [H&E Stain; Medium Power]. Meningioma of the lung is histologically indistinguishable from its meningeal counterpart. This example shows the classic multinodular whorled pattern, with spindled to epithelioid cells with abundant eosinophilic cytoplasm and open chromatin with punctate nucleoli. Psammoma bodies may be present. Immunohistochemical stains for EMA, vimentin, and progesterone receptor are routinely positive, while keratin stains are negative. In the lung, this rare tumor is more often a metastasis from a meningeal primary than a primary neoplasm. In small biopsies, the features may suggest solitary fibrous tumor (STAT6-positive, EMA-negative), synovial sarcoma (CD99+, bcl-2+, EMA+), or a granuloma (CD68+; negative for EMA and PR).

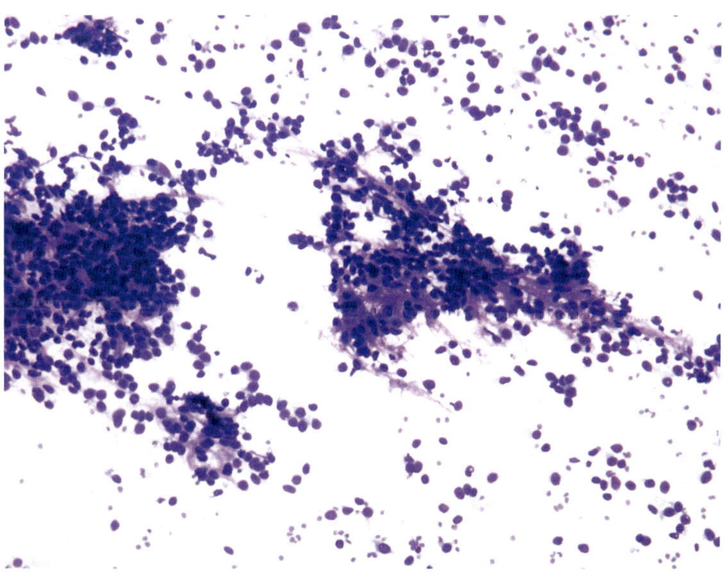

Figure 7.8a — Solitary Fibrous Tumor, Fine Needle Aspiration [Diff-Quik Stain; Low Power]. In the thoracic cavity, solitary fibrous tumor most commonly arises from the visceral pleura, and has been described in the mediastinum and trachea, but only very infrequently within the lung parenchyma proper. Solitary fibrous tumor varies greatly in size from a few centimeters to greater than 15 cm, and occurs over a broad age range; most occur in the sixth to seventh decade. In addition to being discovered incidentally, patients may present with nonspecific symptoms. Since the histopathology contains hyper- and hypocellular zones, aspiration smears vary in cellularity from only modestly cellular to containing 3-dimensional hypercellular clusters imitating a sarcoma. The ropy collagen that is often present in tissue can sometimes be captured in cytologic smears. Metachromatic collagen fibers intersect among a uniform population of cells in these two clusters. Single cells with rounded nuclei containing only wispy strands of cytoplasm are dispersed in a clean smear background.

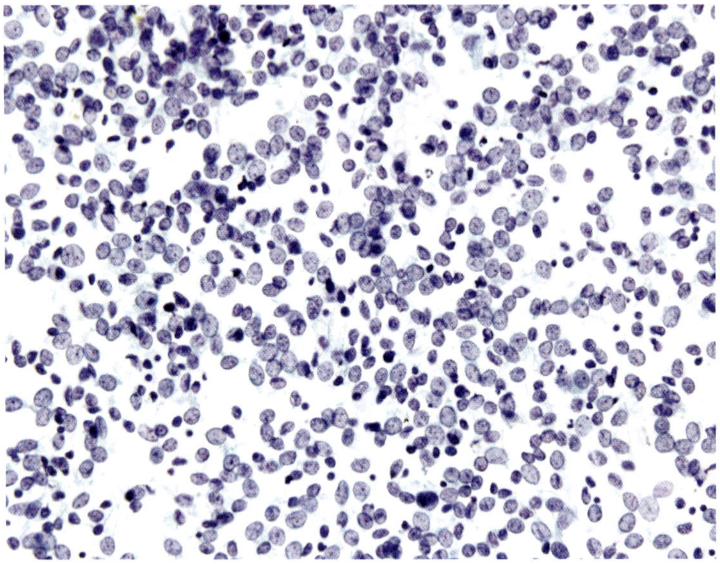

Figure 7.8b — Solitary Fibrous Tumor, Fine Needle Aspiration [Pap Stain; Low Power]. Oval nuclei show extreme uniformity and hypochromasia with some having incomplete nuclear grooves. Cell cytoplasm is barely perceptible. Small lymphocytes are scattered among these fibroblastic cells. Malignant solitary fibrous tumor is defined primarily by mitotic activity. Since accurate mitotic counts are not possible cytologically, definitive statements regarding malignancy for solitary fibrous tumor are not possible. Cytologic images such as this one are easily confused for synovial sarcoma, malignant peripheral nerve sheath tumor, and desmoplastic round cell tumor.

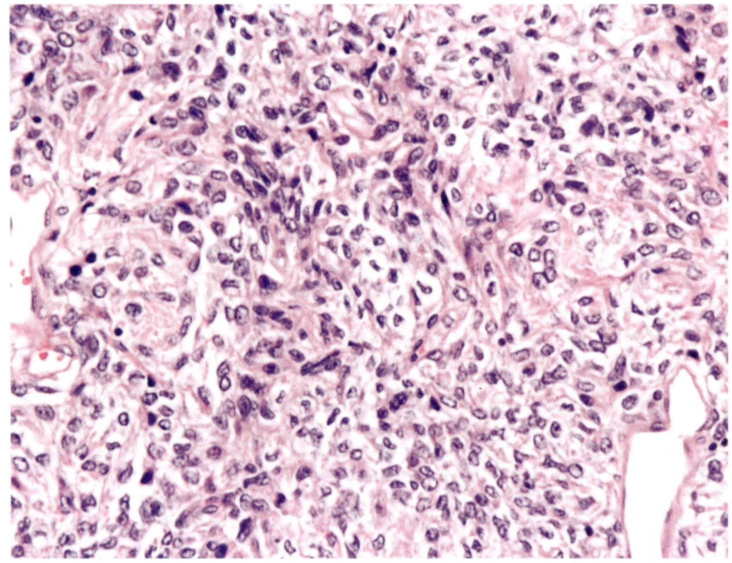

Figure 7.8c — Solitary Fibrous Tumor, Core Needle Biopsy [H&E Stain; Medium Power]. Stromal collagen is evident in this pleural core needle biopsy. Aspirates from these foci of extensive hyalinization are hypocellular due to the inability of a fine needle to extract cells from this matrix. Note that the uniform hypochromic nuclei mirror their appearance in the prior cytologic image. The branching vascular pattern (so-called hemangiopericytomatous), which is so helpful in recognizing solitary fibrous tumor, is absent from cytologic smears. Solitary fibrous tumor has been more readily recognizable in recent years due to the relatively high sensitivity (greater than 95% positive staining) and specificity of STAT6 immunostaining. These neoplasms are also CD34, bcl-2, and CD99 positive.

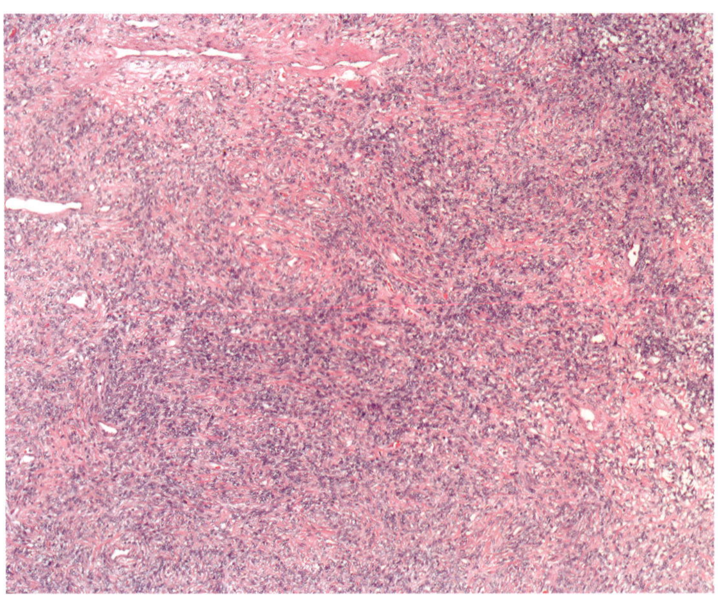

Figure 7.9a — Solitary Fibrous Tumor, Resection [H&E Stain; Low Power]. The characteristic low power appearance of solitary fibrous tumor includes marked variation in cellularity, with fibroblast-like tumor cells arranged in fascicles, storiform arrays, or a "patternless" pattern. The collagenous stroma ranges from attenuated fibrils to a denser, more keloidal pattern; some examples have patches of myxoid stroma. Vasculature is prominent, with a branching pattern classically described as "staghorn"-type vasculature. Perivascular hyalinization is common. Solitary fibrous tumors typically harbor an intrachromosomal inversion of chr 12 which results in the gene fusion *NAB2-STAT6;* the associated overexpression of STAT6 can be detected by immunohistochemistry (see Figure 7.9c). At low power the features may suggest a nerve sheath tumor or other mesenchymal neoplasm.

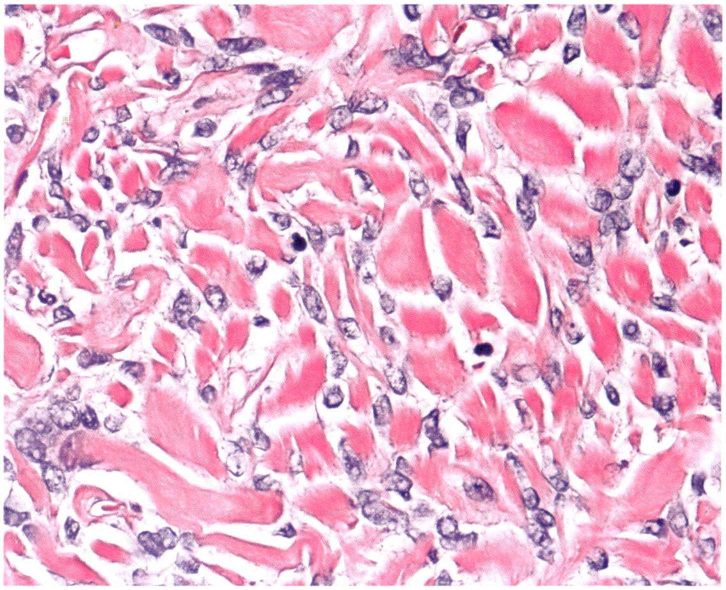

Figure 7.9b — Solitary Fibrous Tumor, Resection [H&E Stain; High Power]. Keloidal collagen dominates this field. The tumor cells are bland, with indistinct cytoplasmic borders and vesicular nuclei with small or indiscernible nucleoli. Solitary fibrous tumors have fewer than 3 mitoses/2 mm^2, and necrosis is uncommon in the absence of trauma (e.g., torsion of the pedicle; prior biopsy). Differential diagnostic considerations for this peripheral/pleural lesion include primary or metastatic synovial sarcoma (EMA+; *S18-SSX* fusion gene detectable in nearly all, due to t(X;18)(p11;q11); sarcomatoid mesothelioma (keratin expression; CD34-, STAT6-; characteristic imaging features); and nerve sheath tumors (S100+, STAT6-, CD34-).

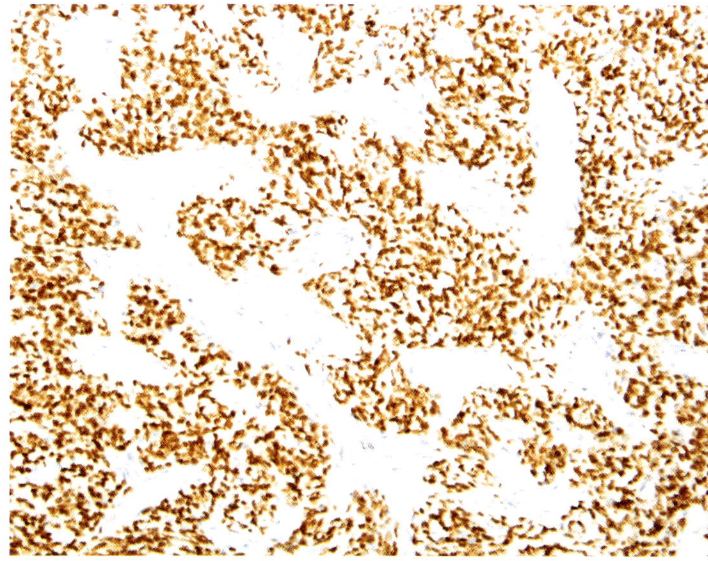

Figure 7.9c — Solitary Fibrous Tumor, Resection [Immunohistochemical Stain for STAT6; High Power]. Strong, diffuse nuclear expression of STAT6 is present in greater than 95% of cases and is highly specific. The staghorn-type vasculature is well delineated by the irregular sheets of STAT6-positive tumor cells. Stains for CD34, bcl-2, and CD99 are also routinely positive. Occasional cases of solitary fibrous tumor show some expression of actins, desmin, keratins, EMA, or S100; a panel of stains that includes STAT6 is therefore optimal for establishing the diagnosis.

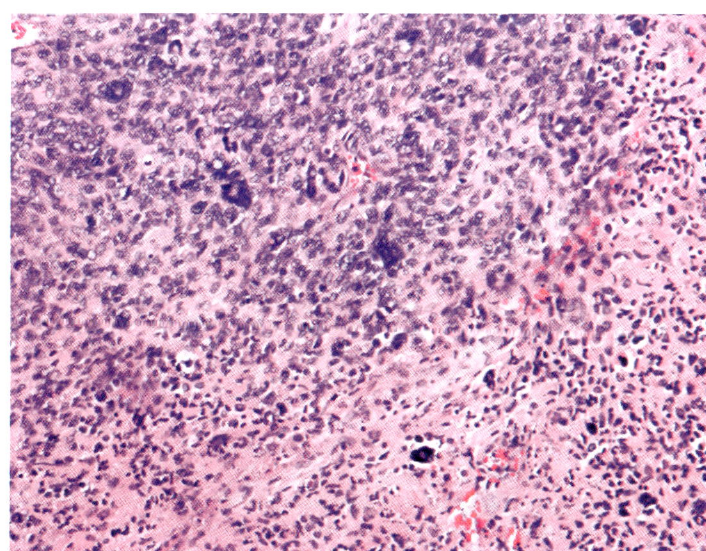

Figure 7.9d — Malignant Solitary Fibrous Tumor, Resection [H&E Stain; High Power]. This malignant solitary fibrous tumor, recurring for the third time with chest wall invasion, shows marked cytologic atypia, with a zone of necrosis at the lower right. Tumor necrosis, atypia, and large size suggest a potential for malignant biology, but a mitotic rate of greater than 4/2 mm^2 has been shown to be the most reliable predictor of aggressive behavior. Approximately 10% of all solitary fibrous tumors recur locally, while the rate of metastasis is about 5%. Even very bland lesions may metastasize on occasion; histology alone is not sufficient to reliably determine malignant potential.

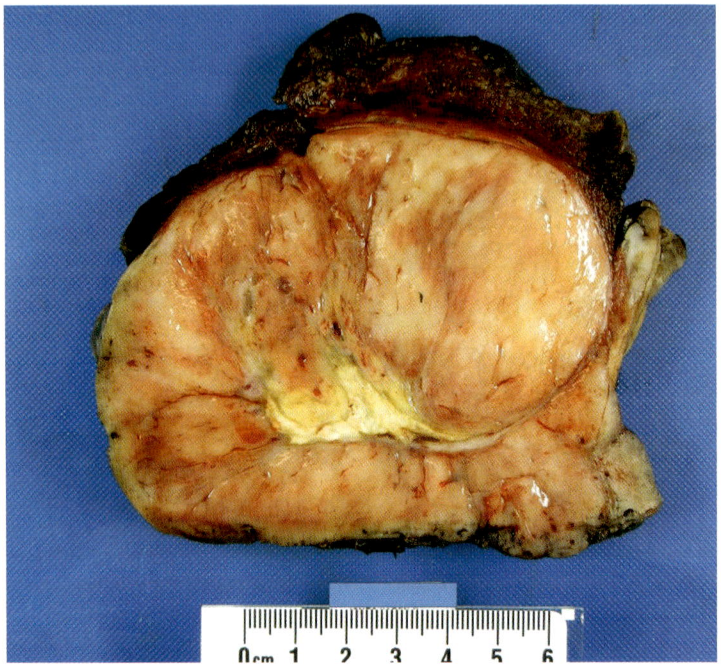

Figure 7.9e — Solitary Fibrous Tumor, Resection [Gross Examination]. Although reported throughout the pleural cavity, solitary fibrous tumors most often arise from the visceral pleura, most likely from submesothelial mesenchyme. They are often large (greater than 10 cm), and pedunculation is common. The cut surface is tan-white and ridged or whorled, and shows sharp circumscription, with expansile compression of the adjacent lung.

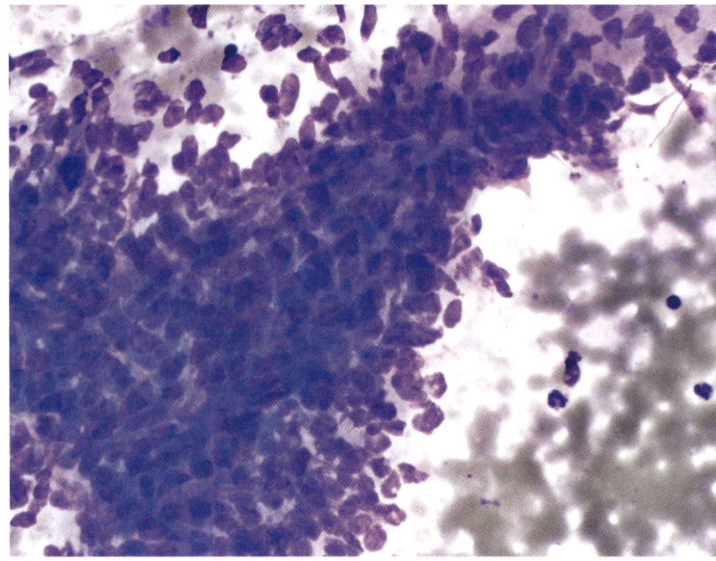

Figure 7.10a — Adult Fibrosarcoma, Fine Needle Aspiration [Diff-Quik Stain; High Power]. The neoplastic cells are present singly as well as in a 3-dimensional fragment. The cells have indistinct cytoplasm and the nuclei are spindle or oval shaped. Because the cells lack any specific cytomorphologic differentiation, ancillary studies are required to further classify this "malignant spindle cell neoplasm" as a sarcoma or carcinoma.

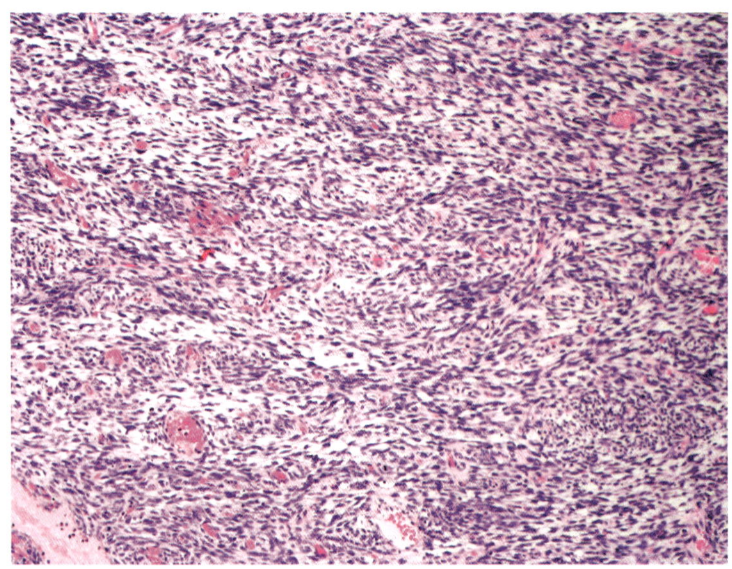

Figure 7.10b — Adult Fibrosarcoma, Biopsy [H&E Stain; Low Power]. This section demonstrates the classic "herringbone" pattern seen in adult fibrosarcoma. While fibrosarcoma used to be the most common sarcoma, with the advent of immunohistochemical and molecular methods to characterize sarcomas, it has become a rare diagnosis. The diagnosis of adult fibrosarcoma is one of exclusion; a sarcoma must not demonstrate a specific differentiation on ancillary studies. The sarcoma must also lack pleomorphism, which would otherwise make it a pleomorphic sarcoma.

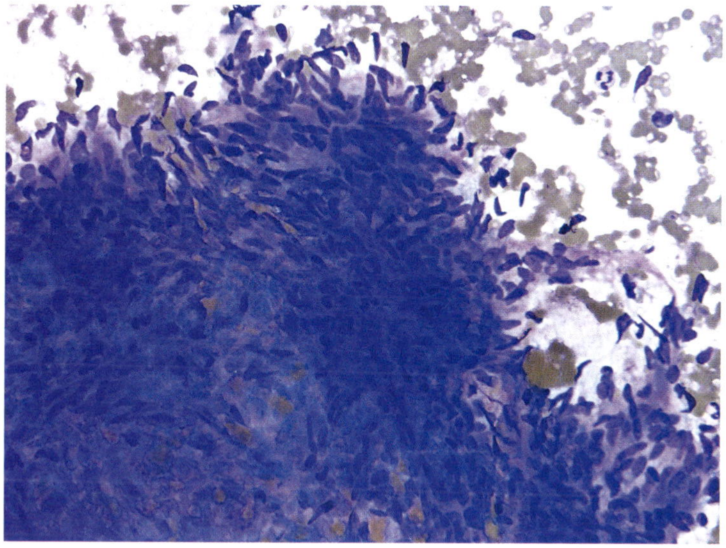

Figure 7.11a — Synovial Sarcoma, Fine Needle Aspiration [Diff-Quik Stain; Medium Power]. Synovial sarcoma involves the lung most often as a manifestation of metastatic disease. Primary pulmonary synovial sarcoma may be intrapulmonary or pleural based upon the lung being the most common organ-based site for primary synovial sarcoma. Smears of synovial sarcoma are highly cellular. This 3-dimensional hypercellular spindle cell cluster is typical, showing a uniformly sized population of nuclei with minimal irregularity and no pleomorphism. Except for its poorly differentiated variant, which is a round cell malignancy, synovial sarcoma is characterized by cellular spindle cell monotony. Because several other primary spindle cell malignancies of the lung enter into the differential diagnosis, such as pulmonary blastoma, solitary fibrous tumor, leiomyosarcoma, malignant peripheral nerve sheath tumor, and, in the pleura, sarcomatoid mesothelioma, ancillary testing is necessary for definitive diagnosis. Fluorescence in situ hybridization analysis using the synovial sarcoma18 probe [t(X;18)(p11.2;q11.2)] is specific for synovial sarcoma, and has been applied successfully to smears and to cell block preparations to confirm the diagnosis of synovial sarcoma.

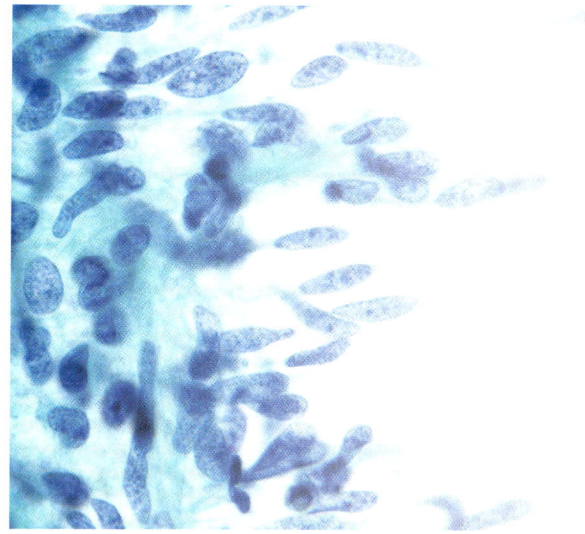

Figure 7.11b — Synovial Sarcoma, Fine Needle Aspiration [Pap Stain; High Power]. Although synovial sarcoma is subdivided histologically into monophasic and biphasic forms, this division is rarely appreciated in cytologic smears. With the monophasic type being most common, smears reveal elongated and ovoid isomorphic nuclei, evenly dispersed nucleoplasm, and thin delicate short cytoplasmic processes as in this high-power image. Typical for synovial sarcoma is the absence of nuclear pleomorphism, macronucleoli, and individual cell necrosis. Immunostaining for TLE-1 is relatively specific, and readily performed on cell blocks.

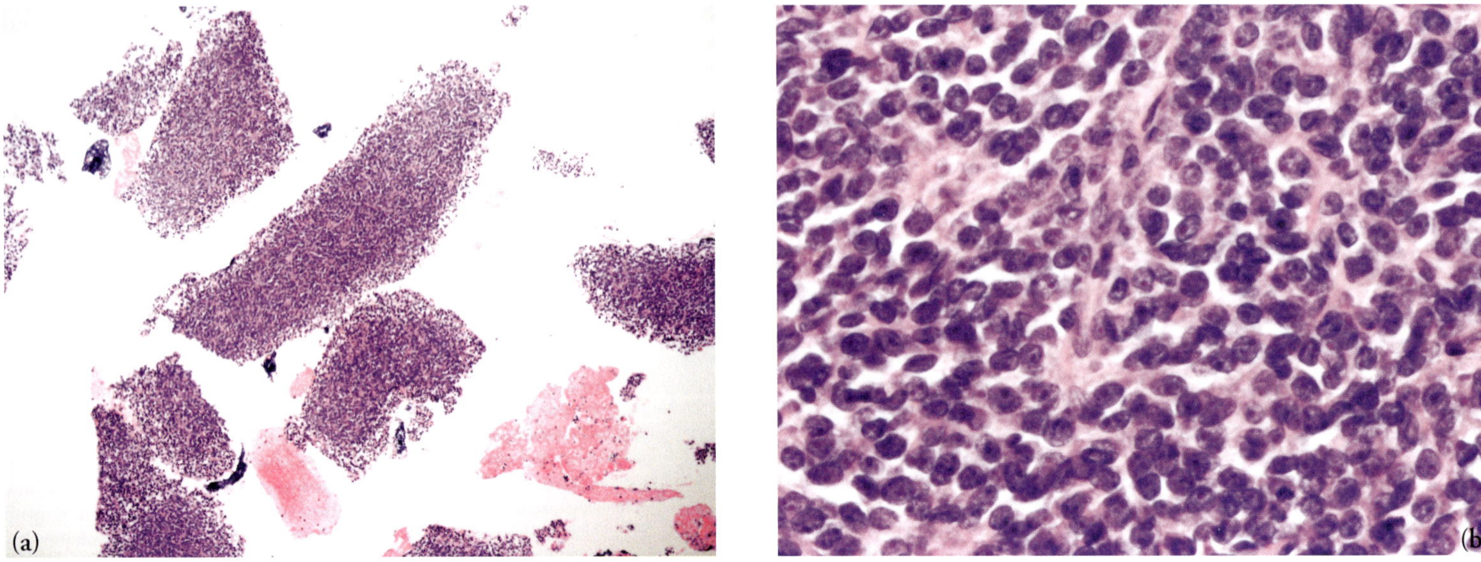

Figure 7.12(a, b) — Synovial Sarcoma, Fine Needle Aspiration [H&E Stain; Low and High Powers]. This cell block preparation shows sampling of a very cellular synovial sarcoma; in this case, the tumor cells appear entirely epithelioid and may resemble other small round blue cell tumors. Note how monotonous the tumor cells appear; this is a common finding in translocation sarcomas. At low magnification, the tumor cell sheets are interrupted by randomly distributed capillaries. Unless this is a recurrence, immunohistochemical and/or molecular studies are required to confirm the diagnosis.

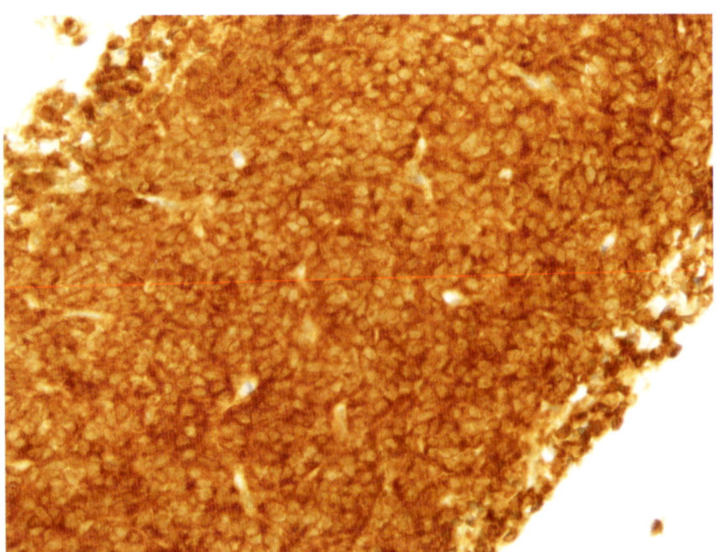

Figure 7.12c — Synovial Sarcoma, Fine Needle Aspiration [Bcl-2 Immunohistochemical Stain; Medium Power]. Expression of bcl-2 can typically be detected in both spindled and epithelioid components of synovial sarcoma. Here, the tumor cells are diffusely positive. TLE-1 also appears to be an excellent marker for synovial sarcoma, with one study showing expression in 97% of synovial sarcomas and much less frequently in other sarcomas.

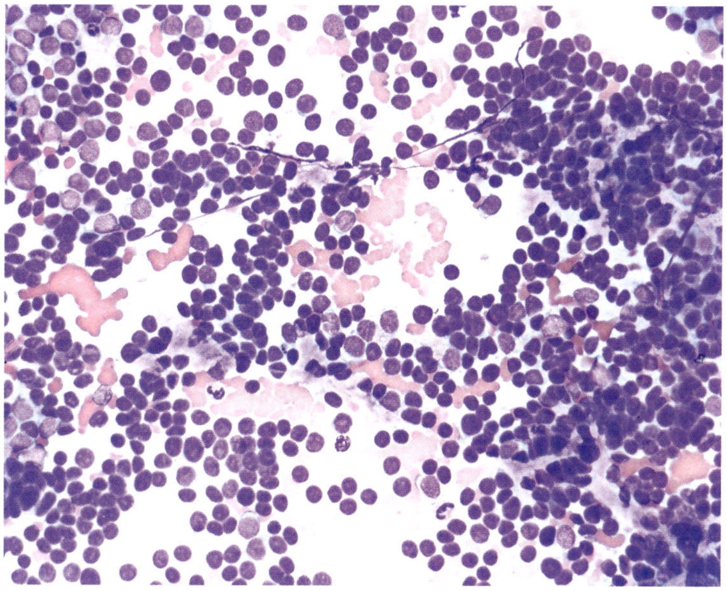

Figure 7.13a — Primitive Neuroectodermal Tumor, Fine Needle Aspiration [Diff-Quik Stain; Medium Power]. Primitive neuroectodermal tumor is primarily a tumor of the thoracopulmonary region with involvement of the ribs, pleura, and lung. It is currently considered a member of the Ewing sarcoma "family of tumors" due to its reciprocal t(11;22)(q24;q12) chromosomal translocation, and the absence of any clinical relevance for the degree of neural differentiation that may be present. It is largely confined to patients less than 30 years of age. The cytopathology is essentially that described for Ewing sarcoma. Smears are highly cellular due to the absence of stroma in this neoplasm with a single cell and clustered pattern of cell distribution. This neoplasm is archetypical for the "malignant small round cell tumor" category of tumors. Uniformly sized cells have rounded to slightly irregular nuclei, indistinct nucleoli, and meager amounts of cytoplasm, though some cases contain cells with visible cytoplasmic glycogen-filled vacuoles.

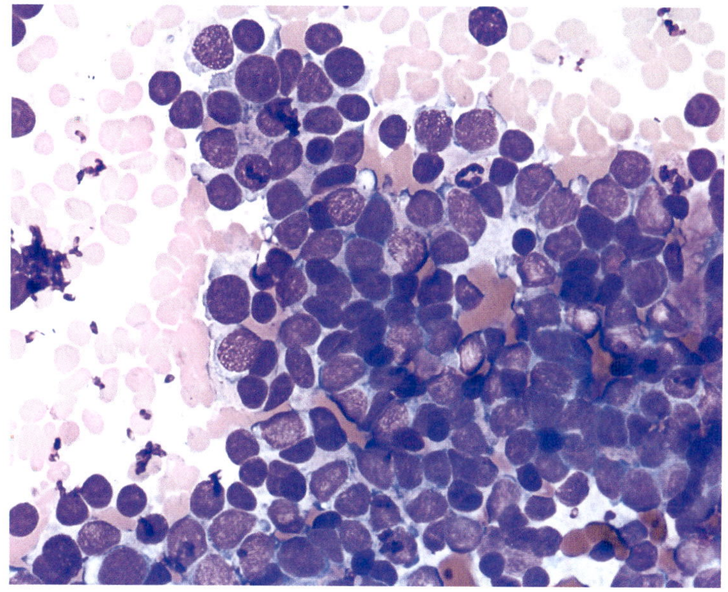

Figure 7.13b — Primitive Neuroectodermal Tumor, Fine Needle Aspiration [Diff-Quik Stain; High Power]. These monomorphic cells usually are in flat sheets, but cases with more pronounced neural differentiation may show rosette formations. Nuclear molding is not unusual. Due to the absence of cellular differentiating features, ancillary testing is an absolute must for definitive diagnosis. CD99 and FLI-1 immunostains are positive, but not unequivocally specific. Neural markers such as PGP 9.5, neurofilament, Leu-7, and synaptophysin may be positive in cases with greater neural differentiation. Fluorescence in situ hybridization testing for *EWSR1* gene rearrangement occurs in about 95% of cases. Poorly differentiated synovial sarcoma, metastatic alveolar rhabdomyosarcoma, non-Hodgkin lymphoma, and mesenchymal chondrosarcoma all enter into the differential diagnosis when such lesions occur in the lung and thorax of children and young adults.

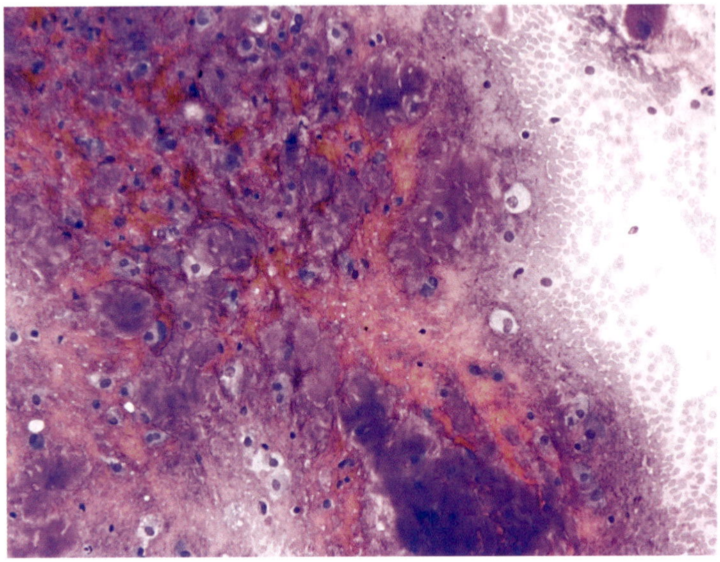

Figure 7.14a — Chondrosarcoma, Fine Needle Aspiration [Diff-Quik Stain; Medium Power]. The field contains copious magenta-colored matrix material and scattered neoplastic cells with round nuclei and abundant blue, irregularly shaped cytoplasm. Some neoplastic cells are embedded in matrix material while others are present individually in the field. Chondrosarcoma may be a metastatic tumor to the lung, or may directly invade the lung from the axial skeleton.

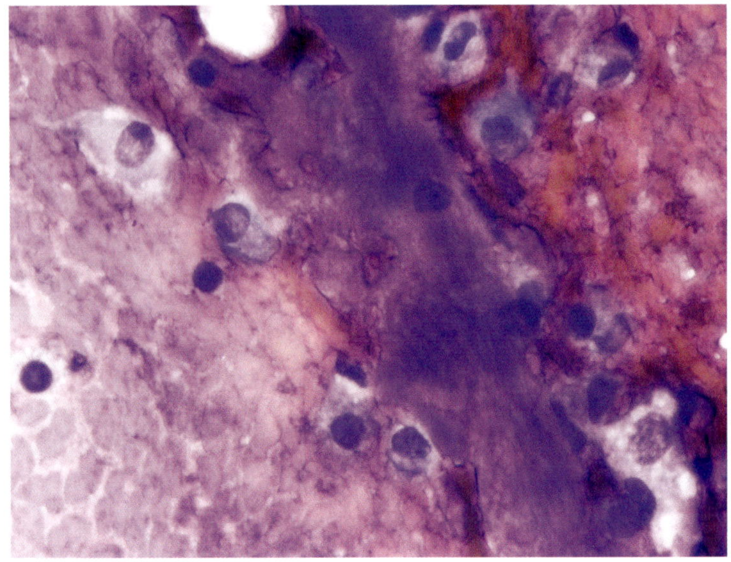

Figure 7.14b — Chondrosarcoma, Fine Needle Aspiration [Diff-Quik Stain; Medium Power]. Neoplastic cells are seen within and adjacent to magenta-colored matrix material. The differential includes hamartoma and pleomorphic adenoma; clinical history and radiologic data should help greatly in this instance. Some cells have irregular nuclear borders, which would be unusual for a pleomorphic adenoma. It is difficult to definitively identify the matrix material as chondroid in this instance.

Figure 7.15a — Pleural Angiosarcoma, Fine Needle Aspiration [Diff-Quik Stain; Medium Power]. As with most sarcomas, angiosarcoma (AngioS) when it involves the lung and/or pleura does so as metastatic deposits from a known soft tissue, breast, or cutaneous primary. This enables a specific cytologic diagnosis in a high percentage of cases when cytologic aspirates can be compared with prior tissue specimens. However, primary pulmonary AngioS is extremely rare, and the subject of case reports. In this latter instance, immunophenotyping is necessary for a specific diagnosis. For primary pleural AngioS, diffuse thickening mimics the radiologic appearance of malignant mesothelioma. AngioS can exhibit a variety of shapes including spindle, pleomorphic, and epithelioid cytomorphology, thereby imitating sarcomatoid carcinoma, malignant melanoma, and sarcomatoid mesothelioma. Of course, the anastomosing vascular channels seen in tissue sections are missing in cytologic smears. This particular image from an aspirate of a pleura-based mass shows predominantly epithelioid malignant cells accompanied by a mixed inflammatory infiltrate. Typical of most sarcomas, the smeared cells have a dual single cell and clustered distribution on the slide.

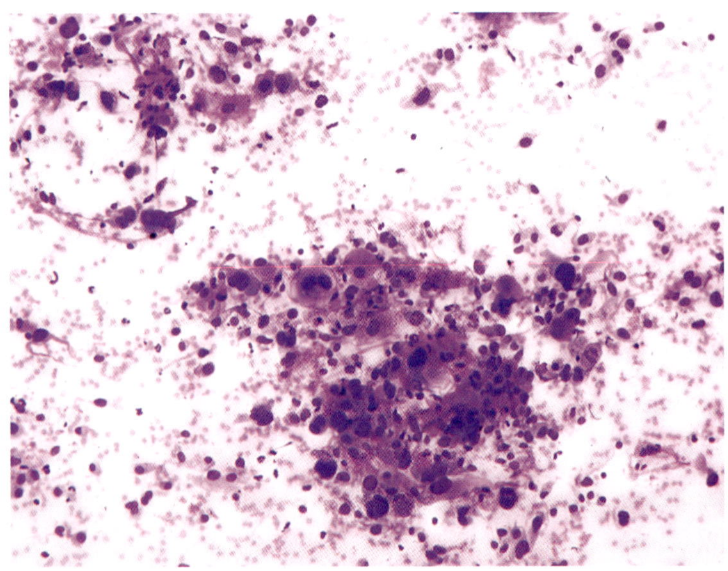

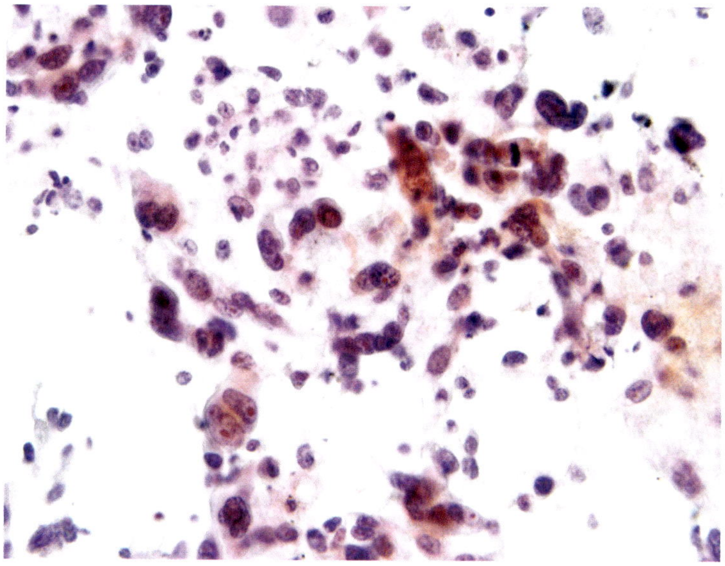

Figure 7.15b — Pleural Angiosarcoma, Fine Needle Aspiration [Pap Stain; High Power]. Single and multinucleated malignant cells are loosely gathered together in this image. Closer inspection highlights the marked nuclear pleomorphism and membrane irregularity, open vesicular dispersion of nucleoplasm, and presence of markedly enlarged nucleoli. Intranuclear cytoplasmic pseudoinclusions and cytoplasmic emperipolesis by inflammatory cells can also be seen, but are not specific features of AngioS. Immunophenotyping for endothelial differentiation is relatively specific nowadays. Positive staining using antibodies to both CD31 and ERG are the most reliable combination, but CD34, WT 1, and FLI-1 are also positive in a high percentage of vascular neoplasms. It must be remembered that pan-cytokeratin staining is positive in a high percentage of AngioS, particularly those with epithelioid morphology. Survival for individuals with primary or metastatic pulmonary or pleural AngioS is usually measured in months.

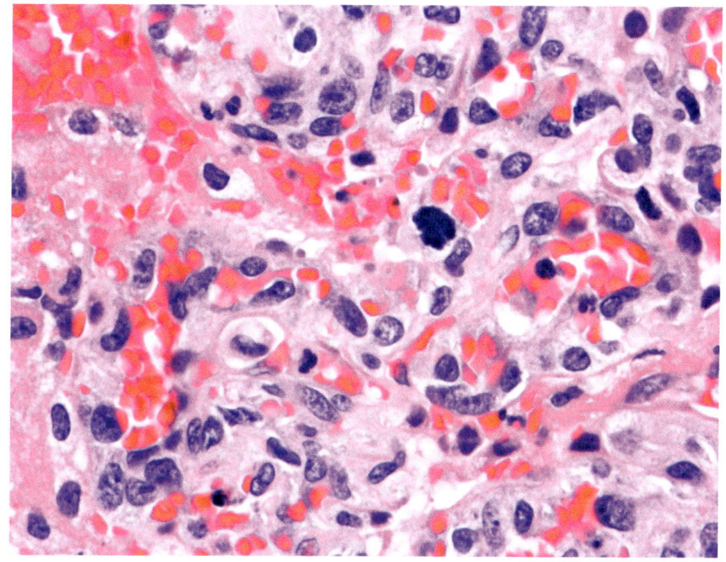

Figure 7.15c — Angiosarcoma, Resection [H&E Stain; Low Power]. At low power, this angiosarcoma shows aggregates of red blood cells and fibrin, with admixed islands of hyperchromatic spindle cells, features suggestive of acute and organizing alveolar hemorrhage with reactive changes. However, by imaging, this large mass lesion involved the chest wall as well as the lung parenchyma. Consolidation and mass effect are often associated with angiosarcoma, although it is believed to arise from subpleural mesenchyme, and is therefore classified by the World Health Organization with the pleural tumors.

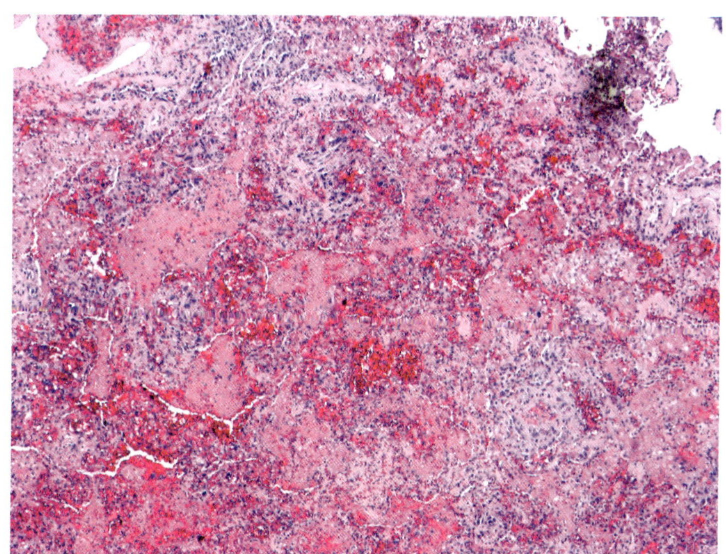

Figure 7.15d — Angiosarcoma, Resection [H&E Stain; High Power]. Higher magnification reveals marked pleomorphism, frequent mitoses, and large metachromatic nucleoli. There are multiple small vascular spaces filled with red cells, and some tumor cells contain intracytoplasmic red cells. Metastatic angiosarcoma has similar features, and must be excluded by history and imaging.

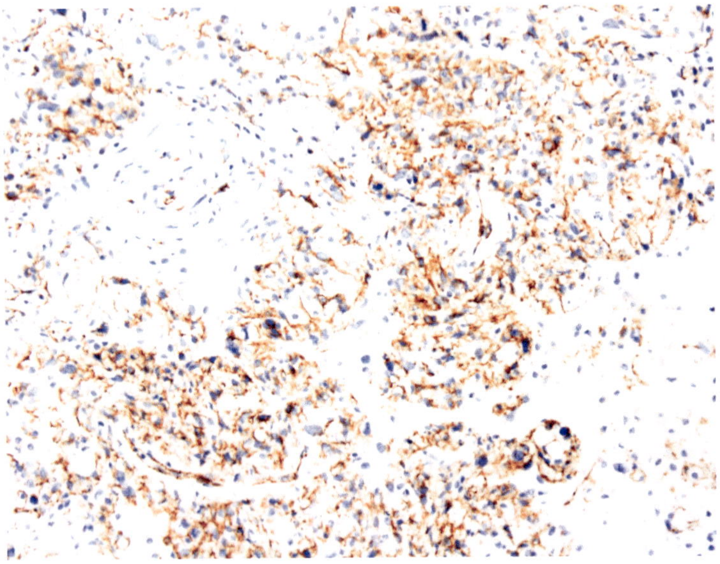

Figure 7.15e — Angiosarcoma, Resection [CD31 Immunohistochemical Stain; Low Power]. An immunostain for CD31 shows strong and uniform cytoplasmic expression in the nests of cells between the areas of hemorrhage. CD34 is also routinely expressed, with a similar pattern.

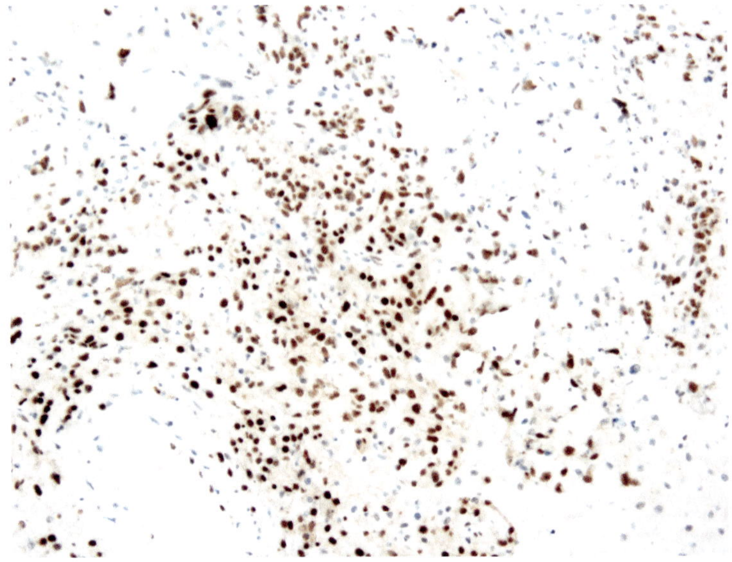

Figure 7.15f — Angiosarcoma, Resection [ERG Immunohistochemical Stain; Low Power]. This tumor shows the characteristic strong and uniform staining for ERG. The nuclei of angiosarcoma are positive for ERG in greater than 95% of cases, making ERG the most sensitive marker for endothelial differentiation currently in use; it is also relatively specific. Some angiosarcomas show patchy keratin expression, a potential pitfall in a small biopsy.

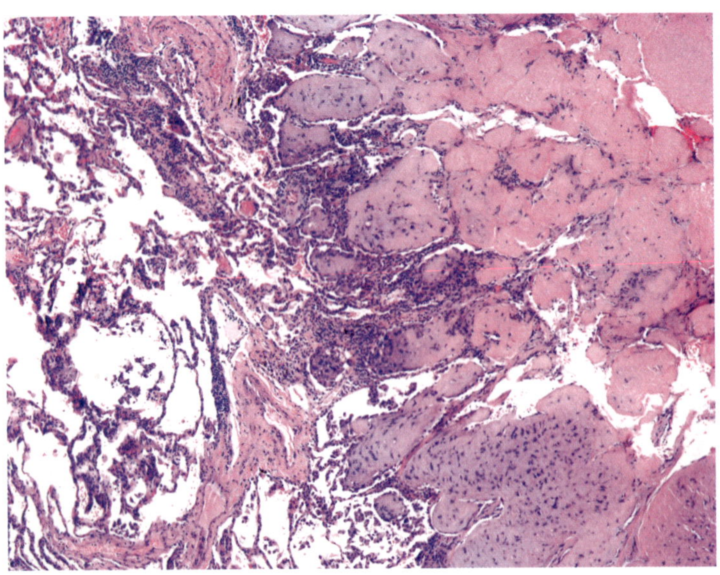

Figure 7.16a — Epithelioid Hemangioendothelioma, Biopsy [H&E Stain; Low Power]. This tumor is characteristically intraparenchymal and peripheral, with lobulated/nodular architecture that is intra-alveolar at the periphery. Individual nodules are round to oval, with sclerotic centers and increased cellularity at the edges. Tumors that extend to the pleura and elicit reactive pleural thickening may be confused with malignant mesothelioma. The low power features may also mimic old granulomatous disease, organizing infarct, amyloidoma (Congo red-positive), or nonspecific subpleural scarring, all of which lack nuclear atypia on high power.

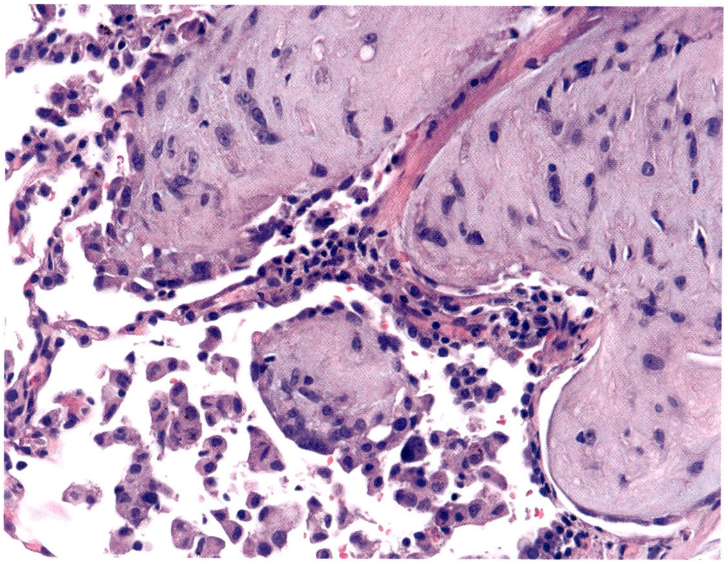

Figure 7.16b — Epithelioid Hemangioendothelioma, Biopsy [H&E Stain; High Power]. The neoplastic cells show mild to moderate nuclear atypia and are embedded as strands, solid nests, and single cells in the eosinophilic stroma. An intracytoplasmic lumen is present (top center); elsewhere, some of these lumina contained red blood cells. Alternative stromal patterns include chondroid, myxomatous, and mucinous, and calcification and ossification are sometimes present. The differential diagnosis is broad, and positive stains for CD31, CD34, and FLI-1/ERG are crucial in identifying this lesion and distinguishing it from a broad range of benign and malignant mimics (hamartoma, sclerosing pneumocytoma, mucinous adenocarcinoma, malignant mesothelioma, angiosarcoma). A characteristic fusion gene associated with epithelioid hemangioendothelioma (*WWTR1-CAMTA1*) has been demonstrated.

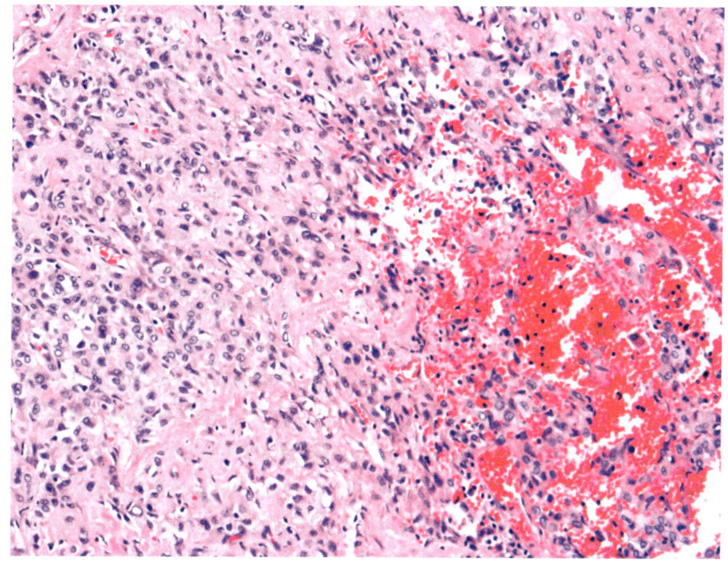

Figure 7.17a — Sclerosing Pneumocytoma, Resection [H&E Stain; Low Power]. This field shows three of the four patterns observed in sclerosing pneumocytoma: solid growth at the upper left, sclerotic at the lower left, and hemorrhagic at the right. Elsewhere, a pseudopapillary pattern was also present. This benign neoplasm, classified in the "Adenomas" category in the World Health Organization system, is derived from pneumocytes, and most often presents as a solitary circumscribed mass in a middle-aged woman. Given its rarity, mixed growth patterns, and moderate cellular pleomorphism, sclerosing pneumocytoma is a close histologic and immunohistochemical mimic of adenocarcinoma, and probably cannot be diagnosed with certainty on a small biopsy.

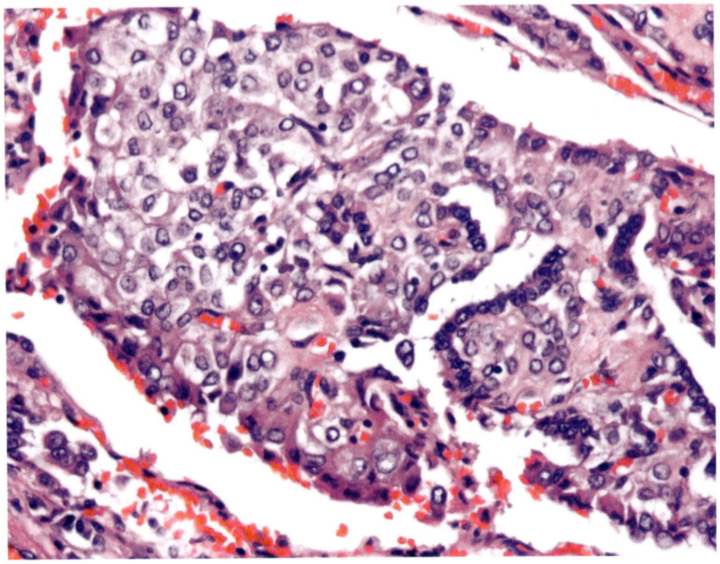

Figure 7.17b — Sclerosing Pneumocytoma, Resection [H&E Stain; High Power]. This pseudopapilla lacks a fibrovascular core; instead, it is composed of the dual cell population that characterizes sclerosing pneumocytoma: cuboidal surface cells and stromal round cells, both neoplastic. The cuboidal cells have morphologic features of reactive type II pneumocytes, including apical snouts, small punctate nucleoli, and occasional intranuclear pseudoinclusions. The underlying round cells have vacuolated cytoplasm with well-defined borders; the nuclei have finely granular chromatin, with inapparent nucleoli.

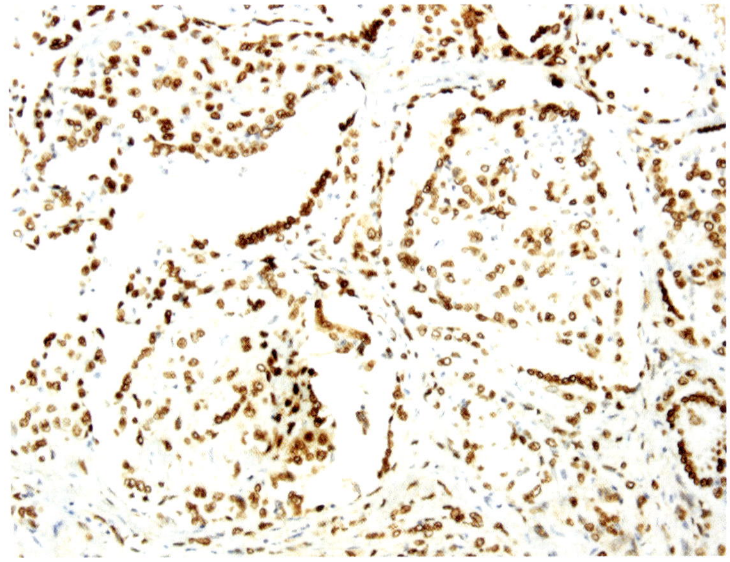

Figure 7.17c — Sclerosing Pneumocytoma, Resection [TTF-1 Immunohistochemical Stain; Low Power]. An immunostain for TTF-1 confirms the pneumocytic phenotype of both the surface cells and the round cells. The surface cuboidal cells typically express TTF-1, pan-cytokeratin, CAM5.2, EMA, CK7, napsin A, and surfactant markers. The round cells express TTF-1 and EMA, and are only focally positive for CAM5.2 and CK7; they are usually negative for pan-cytokeratin; surfactant markers are negative, and napsin may be weakly positive or negative.

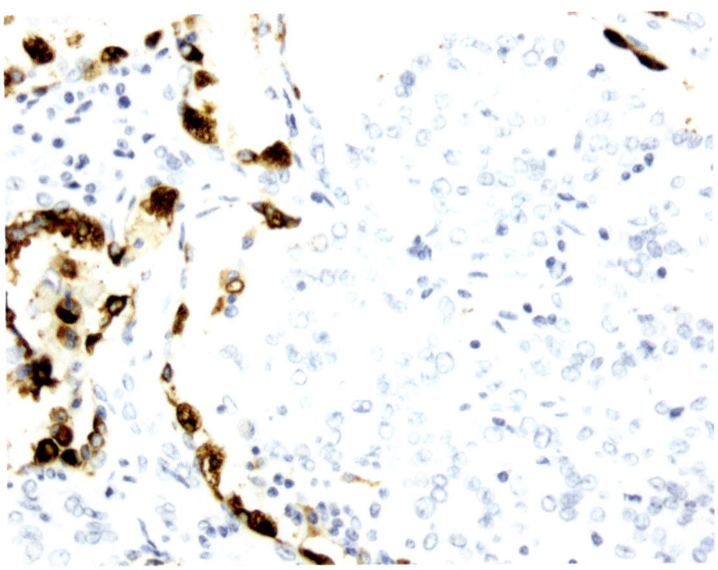

Figure 7.17d — Sclerosing Pneumocytoma, Resection [Napsin A Immunohistochemical Stain; High Power]. This stain for napsin A shows differential staining of the two cell populations in sclerosing pneumocytoma:The cuboidal cells are strongly positive, while the round cells are negative. Prior to the general availability of immunohistochemical staining, the presence of blood lakes led to the conclusion that this was a vascular neoplasm, hence the now-obsolete name "sclerosing hemangioma." Immunostains for vascular markers (ERG, CD31, CD34, factor VIII) are routinely negative.

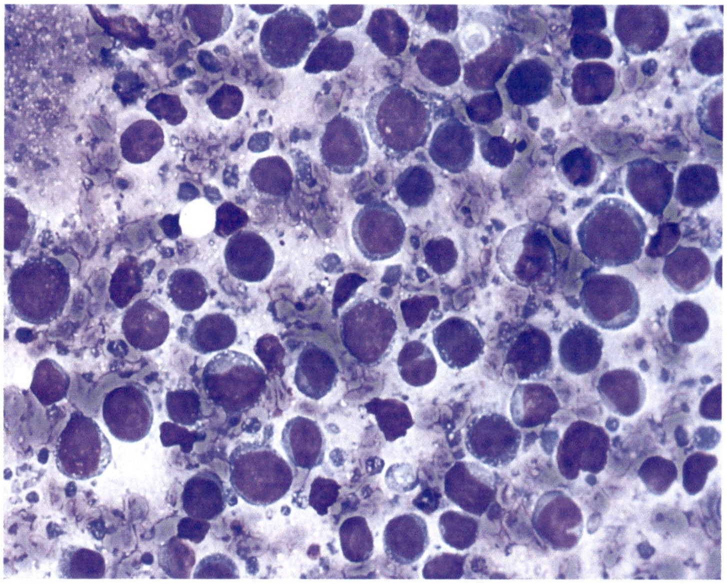

Figure 7.18a — Large Cell Lymphoma, Fine Needle Aspiration [Diff-Quik Stain; High Power]. Primary non-Hodgkin lymphoma of the lung is rare, but secondary involvement is not uncommon, being encountered in about a quater of non-Hodgkin lymphoma cases. The majority of primary pulmonary non-Hodgkin lymphomas are examples of extranodal marginal zone lymphoma, a small cell low-grade neoplasm. However, most cytopathology specimens of pulmonary non-Hodgkin lymphoma are those of diffuse large B-cell lymphoma (DLBL), of which this image is an example. Typical of all forms of non-Hodgkin lymphoma, smears are hypercellular. They display a singly dispersed (dissociated) population of more or less monotonous large lymphocytes. These show smooth nuclear outlines with occasional nuclear clefts, coarse chromatin, one or more visible nucleoli, and a minimal amount of deep blue cytoplasm. Occasional cells contain cytoplasmic vacuoles. Innumerable bluish cytoplasmic fragments (so-called "lymphoglandular bodies") are seen and are a key cytologic feature of all lymphoid lesions–benign and malignant.

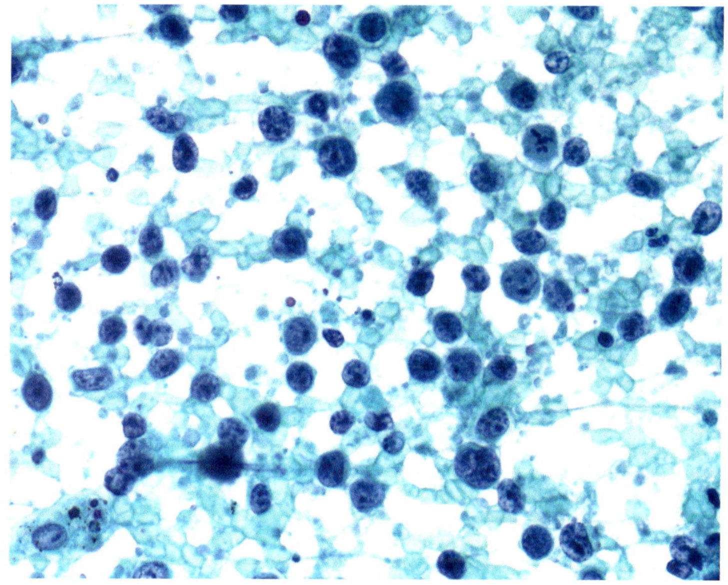

Figure 7.18b — Large Cell Lymphoma, Fine Needle Aspiration [Pap Stain; High Power]. This Papanicolaou stain highlights nuclear detail of lymphocytes with coarse irregular chronic clumping. However, unlike Romanowsky-stained smears, the lymphoglandular bodies are often obscured by the intact red cells as in this image. A tingible-body macrophage (TBM) is at the extreme lower left. TBMs are not uncommon in high-grade non-Hodgkin lymphomas, and are not a guarantee of a benign reactive lymphoid population. Because this image resembles that of a malignant small rounded cell neoplasm, nonlymphoid neoplasms of the lung, such as small cell neuroendocrine carcinoma, melanoma, and even sarcoma, need to be excluded. Aspirates and broncoalveolar lavage specimens of pulmonary non-Hodgkin lymphoma lend themselves easily to immunophenotyping by flow cytometry analysis for definitive diagnosis.

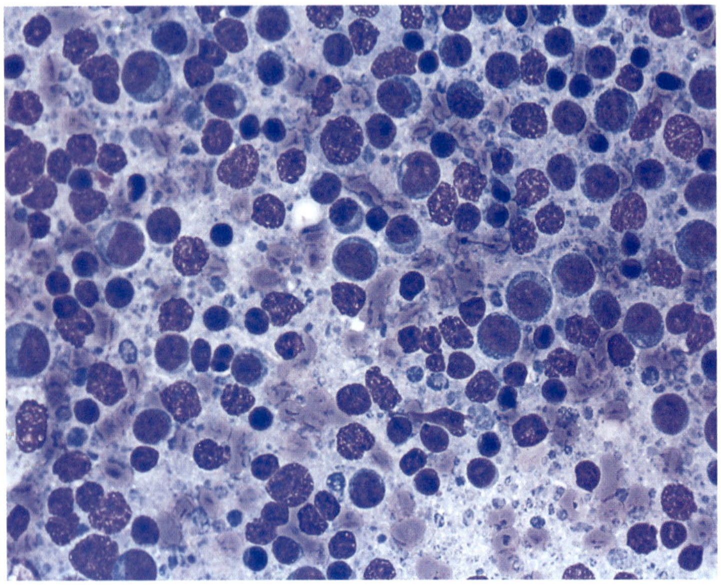

Figure 7.18c — Large Cell Lymphoma, Fine Needle Aspiration [Diff-Quik Stain; High Power]. This image of large cell lymphoma has a greater degree of polymorphism. Although large lymphocytes seem to predominate, enough of a cytologic spectrum composed of small lymphocytes and plasmacytoid lymphocytes is present to mimic a benign process. Because background lymphoglandular bodies are so numerous, a nonlymphoid lesion is largely excluded. Without ancillary testing such as flow cytometry, however, this image could be mistaken easily for a reactive lymphoid condition. Transplant patients are prone to develop posttransplant lymphoproliferative disorder that can be morphologically identical to pulmonary large cell non-Hodgkin lymphoma. Thus, the clinical context of the patient must be considered, and in posttransplant patients testing for Epstein–Barr virus is warranted.

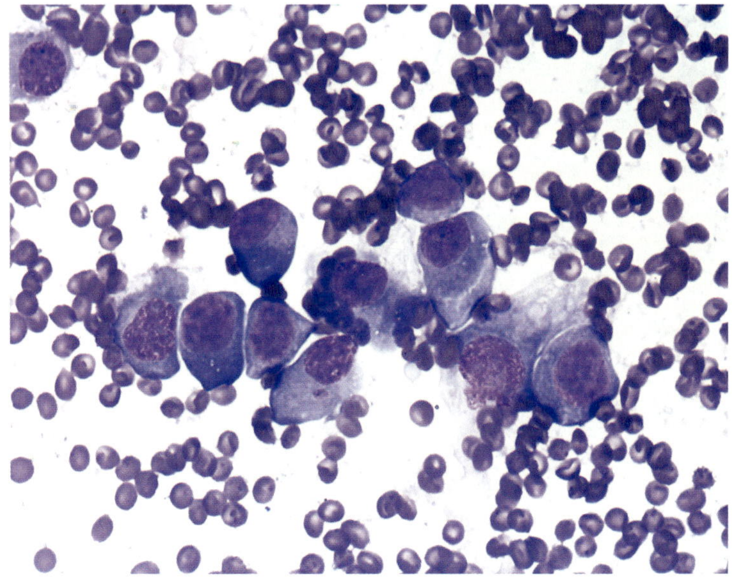

Figure 7.19 — Plasma Cell Myeloma, Fine Needle Aspiration [Diff-Quik Stain; High Power]. Involvement of the lung by plasma cell neoplasia is most often encountered in patients with known multiple myeloma as part of their systemic disease. Primary plasma cell myeloma (plasmacytoma) is rare. In patients with multiple myeloma, the radiologic appearance may be of a diffuse infiltrate, or, more commonly, multiple pulmonary nodules. The large plasmablastic cells in this image show eccentric placement of cell nuclei and enlarged, coarsely granular nuclei, but no perinuclear cytoplasmic hof. Large B-cell lymphoma with plasmacytoid differentiation may appear similar. Thus, definitive diagnosis can be achieved by demonstrating monotypic cytoplasmic immunoglobulin and immunohistochemical expression of CD138, VS38c, and CD38.

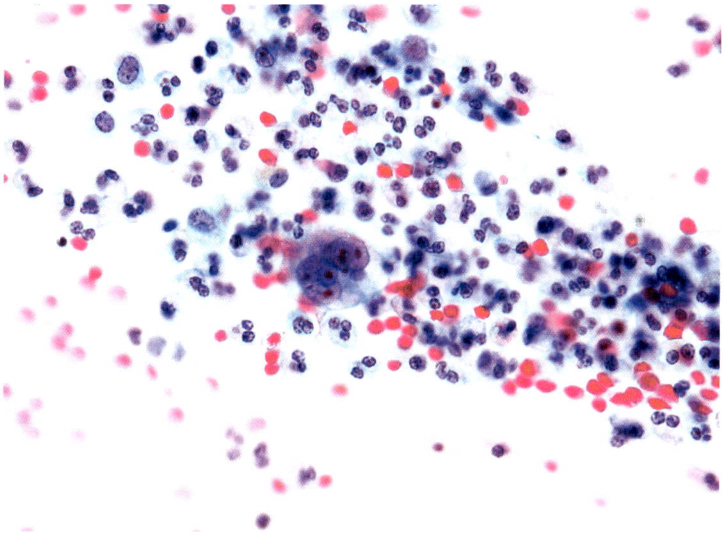

Figure 7.20a — Hodgkin Lymphoma, Fine Needle Aspiration [Pap Stain; High Power]. Hodgkin lymphoma is rarely found on fine needle aspiration of lung lesions. Here, a single yet highly atypical Reed-Sternberg cell is seen among mixed inflammatory cells. The cell is multinucleated and contains multiple prominent nucleoli. These individual cells are easily missed among the numerous inflammatory cells; if seen, they may be mistaken for a poorly differentiated carcinoma or atypical-appearing multinucleated giant cell.

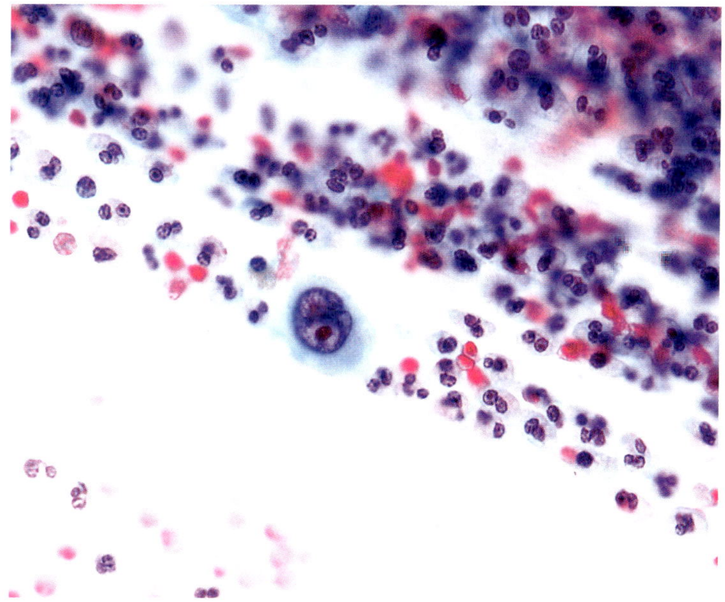

Figure 7.20b — Hodgkin Lymphoma, Fine Needle Aspiration [Pap Stain; High Power]. A single Reed-Sternberg is seen with its classic appearance, a binucleated large cell with two prominent nucleoli and abundant cytoplasm. The two nuclei appear to be mirror images of one another. This appearance may also be seen with a metastatic melanoma, though the presence of rare atypical cells in a background of mixed inflammation should always suggest consideration of Hodgkin lymphoma.

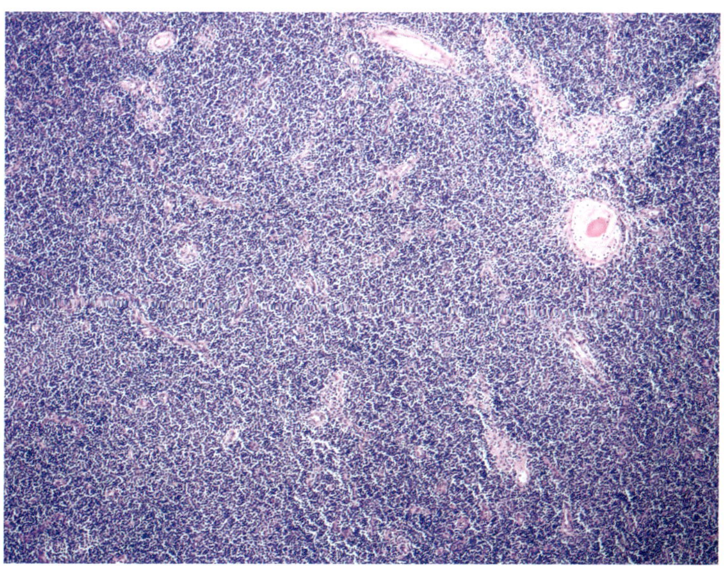

Figure 7.21a — Chronic Lymphocytic Leukemia/Small Lymphocytic Lymphoma, Level 4 Lymph Node Dissection [H&E Stain; Low Power]. This 1.6-cm lymph node from level 4 was one of numerous large nodes dissected at multiple levels during a lung cancer resection. The node is negative for carcinoma, but the normal follicular architecture is absent at low power. Lymph node dissections that generate larger and/or more numerous nodes than usual should raise suspicion for involvement by a small lymphocytic neoplasm, which may or may not have been previously diagnosed.

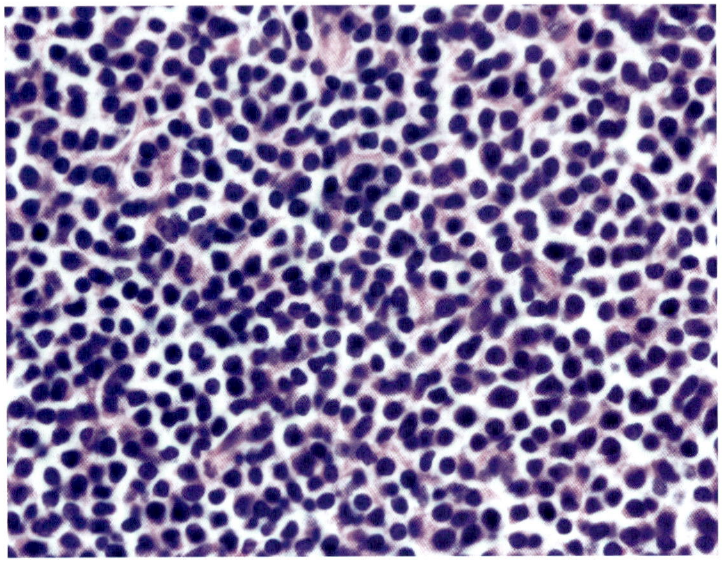

Figure 7.21b — Chronic Lymphocytic Leukemia / Small Lymphocytic Lymphoma, Level 4 Lymph Node Dissection [H&E Stain; High Power]. A uniform population of small lymphocytes replaces the usual mix of lymphocytes, plasma cells, and pigment-laden histiocytes that comprise the normal/reactive follicular elements of a mediastinal node.

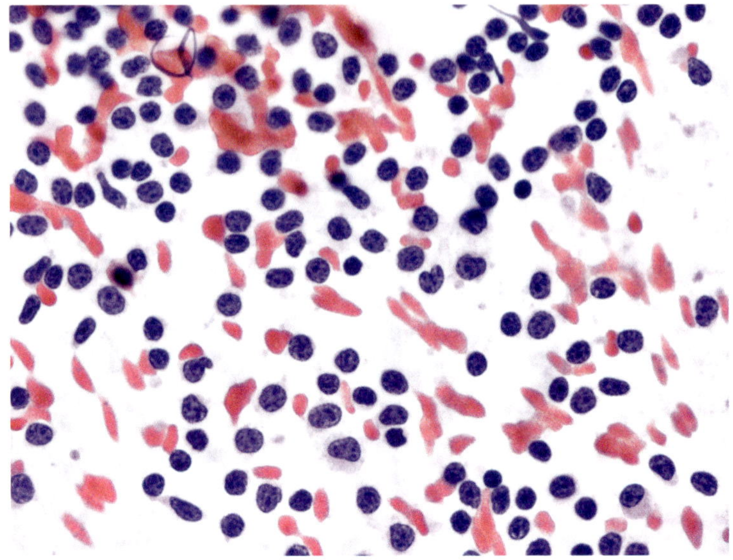

Figure 7.22a — Mucosa-Associated Lymphoid Tissue Lymphoma, Fine Needle Aspiration [Pap Stain; Medium Power]. The field contains numerous small cells with a narrow rim of cytoplasm, nuclear border irregularities, and coarse chromatin. Small lymphomas are challenging to identify by cytomorphology alone, as a monotonous population of lymphoma cells may be intermixed with a polymorphous population of benign lymphoid cells. Furthermore, many small lymphomas do not necessarily appear monotonous. One must prove clonality within the population, through molecular studies, flow cytometry, and/or immunohistochemistry.

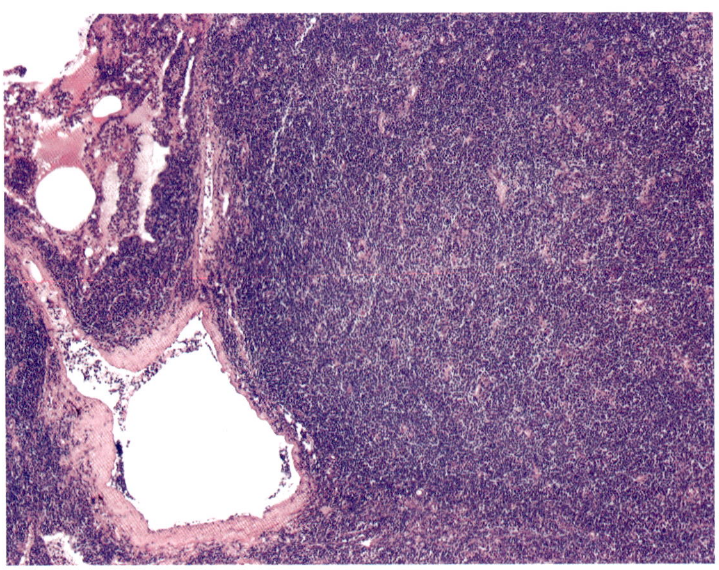

Figure 7.22b — Marginal Zone Lymphoma of Mucosa-Associated Lymphoid Tissue, Biopsy [H&E Stain; Low Power]. "MALToma" is a B-cell neoplasm, characterized by a diffuse and vaguely nodular neoplastic lymphoid infiltrate associated with bronchovascular bundles. The tumor effaces lung architecture and extends into distal air spaces. Foci of residual reactive follicles of bronchus associated lymphoid tissue may be associated. At low power, small cell carcinoma and metastatic small blue cell tumors enter the differential.

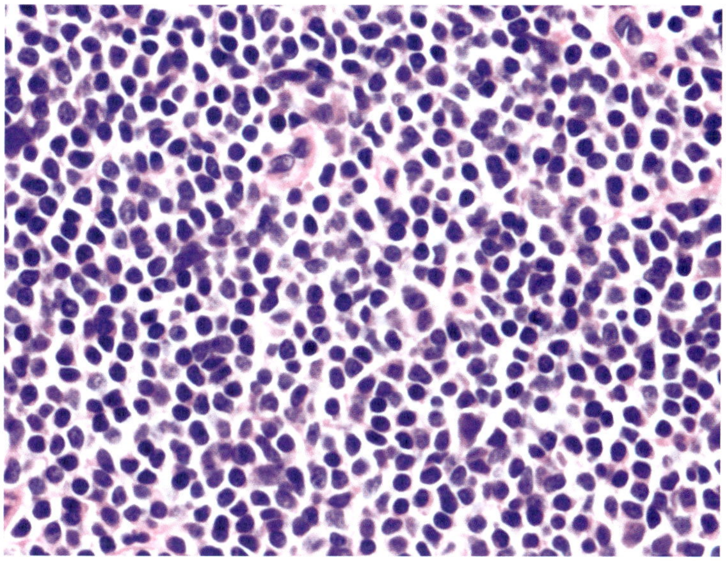

Figure 7.22c — Marginal Zone Lymphoma of Mucosa-Associated Lymphoid Tissue, Biopsy [H&E Stain; High Power]. Mucosa-associated lymphoid tissue lymphoma is composed of small lymphoid cells with condensed chromatin, irregular nuclei, indistinct nucleoli, and a variable amount of pale cytoplasm. Admixed are few scattered larger cells with round nuclei, vesicular chromatin, and prominent nucleoli. There is no necrosis, and mitoses are not present. Flow cytometry or immunohistochemical staining typically shows expression of CD20 and bcl-2, with negative stains for CD5 and CD10. Inclusion of a keratin stain on an initial panel will allow exclusion of small cell carcinoma.

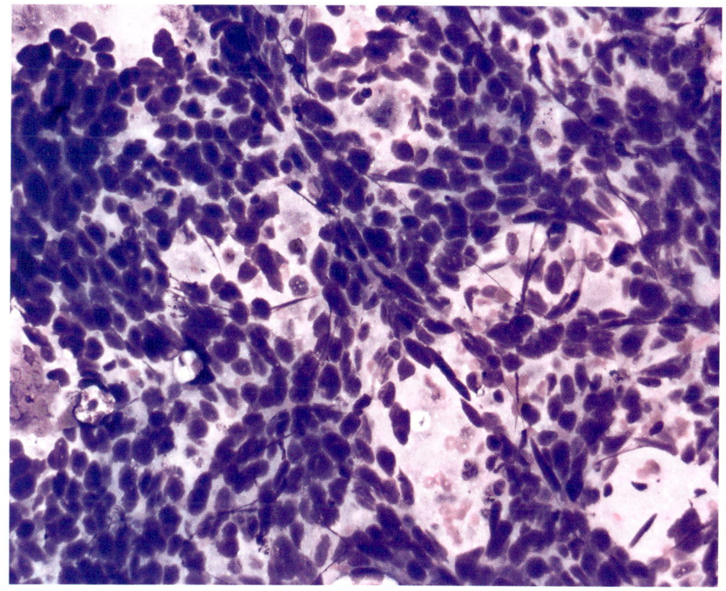

Figure 7.23a — Metastatic Alveolar Rhabdomyosarcoma, Fine Needle Aspiration [Diff-Quik Stain; Medium Power]. This fine needle aspirate is composed of a uniform population of small, blue cells. The cells are primarily plump and vaguely epithelioid, with a hint of a fine, pale blue cytoplasm (best seen to the left). The cells are arranged in sheets with gaps and spaces opening up between the cells. Occasional mitotic figures and apoptotic bodies are seen. The differential diagnosis is broad for such a small round blue cell tumor; this example is of a metastatic alveolar rhabdomyosarcoma. Alveolar rhabdomyosarcomas are characterized by translocations involving FOXO1 and PAX3 or PAX7.

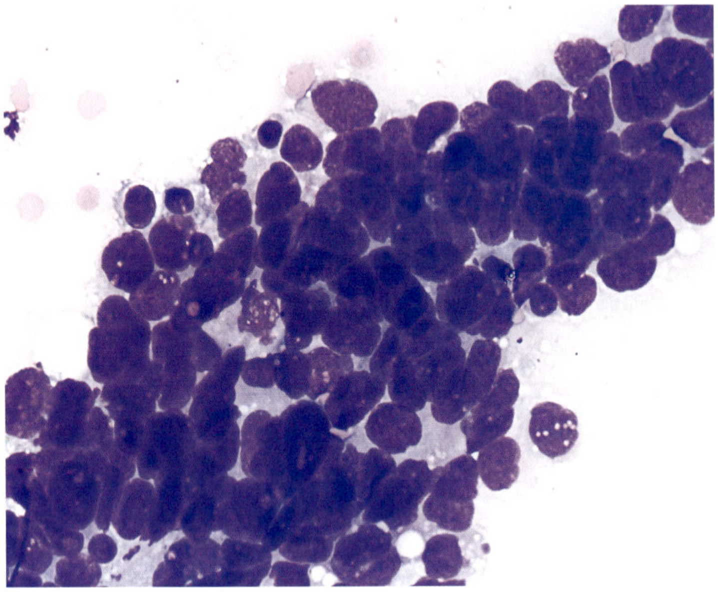

Figure 7.23b — Metastatic Alveolar Rhabdomyosarcoma, Fine Needle Aspiration [Diff-Quik Stain; High Power]. At higher magnification, the cells of metastatic alveolar rhabdomyosarcoma are clustered, primitive-appearing cells with scant eccentric blue cytoplasm visible in a few cells. The chromatin pattern is fine with small nucleoli present. Alveolar rhabdomyosarcoma may be difficult to diagnosis without immunohistochemistry, but does express markers of muscle differentiation (desmin, myogenin, myo-D1) and can also express neuroendocrine markers.

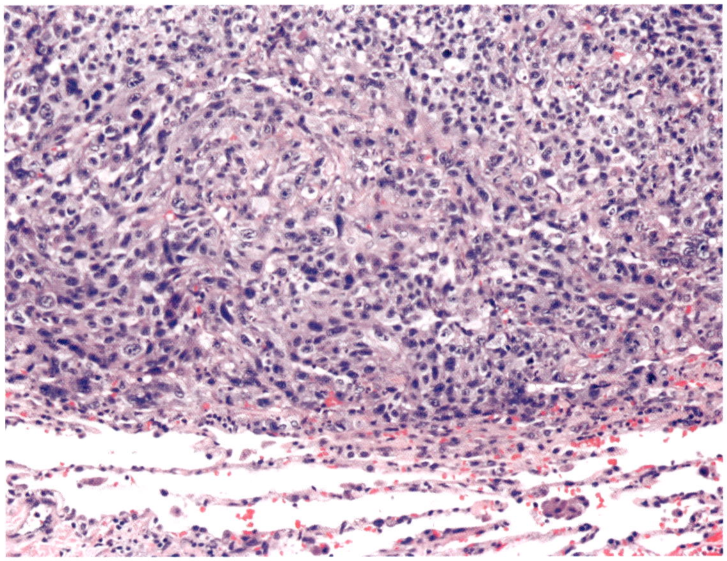

Figure 7.24a — Metastatic Embryonal Rhadomyosarcoma, Resection [H&E Stain; Low Power]. This high-grade "blue cell" tumor metastasis has a sharp border with the lung parenchyma, and lacks an organized growth pattern. Most often, there is a known history of rhabdomyosarcoma, and comparison with the original tumor is often helpful. However, chemotherapy or subclone development may alter the cytology, in which case immunohistochemical stains are useful in confirming muscle differentiation (myo-D1, desmin, myogenin). In alveolar rhabdomyosarcoma, identification of the characteristic t(2;13) or t(1;13) translocation can be useful in confirming the diagnosis.

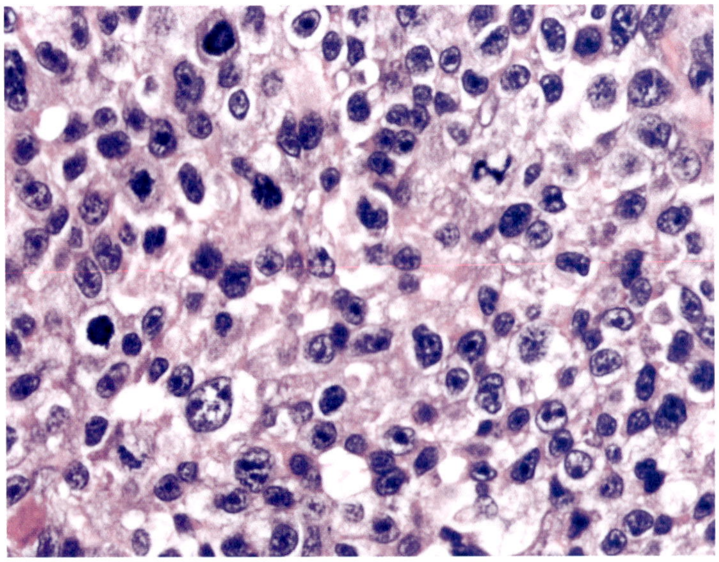

Figure 7.24b — Metastatic Embryonal Rhabdomyosarcoma, Resection [H&E Stain; High Power]. The sarcoma cells have a variable amount of eosinophilic to clear cytoplasm. The nuclei are highly pleomorphic, with frequent prominent nucleoli. Three mitoses are present. In some undifferentiated cases, lymphoma may enter the differential diagnosis, and can be excluded with immunohistochemical stains for lymphoid antigens (CD45, CD3, CD20, PAX5).

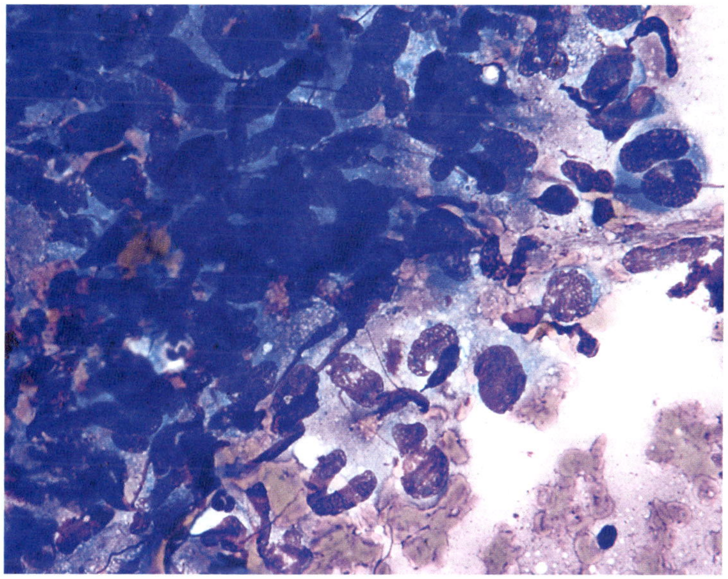

Figure 7.25a — Metastatic Leiomyosarcoma, Fine Needle Aspiration [Diff-Quik Stain; High Power]. Large, pleomorphic cells predominate, with a suggestion of spindle morphology in the upper left. The cells have large, irregular nuclei, multiple nucleoli, blue cytoplasm, and a bloody background. A few binucleate cells are present. The lung is the most frequent site for metastasis of leiomyosarcoma.

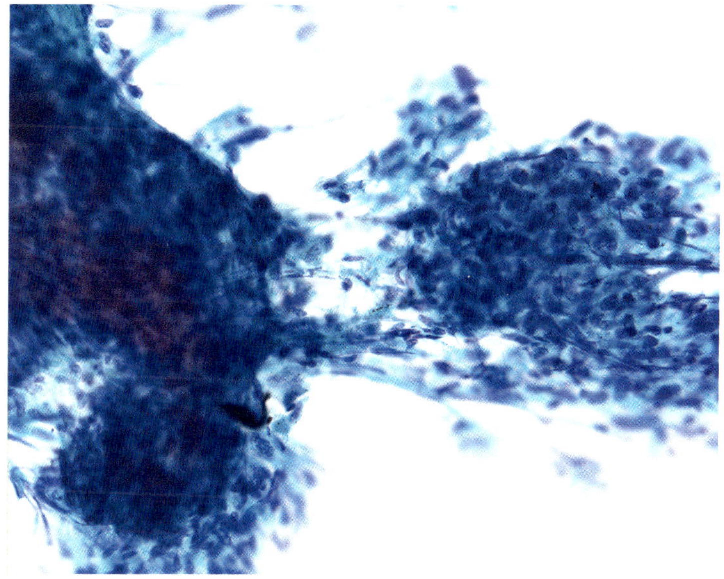

Figure 7.25b — Metastatic Leiomyosarcoma, Fine Needle Aspiration [Pap Stain; Medium Power]. In this Pap-stained aspirate, a spindle cell morphology is more evident, and a suggestion of a fascicular pattern is seen at the left side of this microscopic field. The cells have the same large nuclei and nucleoli, and irregular shapes with binucleated cells are also noted. Leiomyosarcomas may originate in the uterus, or in other soft tissue sites, including within vessels.

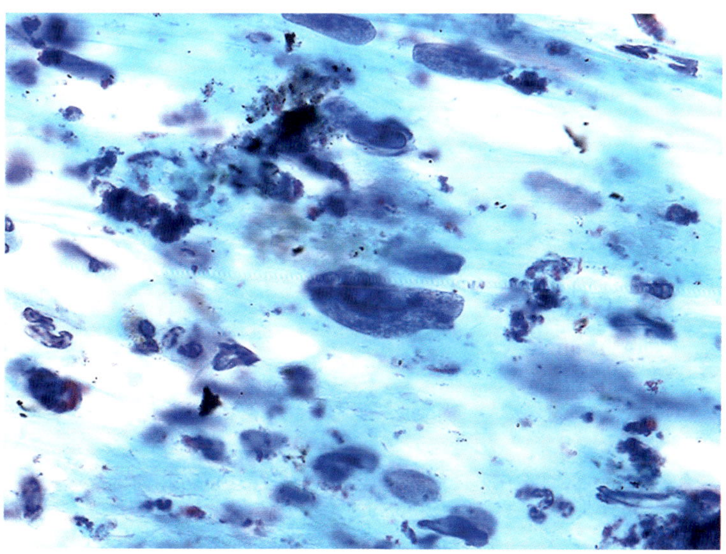

Figure 7.25c — Metastatic Leiomyosarcoma, Fine Needle Aspiration [Pap Stain; High Power]. At high power, hyperchromasia and pleomorphism in the spindled nuclei are readily apparent, as well as inflammatory debris. Uterine leiomyosarcomas are aggressive tumors prone to recurrence and metastasis, even when seemingly confined to the uterus initially.

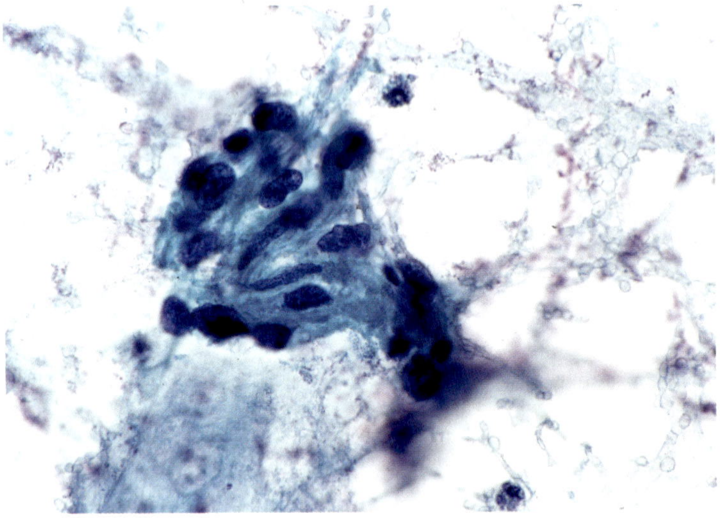

Figure 7.26a — Metastatic Leiomyosarcoma, Fine Needle Aspiration [Pap Stain; High Power]. This small fragment contains cells with pleomorphic, spindled nuclei with dark chromatin and markedly irregular nuclear borders. The cells have elongated shapes but the cytoplasm is otherwise nondescript. The cytomorphological features suggest malignancy, and thus the spindled nature indicates this is either a sarcoma or a sarcomatoid carcinoma. However, in the absence of a history of malignancy, further studies such as molecular testing or immunohistochemistry are required to provide a more definitive diagnosis.

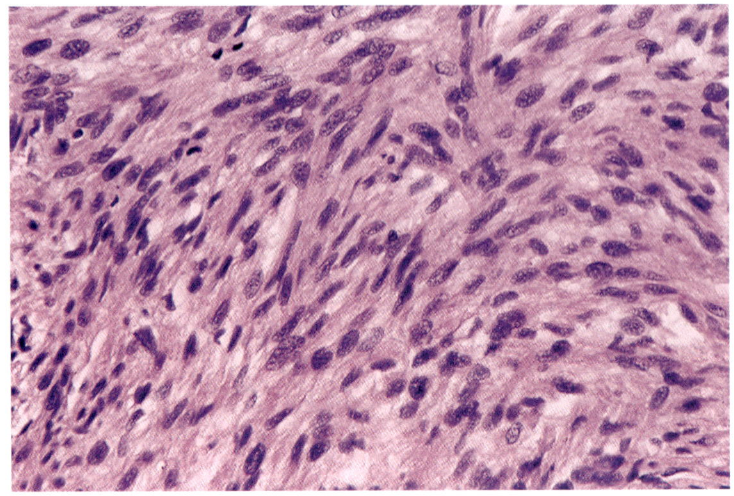

Figure 7.26b — Metastatic Leiomyosarcoma, Fine Needle Aspiration [H&E Stain; High Power]. Spindled cells form streaming and interweaving fascicles; the nuclei are elongated and cigar-shaped due to the rounded tips. The cytoplasmic borders are indistinct, but in some instances a perinuclear vacuole can be identified, which further suggests smooth muscle differentiation. While leiomyosarcoma is one of the more common sarcomas primary to the lung, this patient had a metastatic leiomyosarcoma to the lung from a leg primary.

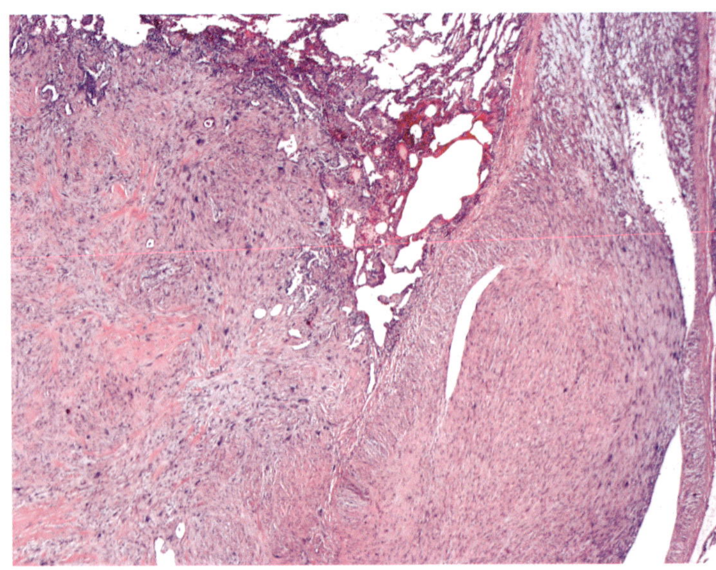

Figure 7.27a — Metastatic Leiomyosarcoma, Resection [H&E Stain; Low Power]. This metastasis from a leiomyosarcoma of soft tissue has a characteristically circumscribed border (top); pleomorphism can be appreciated even at low power. Metastases arrive in the lung most commonly by lymphatic channels or in the systemic venous return and pulmonary arteries; this image shows the likely source artery, to the right of the lesion, with intraluminal and intramural tumor associated with an intimal reaction.

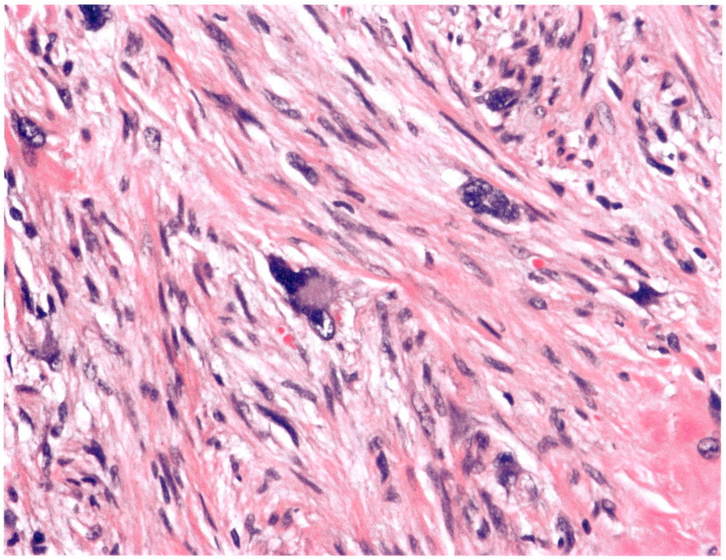

Figure 7.27b — Metastatic Leiomyosarcoma, Resection [H&E Stain; High Power]. The spindle cells are present in fascicles, with several large atypical cells. Metastases are typically multiple, bilateral, and peripheral, but may be solitary, and are sometimes quite large. In the setting of a documented prior primary sarcoma with similar features, such metastases can be diagnosed on H&E alone. In the absence of such a history, differential considerations include primary or metastatic synovial sarcoma (EMA and CAM 5.2+; CD99 and bcl-2+; fusion of SS18 to SSX1 or SSX2) and sarcomatoid carcinoma (keratin +), as well as metastatic spindle cell melanoma (S100+, desmin and actin-).

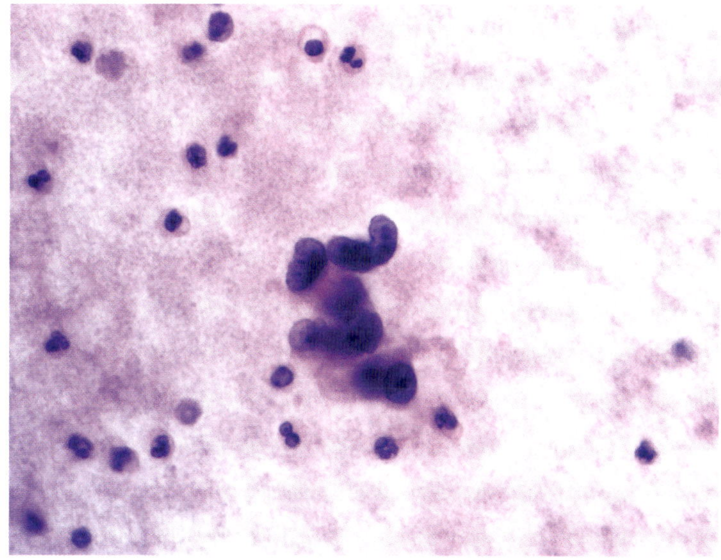

Figure 7.28 — Metastatic Endometrial Stromal Sarcoma, Biopsy Touch Prep [H&E Stain; High Power]. Endometrial stromal sarcoma is an uncommon spindle cell malignancy arising from the endometrial stroma. Without a patient history, it would be difficult to include this entity on an initial differential diagnosis. Here, the nuclei are hyperchromatic and dark, with coarse chromatin and nuclear border irregularities. The malignant cells are often positive for CD10.

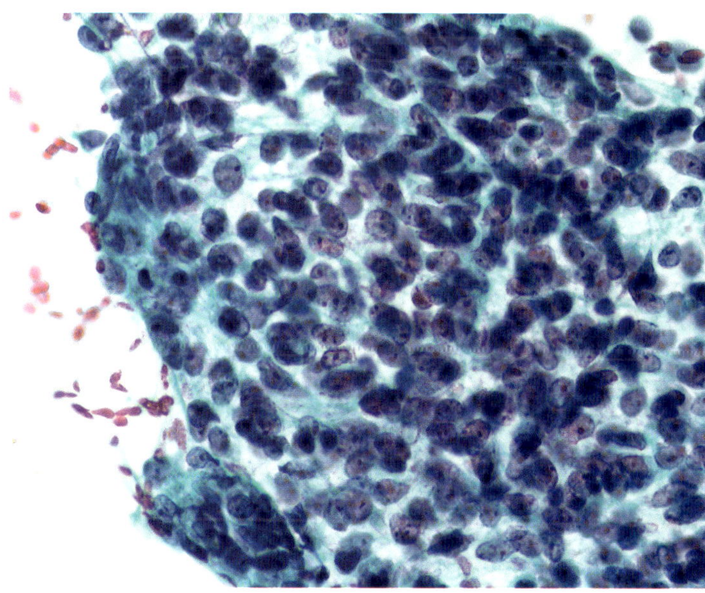

Figure 7.29a — Metastatic Synovial Sarcoma, Fine Needle Aspiration [Pap Stain; High Power]. The tumor cells in this metastatic synovial sarcoma are uniform, spindled, and arranged in whorls and bundles. No epithelial component is visible in this fragment. The cell borders are indistinct, and the nuclei have uneven contours and conspicuous, often multiple nucleoli. Synovial sarcoma typically begins as a soft tissue mass in young adults. The tumors have a biphasic or monophasic appearance, given the presence or absence of an epithelial component.

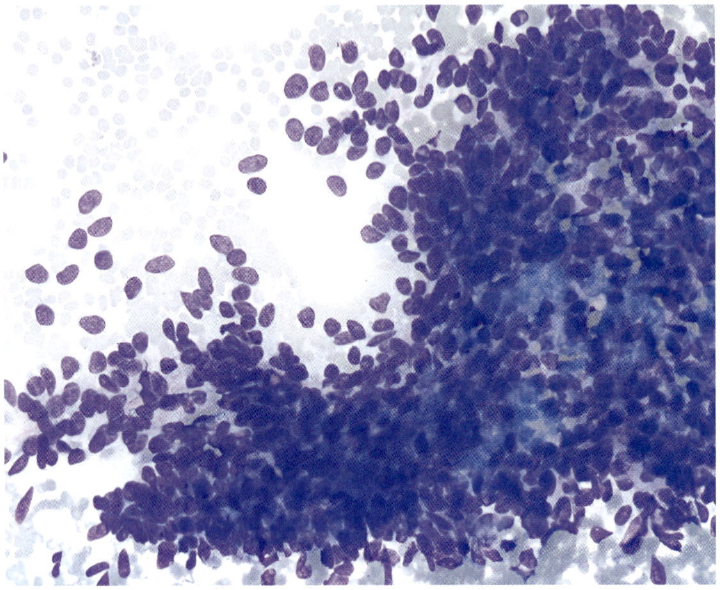

Figure 7.29b — Metastatic Synovial Sarcoma, Fine Needle Aspiration [Diff-Quik Stain; Medium Power]. Diff-Quik staining of a synovial sarcoma shows the spindle cells arranged in bundles. The cells reveal the same indistinct borders and faint, wispy cytoplasm with multiple bare or nearly-bare nuclei at the edge. Synovial sarcoma is a translocation-associated sarcoma with a t(X;18) translocation involving the SYT-SSX1 or SSX2 genes detectable in most cases.

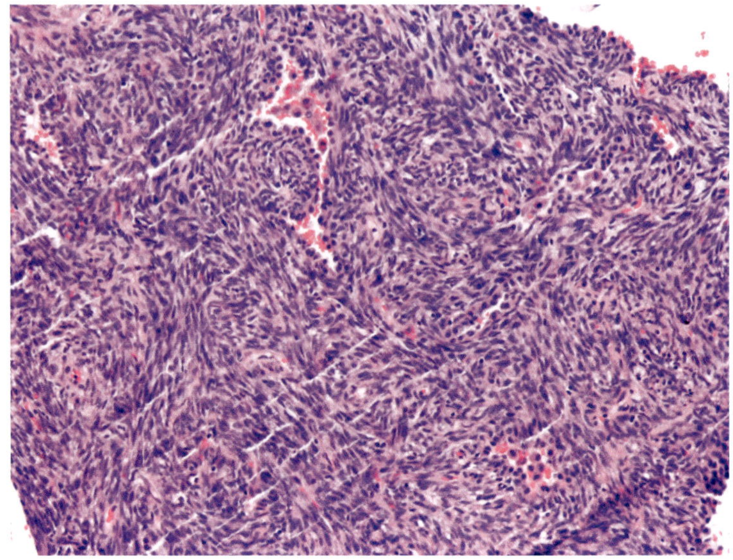

Figure 7.29c — Metastatic Synovial Sarcoma, Biopsy [H&E Stain; Low Power]. The spindle cells of synovial sarcoma are arranged in plump interlacing fascicles or in lobulated nests. The low power appearance of this lesion is monophasic and spindled. The vasculature has a "stag-horn" pattern, a feature synovial sarcoma shares with solitary fibrous tumor. Metastatic synovial sarcoma in the lung is more common than primary pulmonary synovial sarcoma, but the two are morphologically, immunohistochemically, and genetically indistinguishable.

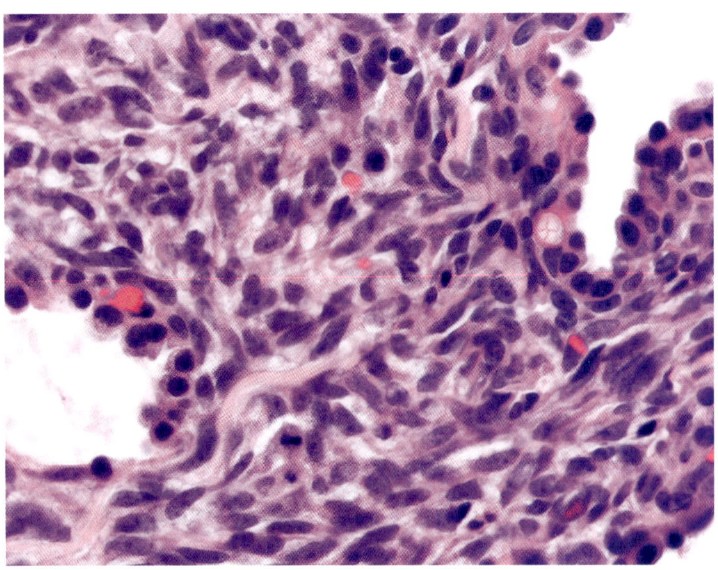

Figure 7.29d — Metastatic Synovial Sarcoma, Biopsy [H&E Stain; High Power]. This field shows the neoplastic spindle cells expanding the pulmonary interstitium; residual alveolar epithelial cells line the open spaces. A mitotic figure is present at the lower left. CK8/18 is positive, at least focally, in most cases, and detection of the t(X;18) translocation with SS18-SSX1 or SSX2 fusion is important in establishing the diagnosis. Differential considerations include primary and metastatic sarcomas, as well as sarcomatoid carcinoma (keratin+).

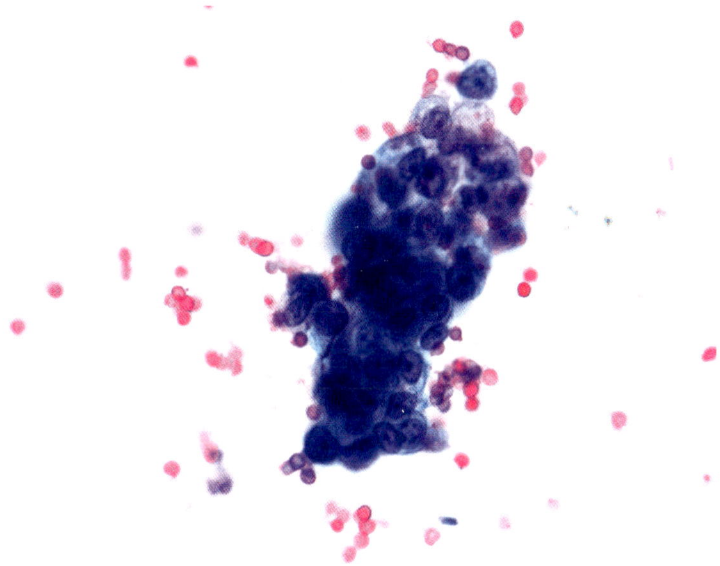

Figure 7.30a — Metastatic Breast Carcinoma, Fine Needle Aspiration [Pap Stain; High Power]. The tumor cells have the finely vacuolated cytoplasm of an adenocarcinoma, and a syncytial arrangement with a hint of glandular architecture in the bottom of the cluster. The nuclei are irregular with prominent nucleoli. Breast cancer is the most common carcinoma in women in the United States, and consideration of metastasis is important, even without a history of a breast tumor.

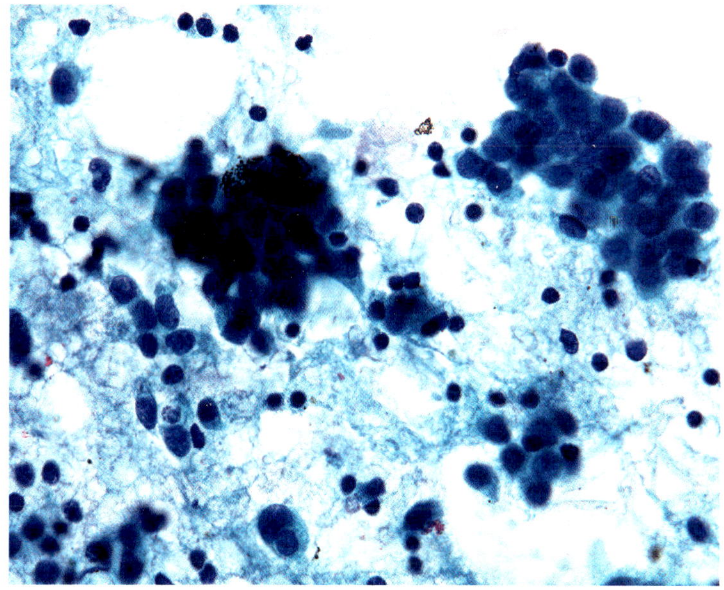

Figure 7.30b — Metastatic Breast Carcinoma, Fine Needle Aspiration [Pap Stain; High Power]. In this image, the tumor cells form both 3-dimensional fragments and discohesive single cells. The cells have high nuclear-to-cytoplasmic ratios but minimal nuclear size variation. This is compatible with although not specific for a breast primary. Because breast cancer is so common, it should be excluded when encountering any CK7 positive adenocarcinoma in a female patient.

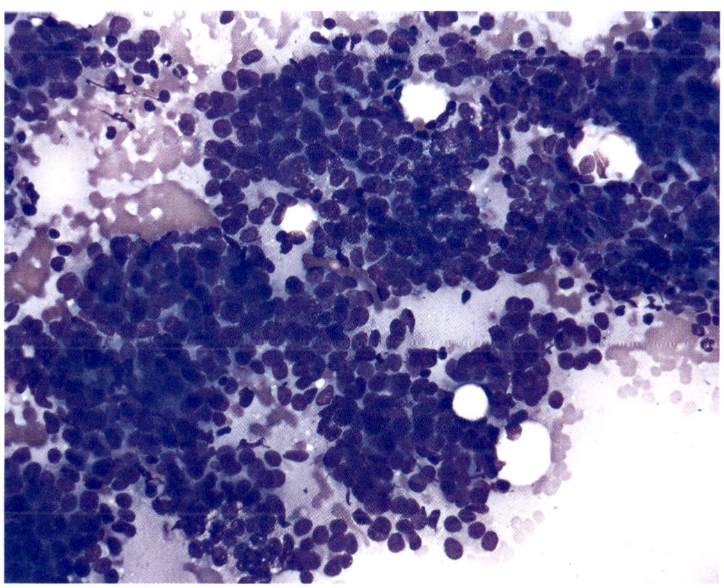

Figure 7.30c — Metastatic Breast Carcinoma, Fine Needle Aspiration [Diff-Quik Stain; Medium Power]. In this Diff-Quik stained smear, the abundant cellularity and syncytial pattern typical of metastatic breast carcinoma are both clearly evident. The tumor cells have fine cytoplasmic vacuoles in areas, and the nuclei are hyperchromatic and enlarged. The fragments form the trabecular pattern that is often seen in breast ductal carcinomas. If possible, a core biopsy or additional passes for creation of cell block material may be warranted to allow the assessment of hormone receptors (ER/PR) as well as HER2/neu status.

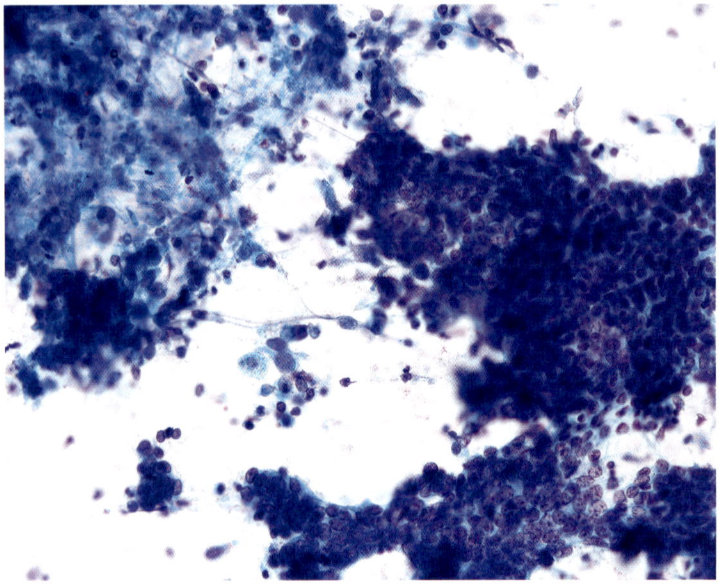

Figure 7.31a — Metastatic Colorectal Adenocarcinoma, Fine Needle Aspiration [Pap Stain; Low Power]. Sheets of malignant cells appear on the right; necrotic and inflammatory debris on the left. The malignant cells have hyperchromatic, large nuclei and a high nuclear-to-cytoplasmic ratio. Metastatic colorectal carcinoma cells are hyperchromatic and necrotic (seen here) and classically form a "picket fence" of palisading tumor cells with elongated nuclei (not seen here).

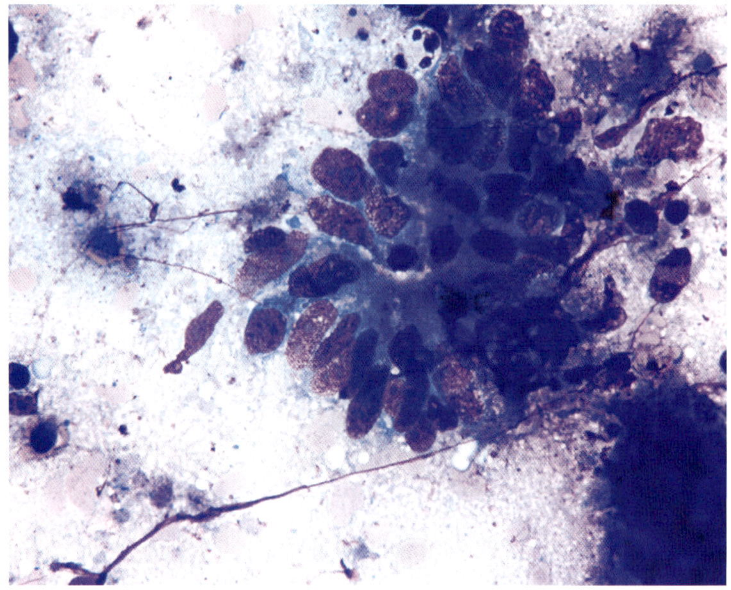

Figure 7.31b — Metastatic Colorectal Adenocarcinoma, Fine Needle Aspiration [Diff-Quik Stain; High Power]. At high power, a cluster of malignant cells is arranged in a glandular-type structure. The cells themselves are elongated, with large oval nuclei and prominent nucleoli. The cells palisade along the edge of the fragment, creating a small "picket fence" pattern. The background may be as helpful as the cytomorphology, with the "dirty necrosis" so often described in colonic adenocarcinomas.

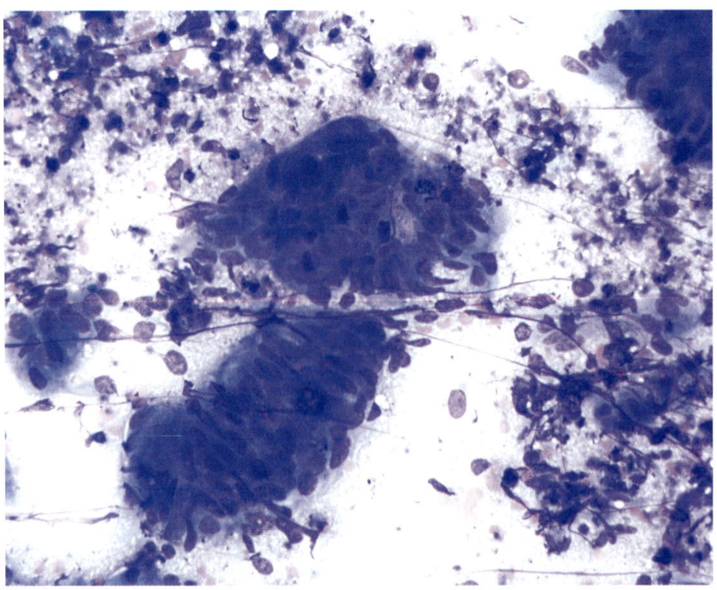

Figure 7.31c — Metastatic Colorectal Adenocarcinoma, Fine Needle Aspiration [Diff-Quik Stain; Medium Power]. The malignant cells at the center of the field recapitulate colon adenocarcinoma in tissue sections: tall cells with hyperchromatic, elongated, overlapping, and pseudostratified nuclei associated with abundant "dirty necrosis" with nuclear and inflammatory debris. Numerous mitotic figures can be seen in the upper cell cluster. Occasionally, primary lung adenocarcinomas will display intestinal differentiation (by morphology and immunohistochemistry); patient history is necessary to differentiate between a primary and metastasis in these situations.

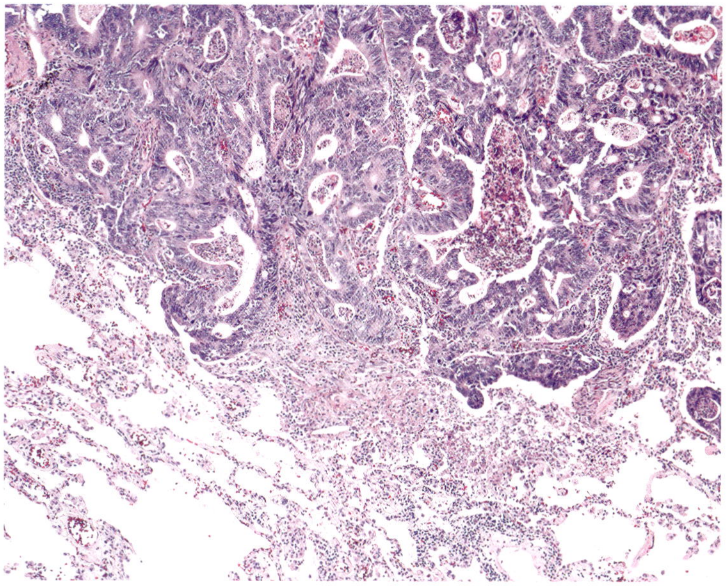

Figure 7.32a — Metastatic Colorectal Adenocarcinoma, Biopsy [H&E Stain; Low Power]. The characteristic gland formation, cribriforming, and nuclear palisading of colorectal adenocarcinoma are well demonstrated in this sharply demarcated metastatic deposit. Immunohistochemical stains for CK20, CDX2, and/or CEA will confirm. In some circumstances it will be important to test such stage IV lesions for MSI, KRAS, and/or BRAF; if tissue is limited and the primary tumor is available for comparison, it may be optimal to omit confirmatory immunohistochemical stains to conserve the tissue for molecular testing.

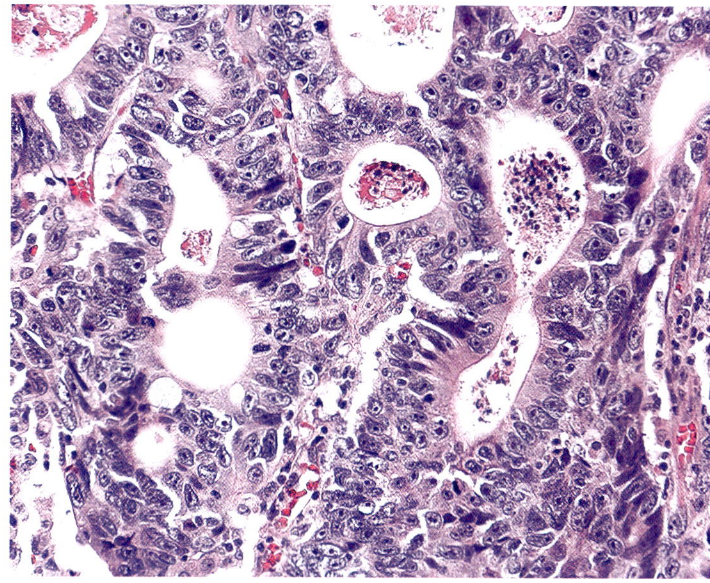

Figure 7.32b — Metastatic Colorectal Adenocarcinoma, Biopsy [H&E Stain; High Power]. At higher power, frequent intraluminal necrosis and prominent magenta nucleoli are readily identified. Pleomorphism, markedly irregular nuclear membranes, and nuclear palisading are additional features that suggest metastasis from colorectal adenocarcinoma. Endometrial endometrioid adenocarcinoma is often histologically similar to colorectal adenocarcinoma, but is typically CK7 and ER+, and negative for CK20, CEA, and CDX2.

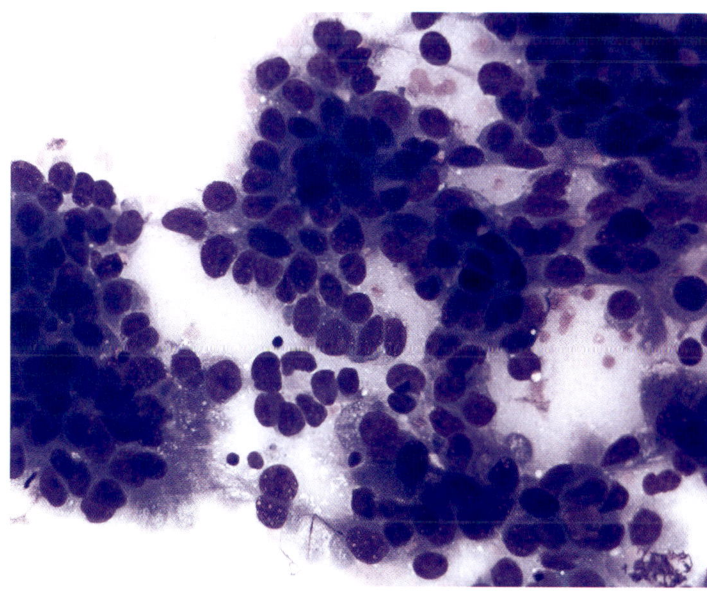

Figure 7.33a — Metastatic Hepatocellular Carcinoma, Fine Needle Aspiration [Diff-Quik Stain; High Power]. The tumor cells are spread across this field in trabecular arrangement and in small 3-dimensional aggregates. Lower center there is the suggestion of an acinus. Endothelial wrapping is not easily identified in this field. The cells are uniform and relatively small in size, possessing finely vacuolated, delicate cytoplasm. Hepatocellular carcinoma most commonly arises in the background of chronic liver disease and cirrhosis.

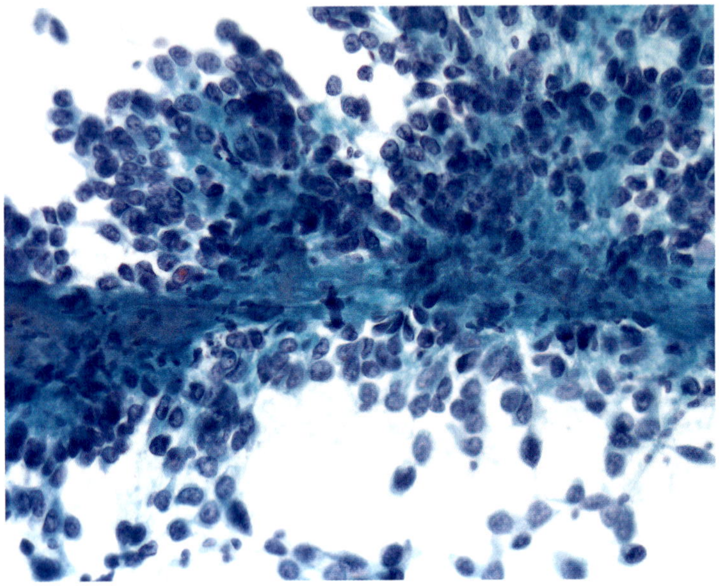

Figure 7.33b — Metastatic Hepatocellular Carcinoma, Fine Needle Aspiration [Pap Stain; High Power]. A vessel traverses the center of this field with the tumor cells splayed to either side. The cells are somewhat discohesive, although the cytoplasm remains intact. Again, the cells are mostly uniform and small in size. A microacinus is present in the upper right of the image. The nuclei resemble those of normal hepatocytes, even with nuclear pseudoinclusions (left). Hepatocellular carcinoma may present in the liver as a single mass, multiple masses simulating metastatic disease, or diffuse liver involvement without a distinct lesion on imaging.

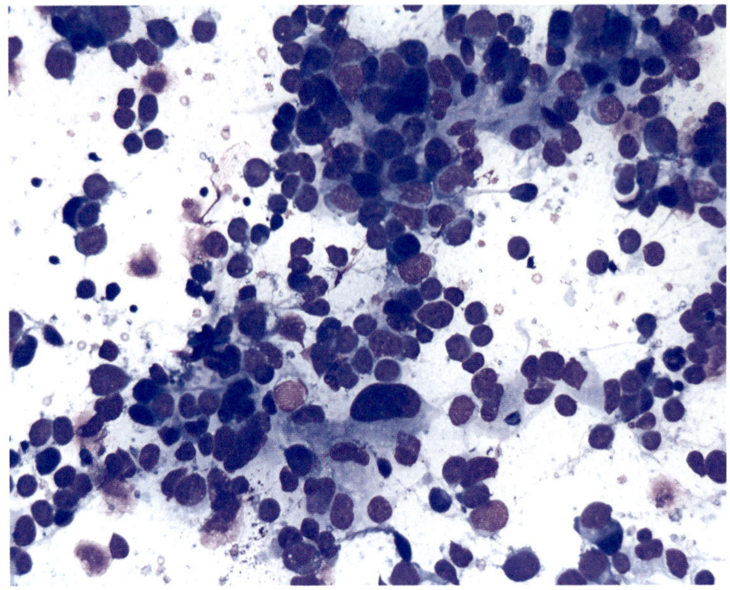

Figure 7.34a — Metastatic Glioblastoma, Fine Needle Aspiration [Diff-Quik Stain; High Power]. The tumor cells are highly pleomorphic and discohesive. There are many stripped nuclei, but the cytoplasm that is present is fibrillary and wispy. Rare lymphocytes are present in the background and give a sense of the tumor cell size. Glioblastoma multiforme rarely metastasizes outside the central nervous system, perhaps because of the strong physical protection of the central nervous system provided by the dura and blood-brain barrier, and also perhaps due to the short survival (median approximately 12 months) after a glioblastoma multiforme diagnosis.

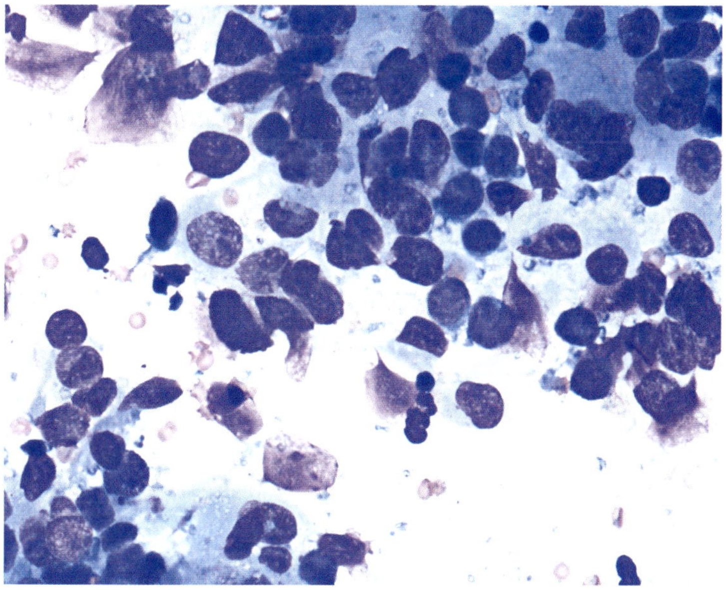

Figure 7.34b — Metastatic Glioblastoma, Fine Needle Aspiration [Diff-Quik Stain; High Power]. At higher magnification, the fibrillary cytoplasm can be appreciated in better detail. Occasional fine cell-to-cell processes are visible. The nuclei are dark, with very coarse chromatin. Glioblastoma multiforme may develop "de novo" or arise from a preceding lower grade astrocytoma. As an astrocytic tumor, glioblastoma multiforme typically expresses GFAP and S100 protein.

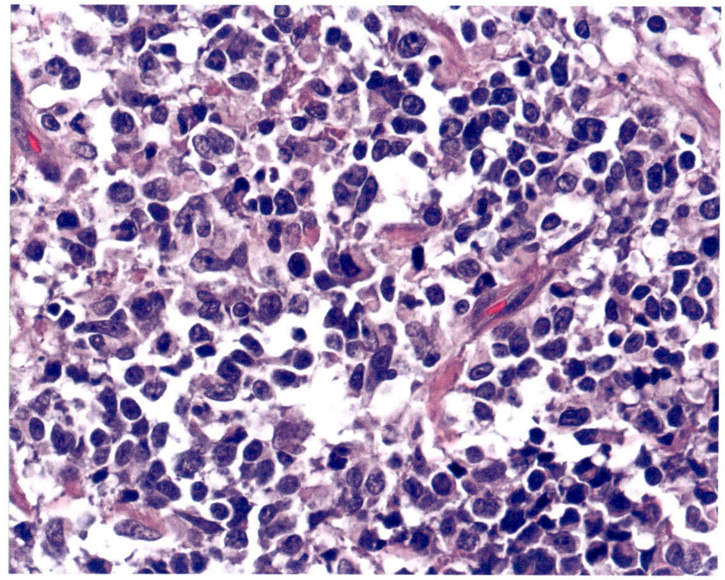

Figure 7.34c — Metastatic Glioblastoma, Fine Needle Aspiration [H&E Stain; High Power]. This anaplastic tumor is composed of pleomorphic undifferentiated cells with varying amounts of cytoplasm and a dyshesive, diffuse growth pattern with a rich vascular supply. Some examples are more spindled, or frankly sarcomatoid. The features of metastatic glioblastoma are similar to those of a wide range of undifferentiated neoplasms, both primary and metastatic. Variable expression of keratins is not uncommon in glioblastoma, and is a pitfall.

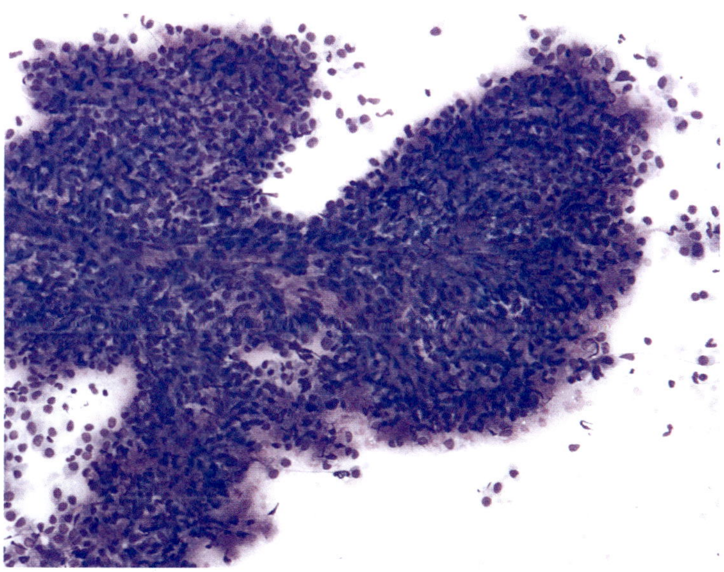

Figure 7.35a — Metastatic Meningioma, Fine Needle Aspiration [Diff-Quik Stain; Low Power]. In this image, plump spindle cells are arranged in fascicles. Fine capillaries are visible in the center of the fragment. Meningiomas are the most common primary brain tumor, and are typically seen in adults. Most tumors are benign (World Health Organization grade I) with very rare metastases reported. A subset (World Health Organization grade II/III) has the potential for aggressive behavior with higher potential for recurrence and distant metastasis.

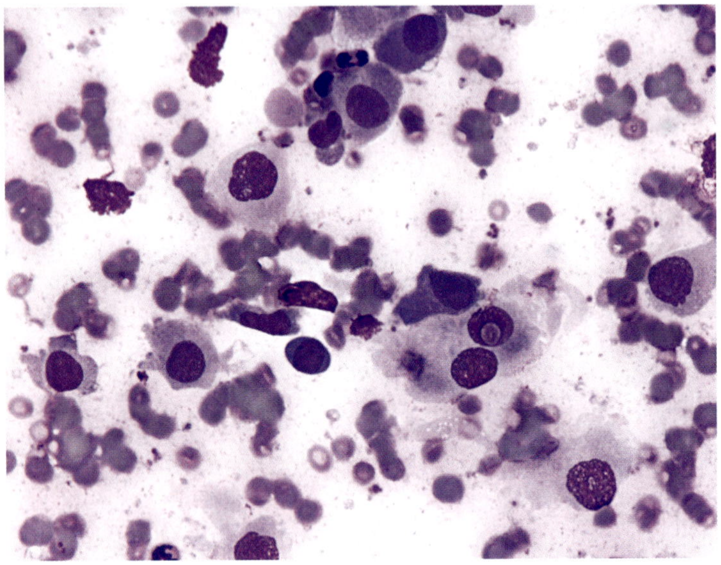

Figure 7.35b — Metastatic Meningioma, Fine Needle Aspiration [Diff-Quik Stain; High Power]. Cytologically, the cells are epithelioid with dense cytoplasm. The nuclei are round to oval with a conspicuous nucleolus. Intranuclear pseudoinclusions, as seen in the center, are a common finding in meningeal tumors. Features of a meningioma that suggest aggressive behavior include infiltrative growth, cellular necrosis, mitosis, and pleomorphism.

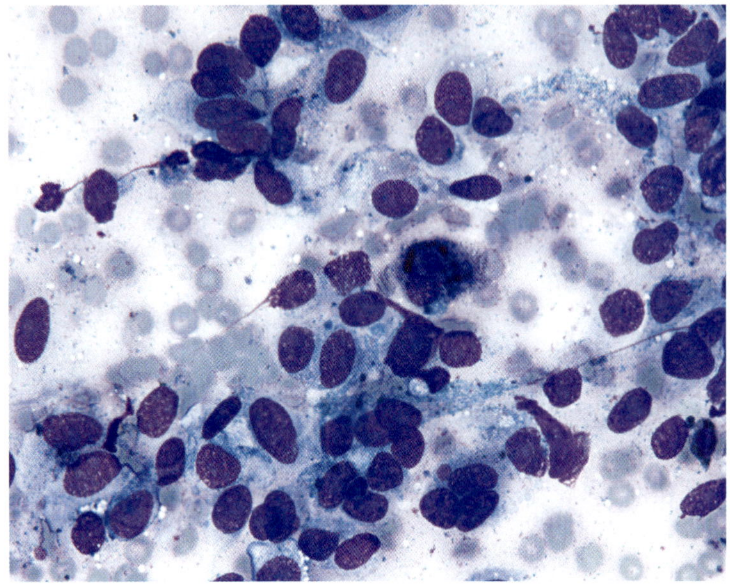

Figure 7.36a — Metastatic Melanoma, Fine Needle Aspiration [Diff-Quik Stain; High Power]. The predominant cells are large, loosely cohesive cells with ovoid nuclei and multiple prominent nucleoli. The background is granular, but in the center are several cells with pale cytoplasm with green-tan cytoplasmic melanin pigment, diagnostic of melanoma. Closer examination reveals this pigment present in many other cells where cytoplasm is appreciable. Metastatic melanoma may present as an isolated metastasis years after the primary lesion was treated.

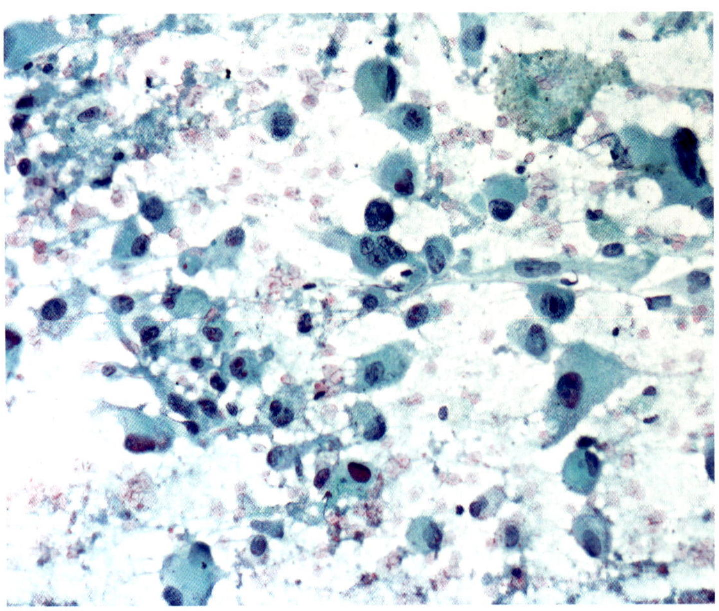

Figure 7.36b — Metastatic Melanoma, Fine Needle Aspiration [Pap Stain; High Power]. Large, pleomorphic, and frankly malignant cells dominate, and cytoplasm is eccentric in many cells, which imparts a rhabdoid appearance. Rare background lymphocytes and endothelial cells are present in the background and may be used for size comparison. The bright red nucleoli are very striking in this image, characteristic of melanoma. Immunohistochemial staining of cell block material for S100, SOX-10, HMB-45, and melan A can be used as aids to the diagnosis.

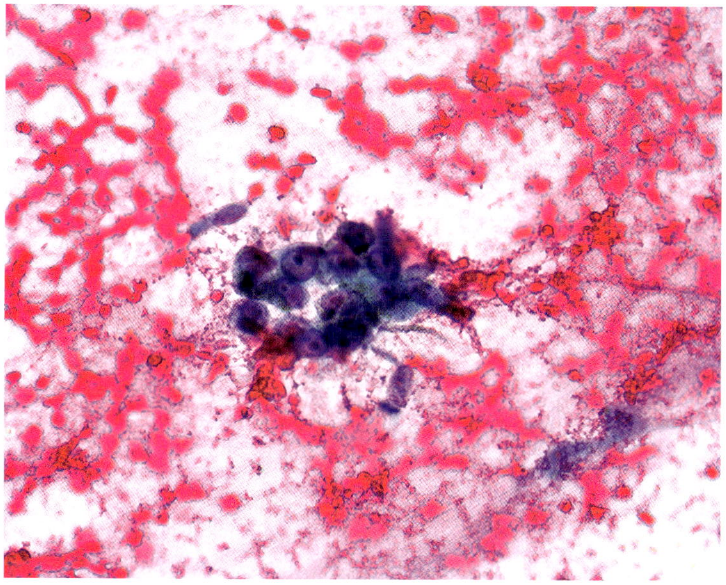

Figure 7.36c — Metastatic Melanoma, Fine Needle Aspiration [Pap Stain; Medium Power]. The tumor cells are plump, epithelioid, and pleomorphic, but the most striking feature here is the large nucleoli. The cell cytoplasm also appears faintly pigmented. These features combined are suggestive of metastatic melanoma. A prior history of melanoma is not always available, but immunohistochemical stains for S100, SOX-10, HMB45, and melan- A (MART1) and negative workup for carcinoma and lymphoma are helpful.

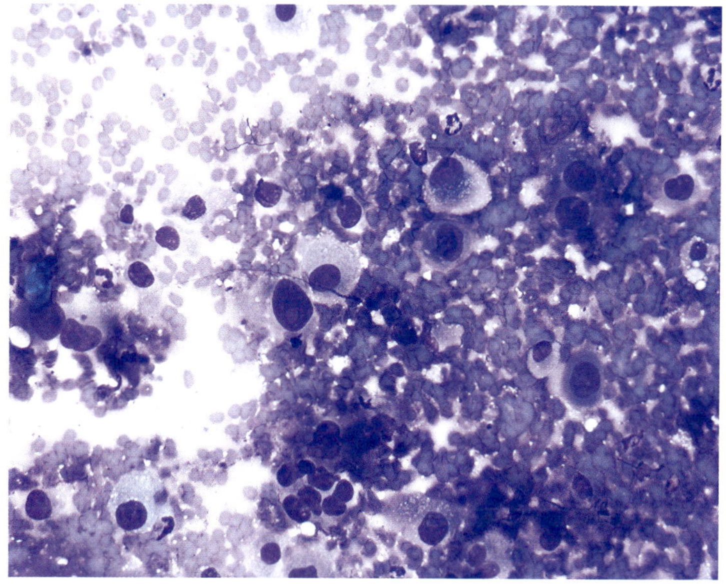

Figure 7.36d — Metastatic Melanoma, Fine Needle Aspiration [Diff-Quik Stain; High Power]. The cells are large and discohesive; even at low power, large nucleoli are visible. Binucleated cells are occasionally seen. Intranuclear pseudoinclusions can be identified, a feature associated with melanoma as well as other neoplasms, such as papillary thyroid carcinoma and bronchoalveolar carcinoma. Risk factors for aggressive disease in primary melanoma lesions include greater depth of invasion (Breslow thickness), vascular invasion, ulceration over the primary, and lymph node status. However, some patients may not have a history of melanoma. In these cases, primary lesions may have involuted after giving rise to metastases.

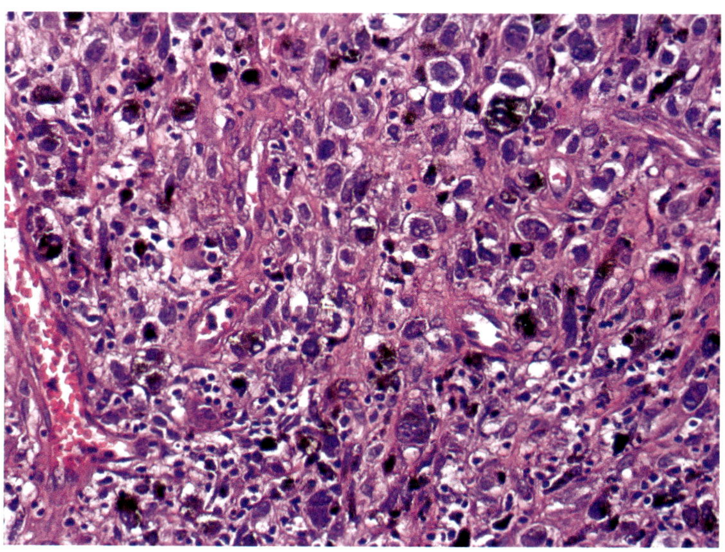

Figure 7.36e — Metastatic Melanoma, Core Biopsy [H&E Stain; High Power]. This metastasis is composed of disorganized sheets of large epithelioid melanocytes with marked nuclear membrane irregularities, frequent prominent nucleoli, and abundant melanin production. In the absence of melanin production, a panel of immunohistochemical markers will allow exclusion of carcinoma, sarcoma, and large cell lymphoma. Metastases resemble the cutaneous primary; thus, the full range of cutaneous melanoma histology may be observed, including epithelioid, nevoid, spindle cell, and desmoplastic patterns. Long-standing and recurrent metastatic lesions of all patterns may dedifferentiate and become indistinguishable from sarcoma, including the loss of melanocytic immunohistochemical markers (e.g., HMB-45, melan A, SOX-10); S100 is rarely lost but is not entirely specific.

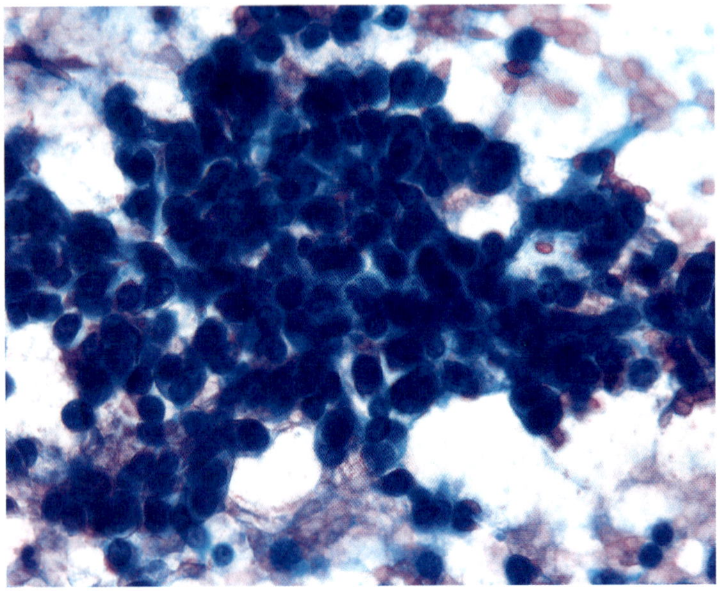

Figure 7.37a — Metastatic Nasopharyngeal Carcinoma, Fine Needle Aspiration [Pap Stain; High Power]. This slide shows an aggregate of tumor cells with large nuclei. The tumor cells themselves have prominent nucleoli. In some instances (not seen here), admixed lymphocytes may be numerous. Without a history or clinical suspicion, the morphology is nonspecific and represents a poorly differentiated epithelioid malignancy. The differential may include diffuse large B-cell lymphoma, large cell neuroendocrine carcinoma, poorly differentiated carcinoma, and melanoma. Nasopharygeal carcinoma is rare in North America, but more common in South China and parts of Africa. It is often associated with Epstein–Barr virus infection.

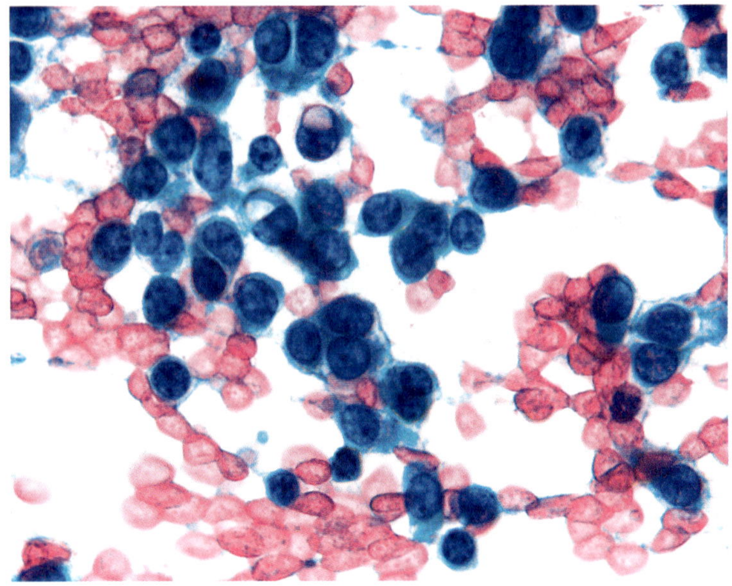

Figure 7.37b — Metastatic Nasopharyngeal Carcinoma, Fine Needle Aspiration [Pap Stain; High Power]. This example of metastatic nasopharyngeal carcinoma is notable for loosely cohesive tumor cells with high nuclear-to-cytoplasmic ratios. Nasopharyngeal carcinoma may be keratinizing or nonkeratinizing, with nonkeratinizing forms being either differentiated or undifferentiated. Its immunohistochemical pattern may overlap with squamous cell carcinoma of the lung; clinical suspicion or the presence of numerous lymphocytes should lead one to perform an in situ hybridization for Epstein–Barr virus.

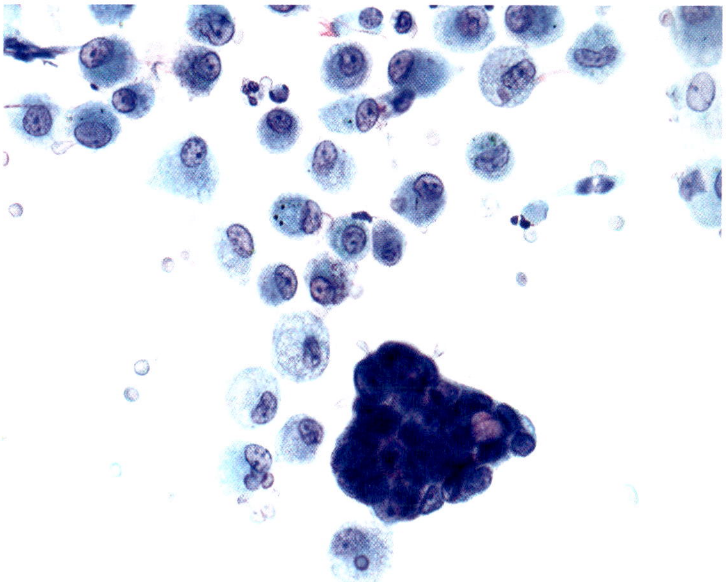

Figure 7.38a — Metastatic Salivary Duct Carcinoma, Fine Needle Aspiration [Pap Stain; High Power]. A single cluster of tumor cells is present in the low center of the field. These cells have high nuclear-to-cytoplasmic ratios, pleomorphic nuclei with open chromatin and prominent nucleoli, and moderate cytoplasm with pink granules. A glandular structure is present to the right within the cluster. In the background lie abundant histiocytes. Salivary duct carcinoma is an uncommon high-grade salivary carcinoma that resembles high-grade breast carcinoma and may present with metastatic disease.

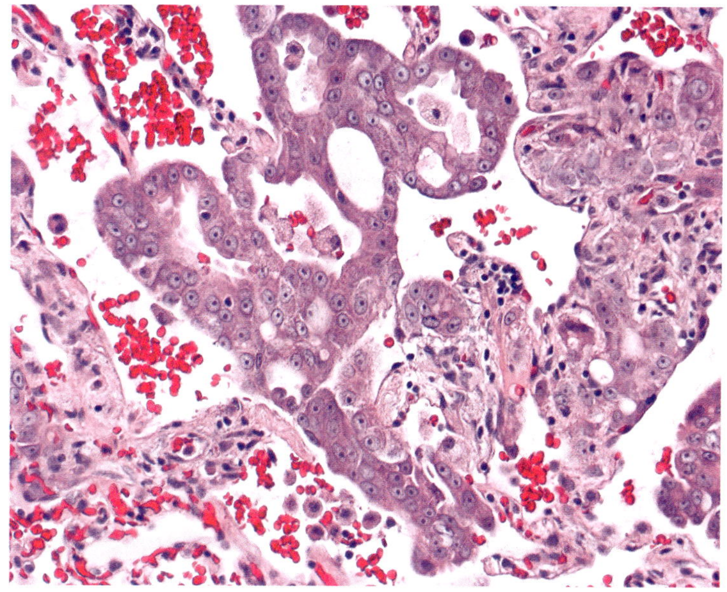

Figure 7.38b — Metastatic Salivary Duct Carcinoma, Biopsy [H&E Stain; High Power]. Lung metastases from salivary gland tumors are uncommon, but salivary duct carcinoma is an often aggressive tumor and may spread to the lungs. This lesion maintains the characteristic features of the primary, including trabecular/cribriform architecture and component cells with eosinophilic cytoplasm, vesicular nuclei, and prominent nucleoli. These tumors closely mimic mammary carcinoma and routinely express GATA-3, Androgen Receptor, ER, HER2, and E-cadherin. In the absence of a documented history of primary salivary duct carcinoma, primary lung cancer (TTF-1 and napsin +; GATA-3 and AR-) enters into consideration, as does breast cancer, which cannot be definitively excluded on morphologic and immunohistochemical grounds alone.

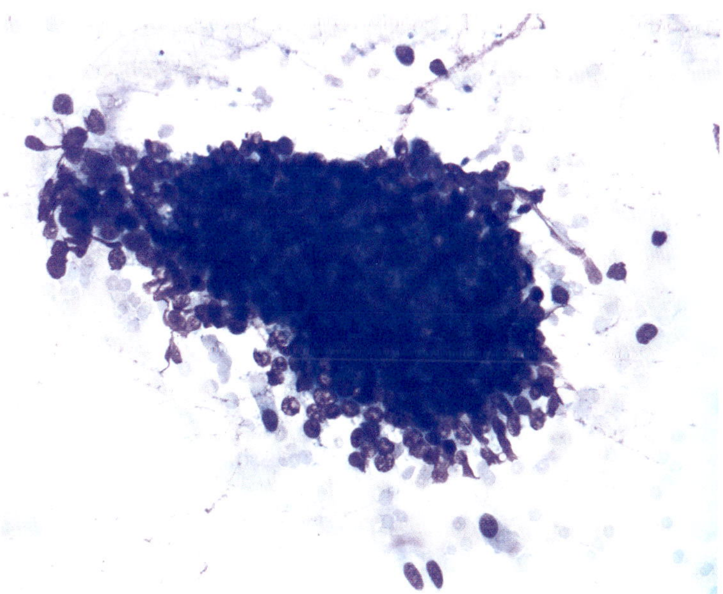

Figure 7.39a — Metastatic Thymoma, Fine Needle Aspiration [Diff-Quik Stain; Medium Power]. The cells are small, tightly clustered, with rounded nuclei and a slender rim of faint cytoplasm. The chromatin is coarse. Rare lymphocytes are present. Thymomas may involve the lung by either direct extension from the mediastinum, or occasionally metastasis.Thymomas are classified by histologic pattern (A, AB, B1, B2, B3, C), although clinical stage is the most important prognosticator.

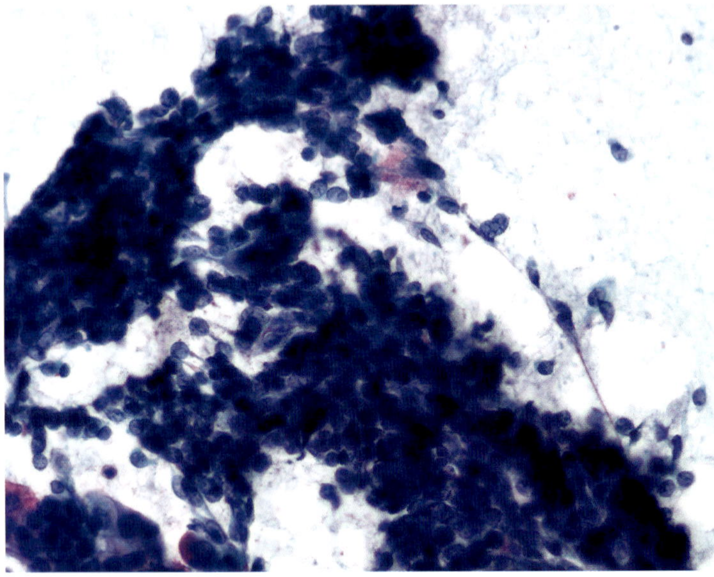

Figure 7.39b — Metastatic Thymoma, Fine Needle Aspiration [Pap Stain; Medium Power]. Sheets and clusters of atypical epithelial cells fill this frame. There is evidence of squamous differentiation in the right side, with intracytoplasmic pink suggesting keratinization and irregular extracellular fragments of keratin. Thymic neoplasms often show squamous differentiation in the epithelial component. The epithelial cells of thymoma are positive for p63 and cytokeratin, while the admixed lymphocytes are immature TdT+ CD3+ T cells.

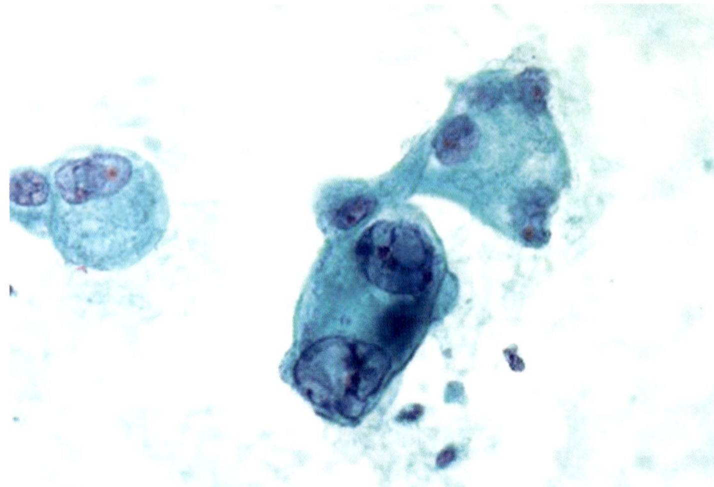

Figure 7.40a — Metastatic Papillary Thyroid Carcinoma, Fine Needle Aspiration [Pap Stain; High Power]. These malignant cells have enlarged nuclei with highly irregular nuclear borders. One cell possesses a feature classically associated with papillary thyroid carcinoma–an intranuclear pseudoinclusion. Some forms of lung adenocarcinoma, such as some neoplasms previously classified as bronchoalveolar carcinoma, are often associated with inclusions and should be included in the differential diagnosis. Because the lung is a common site for metastatic tumors, patient history is critical.

Figure 7.40b — Metastatic Papillary Thyroid Carcinoma, Fine Needle Aspiration [Diff-Quik Stain; High Power]. These oncocytic cells are enlarged, demonstrate striking anisnucleosis, and have abundant cytoplasm. The differential diagnosis includes any lesion in which cells can have oncocytic differentiation; however, in this case the patient had widely metastatic papillary thyroid carcinoma. The cytomorphology of metastases may not always be similar as the primary lesion, although some papillary thyroid carcinomas demonstrate oncocytic differentiation. Papillary thyroid carcinoma typically metastasizes locally to regional lymph nodes and in only rare instances metastasizes to distant organs, such as the lung.

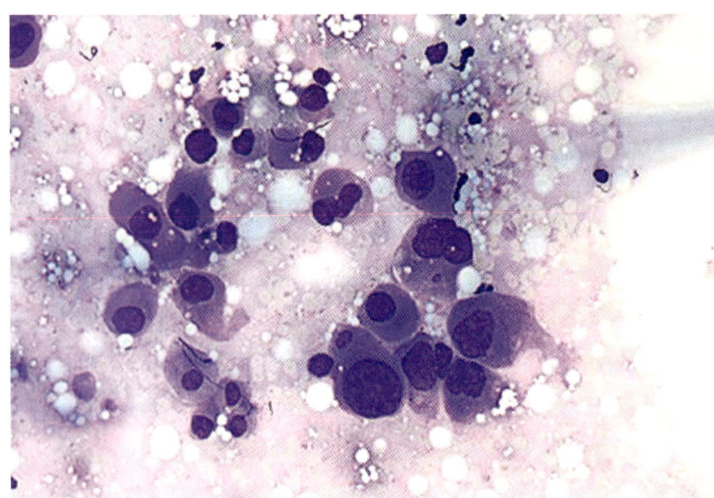

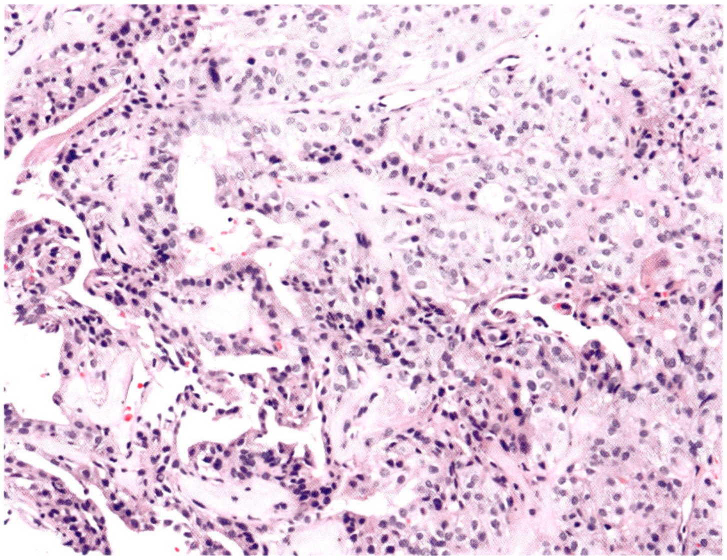

Figure 7.40c — Metastatic Papillary Thyroid Carcinoma, Biopsy [H&E Stain; Low Power]. This transbronchial biopsy shows a tumor with papillary architecture with stromal sclerosis at the left, with a more nested, solid pattern at the right. Primary mixed papillary and solid adenocarcinoma of the lung is the major differential consideration. Nuclear TTF-1 expression is characteristic of both lesions, but stains for napsin A and thyroglobulin will likely distinguish metastatic thyroid carcinoma (thyroglobulin +, napsin A-) from primary lung cancer (napsin A +, thyroglobulin -).

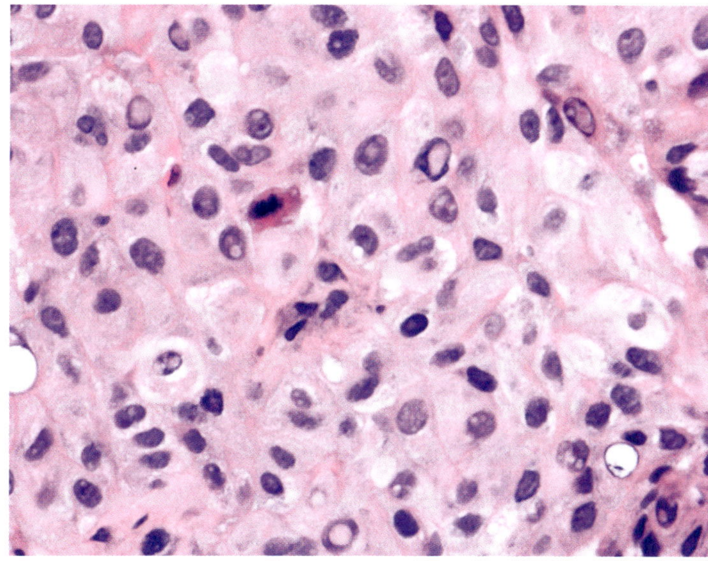

Figure 7.40d — Metastatic Papillary Thyroid Carcinoma, Biopsy [H&E Stain; High Power]. The cells in this solid area show elongated oval nuclei with several intranuclear pseudoinclusions, and a mitotic figure is present. The nuclei are characteristic of papillary thryoid carcinoma, though not specific; many papillary lung tumors have intranuclear pseudoinclusions and/or nuclear grooves.

Figure 7.41a — Metastatic Hurthle Cell Carcinoma, Fine Needle Aspiration [Diff-Quik Stain; Medium Power]. This neoplasm is composed of epithelial cells with finely granular and ample cytoplasm possessing rounded to oval nuclei with prominent nucleoli. The cells show the nuclear variation typical of oncocytic (Hurthle) cells in the thyroid. Hurthle cell carcinoma of the thyroid is a follicular-pattern carcinoma with predominantly Hurthle cells and foci of capsular and/or vascular invasion.

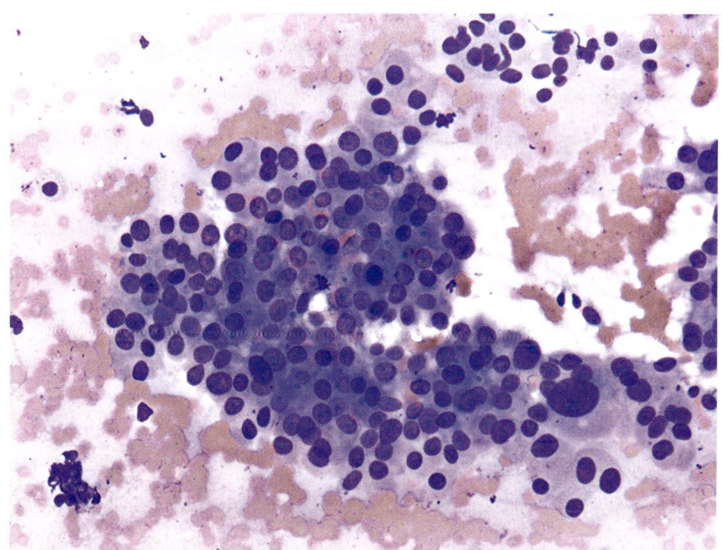

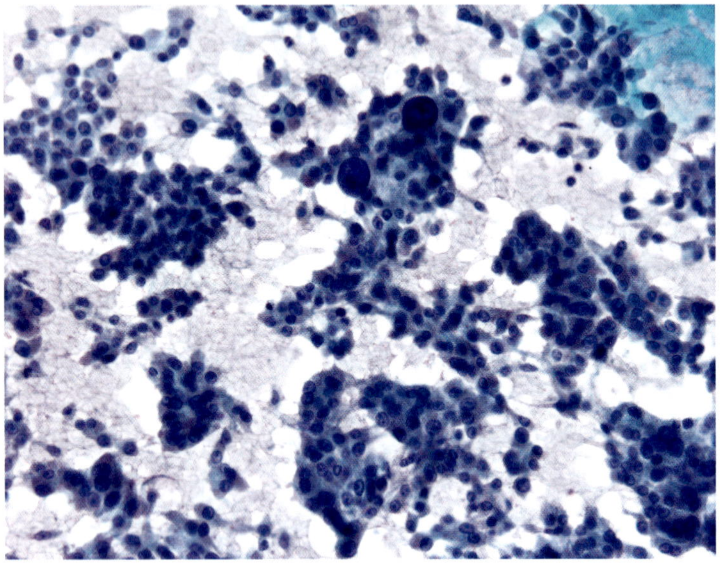

Figure 7.41b — Metastatic Hurthle Cell Carcinoma, Fine Needle Aspiration [Pap Stain; Medium Power]. By Pap stain, the cytoplasmic granules of Hurthle cells that by electron microscopy are revealed to be giant mitochondria are more easily appreciated. In this field, two giant, boulder-like nuclei are in the upper center. Such massive pleomorphism can occasionally be seen in benign Hurthle cell lesions within the thyroid and is not, in and of itself, diagnostic of malignancy. The presence of distant metastasis, as in this case of a lung mass, is diagnostic of malignancy.

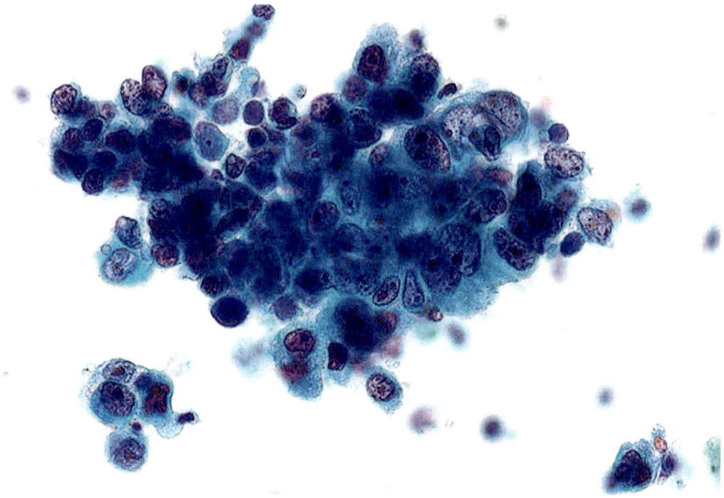

Figure 7.42 — Metastatic Adrenal Cortical Carcinoma, Fine Needle Aspiration [Pap Stain; High Power]. Adrenal cortical carcinoma is uncommon and not usually initially considered when encountering a carcinoma of unknown origin. Immunohistochemical stains compatible with an adrenal origin include melan A (MART1), synaptophysin, and inhibin, though none of these are specific to the adrenal. These carcinomas may have variable cytologic morphologies, but are often discohesive, owing to their neuroendocrine origin. They also typically have moderate-to-marked nuclear pleomorphism and prominent nucleoli; both features are demonstrated in this field.

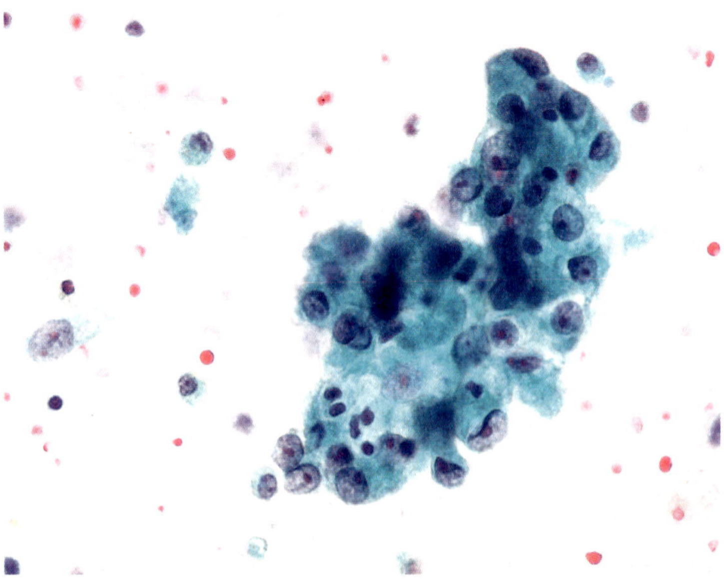

Figure 7.43a — Metastatic Renal Cell Carcinoma, Fine Needle Aspiration [Pap Stain; High Power]. These tumor cells have fluffy and granular appearing cytoplasm, and the cell-cell borders are visible in some areas but appear blurred in others. The nuclei possess somewhat irregular contours and quite prominent nucleoli. Renal cell carcinoma typically affects adults, and is often an incidental finding on imaging performed for other indications.

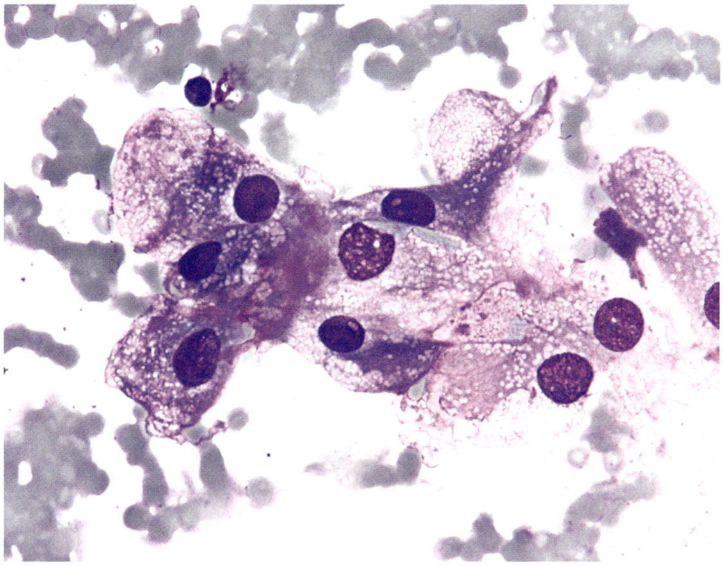

Figure 7.43b — Metastatic Renal Cell Carcinoma, Fine Needle Aspiration [Diff-Quik Stain; High Power]. Diff-Quik stained aspirates from a renal cell carcinoma highlight the abundant, finely vacuolated cytoplasm. In this view, the cell borders are indistinct, and nucleoli are visible in the tumor cells. The cytoplasm becomes clear during tissue fixation and processing, but will not appear so on aspirate smears. Instead, a distinctive feature is the presence of fine vacuoles that contain lipid.

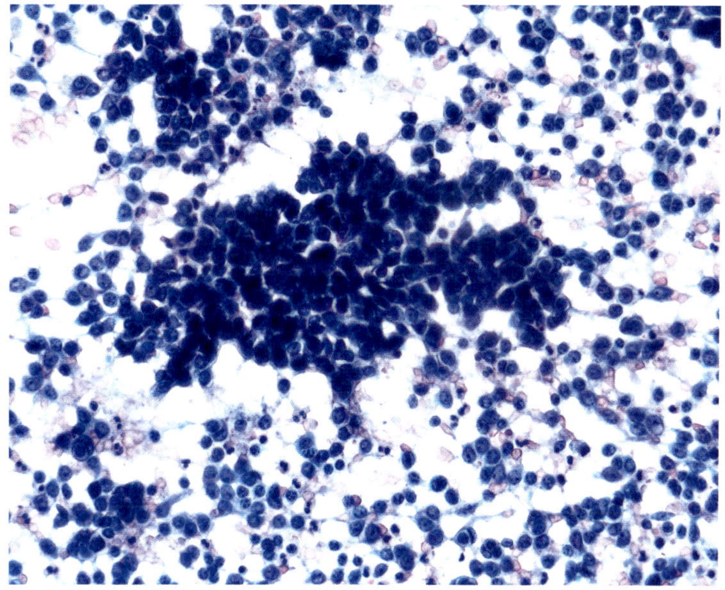

Figure 7.43c — Renal Cell Carcinoma, Fine Needle Aspiration [Pap Stain; Medium Power]. The cells are arranged in loose clusters and sheets with delicate cytoplasmic attachments between cells. There is moderate pleomorphism of the nuclei, and nucleoli are often conspicuous. The cells are mostly small-to-medium in size in renal cell carcinoma.

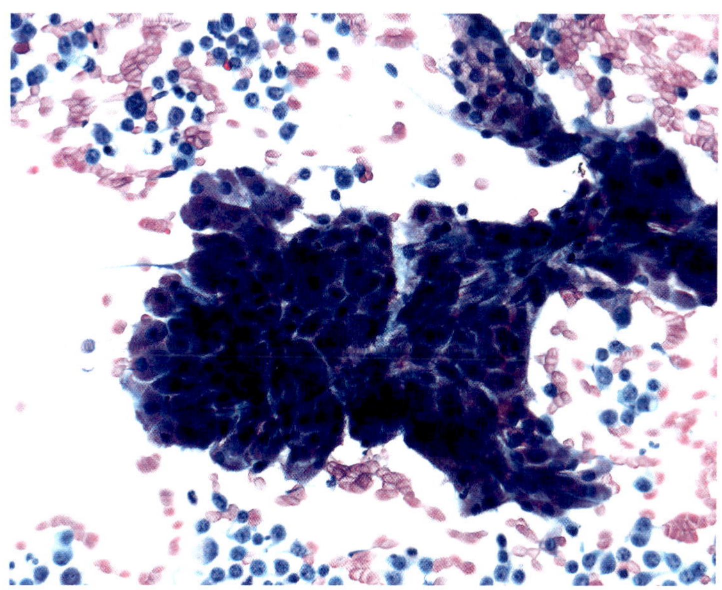

Figure 7.43d — Metastatic Renal Cell Carcinoma, Fine Needle Aspiration [Pap Stain; Medium Power]. The fragment in the center is composed of polygonal, plasmacytoid appearing cells with granular cytoplasm and small, round nuclei. In contrast, the surrounding single cells are less cytoplasm, larger nuclei with coarser chromatin, and scattered cytoplasmic vacuoles. Renal cell carcinoma is typically treated by nephrectomy, even if there is renal vein or vena cava extension, and isolated metastasis is also considered a surgical disease.

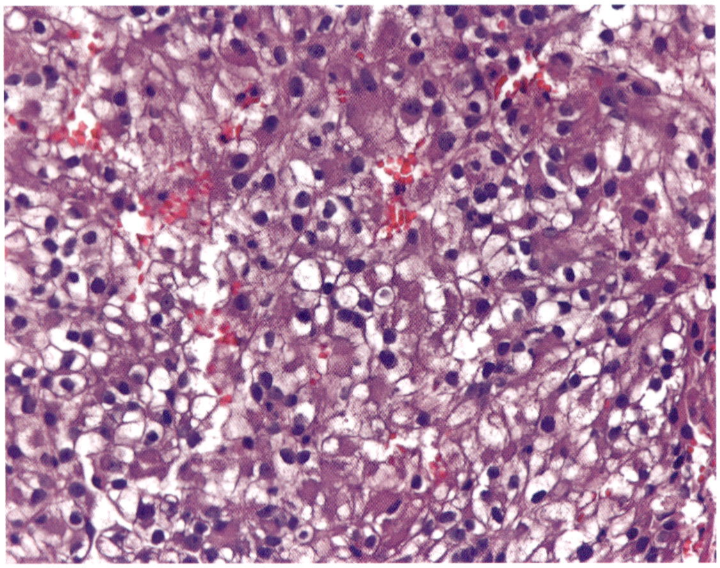

Figure 7.44a — Metastatic Renal Cell Carcinoma, Fine Needle Aspiration [H&E Stain; Medium Power]. A view from a cell block shows the nests of cells with pink to clear cytoplasm often seen in renal cell carcinoma. Red blood cells are scattered throughout as well. Clear cell renal cell carcinoma may be very bloody on aspirates due to its high vascularity.

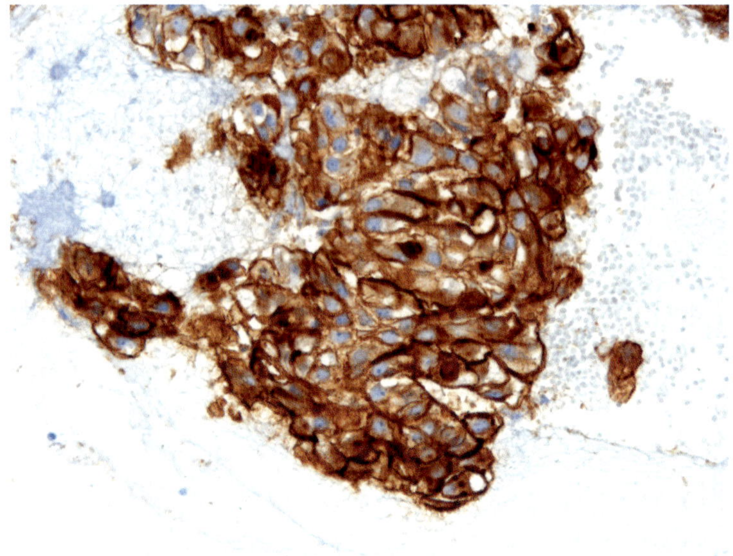

Figure 7.44b — Metastatic Renal Cell Carcinoma, Fine Needle Aspiration [Immunohistochemical Stain for Carbonic Anhydrase -IX; High Power]. Immunohistochemical staining for carbonic anhydrase IX demonstrates a cytoplasmic pattern with membranous accentuation in the tumor cells. This pattern of carbonic anhydrase -IX staining supports clear cell carcinoma. Clear cell renal cell carcinoma is typically negative for CK7 and racemase (AMACR), while papillary RCC shows the inverse pattern of staining.

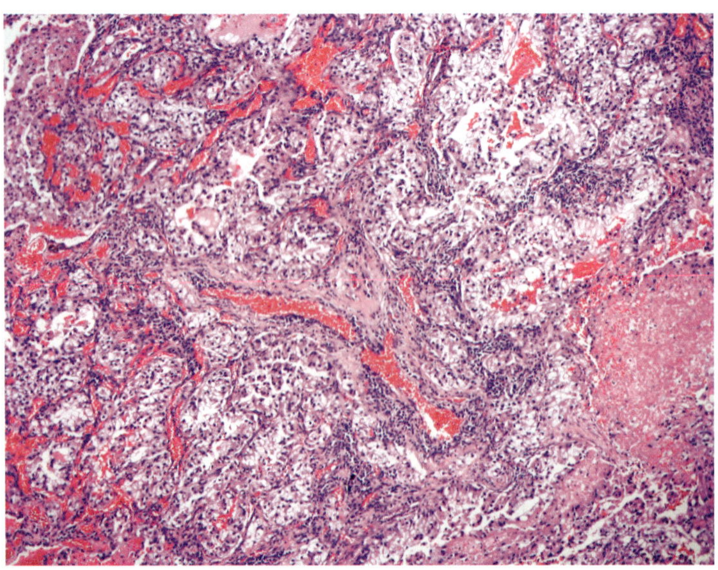

Figure 7.44c — Metastatic Clear Cell Renal Cell Carcinoma, Resection [H&E Stain; Low Power]. This metastasis from a renal cell carcinoma shows a richly vascularized aggregate of nested clear cells. The low power differential additionally incudes fetal-type adenocarcinoma of the lung, as well as metastasis of clear cell carcinoma from other sites (e.g., gynecologic sites).

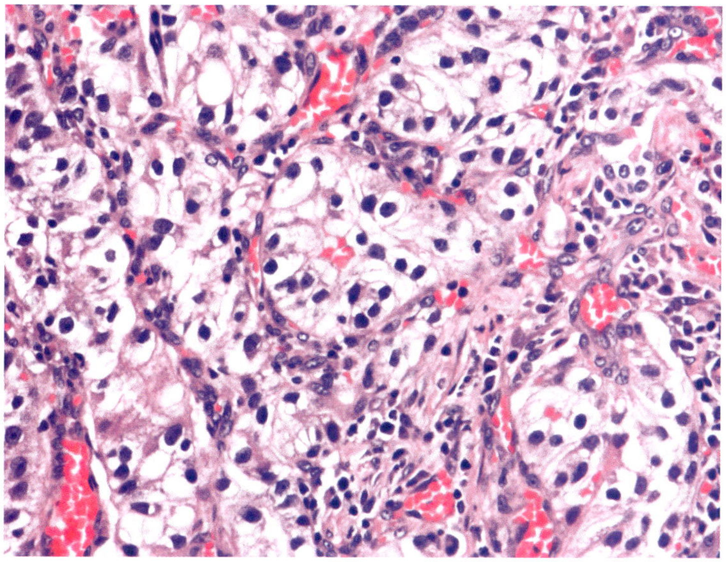

Figure 7.44d — Metastatic Clear Cell Renal Cell Carcinoma, Resection [H&E Stain; High Power]. Higher magnification shows moderately pleomorphic clear cells with disorderly nuclear placement and frequent nucleoli. Immunostains may not be required to make the diagnosis, especially if the classic clear cell morphology is present and the previous kidney lesion is available for review. If the metastasis is of higher grade or the previous is unavailable, a panel of stains may be helpful in recognizing renal origin (PAX8+, carbonic anhydrase -IX+, CD10+, EMA+, vimentin+, CK7-, ER-).

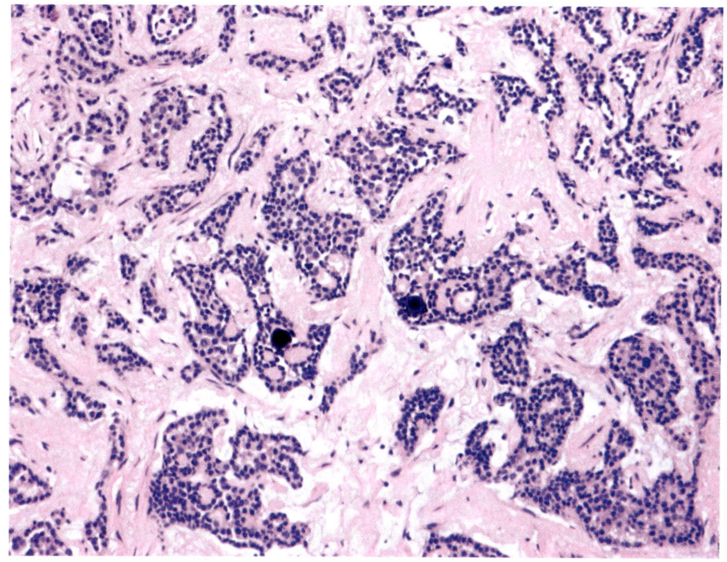

Figure 7.45a — Metastatic Papillary Renal Cell Carcinoma, Resection [H&E Stain; Low Power]. This unusual metastasis is composed of papillae of varying sizes, with sclerotic fibrovascular cores embedded in a dense collagenous stroma. Two psammoma bodies are present (center). Differential considerations include tumors of thyroid and salivary origin, as well as primary papillary adenocarcinoma of the lung (with an unusual appearance). TTF-1 and thyroglobulin stains may be helpful; history and review of a previous lesion are better. This patient's previous renal tumor had an identical appearance.

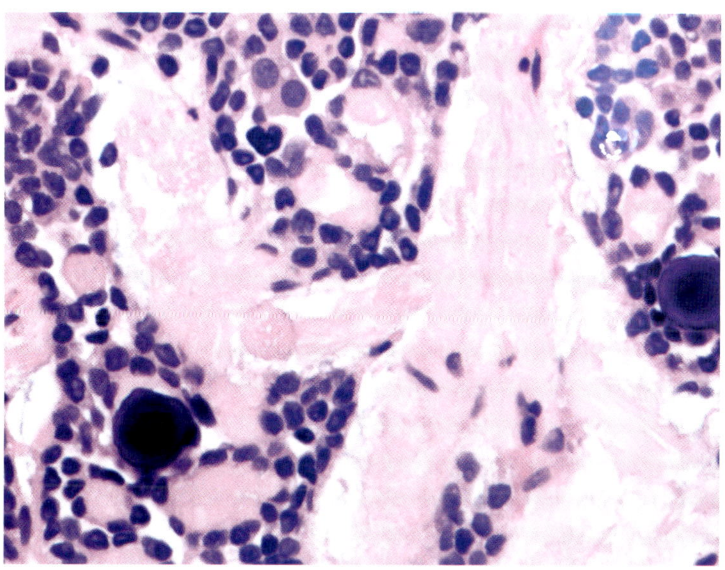

Figure 7.45b — Metastatic Papillary Renal Cell Carcinoma, Resection [H&E Stain; High Power]. Nuclear pleomorphism is apparent at higher power. The two psammoma bodies are surrounded by a rim of tumor cells, and there is notably dense collagen between and within papillae. As in most papillary neoplasms arising from a variety of sites, intranuclear pseudoinclusions may be present.

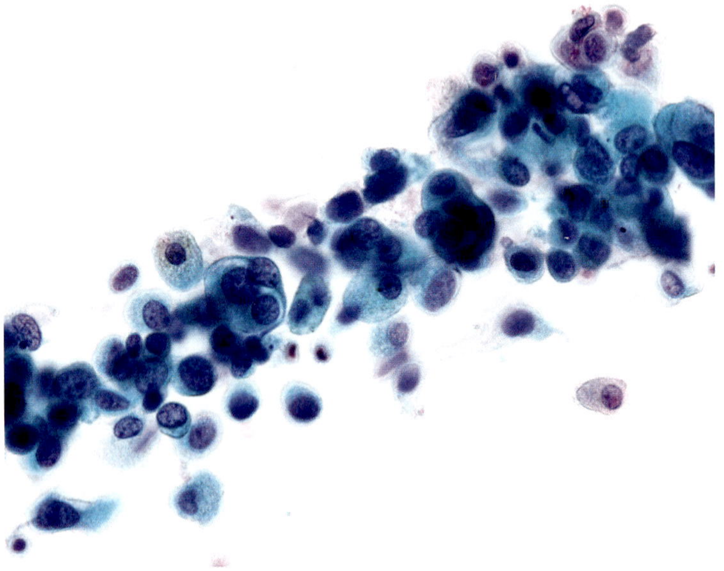

Figure 7.46a — Metastatic Urothelial Carcinoma, Fine Needle Aspiration [Pap Stain; High Power]. Atypical cells cross the image—the nuclei are pleomorphic with coarse chromatin and occasional nucleoli. These cells have finely vacuolated cytoplasm and occasionally a "cell in cell" pattern (entosis) is seen. The prognosis of muscle-invasive urothelial carcinoma is much worse than nonmuscle invasive tumors, with around 50% of patients developing metastasis and a 5-year survival rate of 63% for stage II disease.

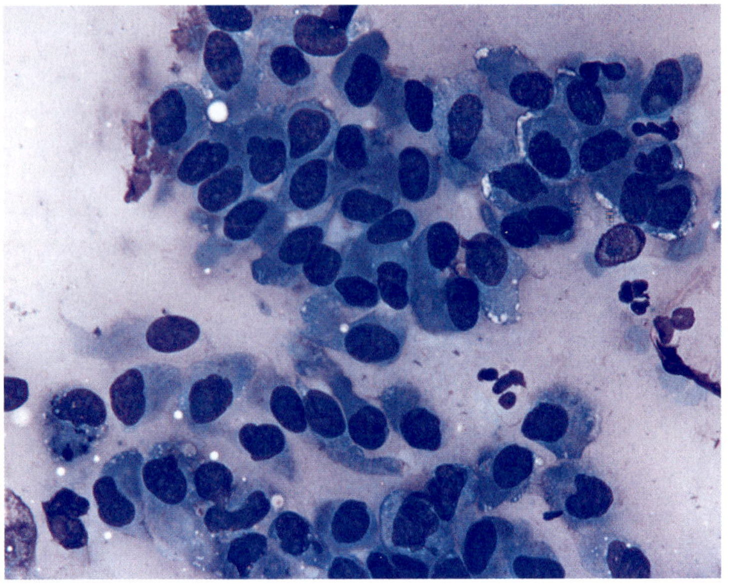

Figure 7.46b — Metastatic Urothelial Carcinoma, Fine Needle Aspiration [Diff-Quik Stain; High Power]. On Diff-Quik, metastatic urothelial carcinoma may have fine cytoplasmic vacuoles, as seen here. The carcinoma cells are loosely aggregated, with cytoplasmic tails evident in the center/center-left. The nuclei are oval with coarse chromatin and scattered folds and nucleoli. Metastatic urothelial carcinoma typically expresses GATA-3 and may also express high molecular weight cytokeratin and p63/p40, which could raise the possibility of squamous cell carcinoma. Urothelial carcinoma is negative for TTF-1 and napsin A.

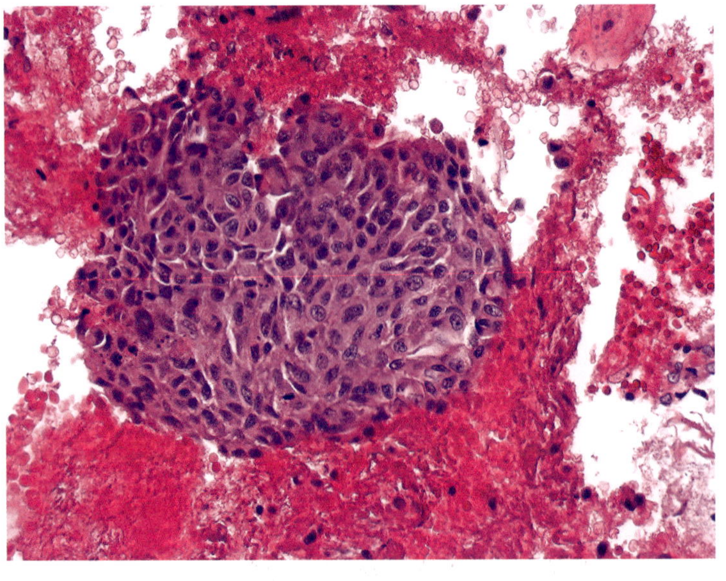

Figure 7.47 — Metastatic Urothelial Carcinoma, Fine Needle Aspiration [H&E Stain; Medium Power]. In this cell block preparation, the tumor cells show similar features: vacuolated cytoplasm, round to oval nuclei with coarse chromatin and nucleoli, and, in this view, several mitotic figures and apoptotic bodies and a bloody background. Urothelial carcinoma can show squamous and/or glandular differentiation, which can make diagnosis difficult. A thorough patient history is indispensable in these situations.

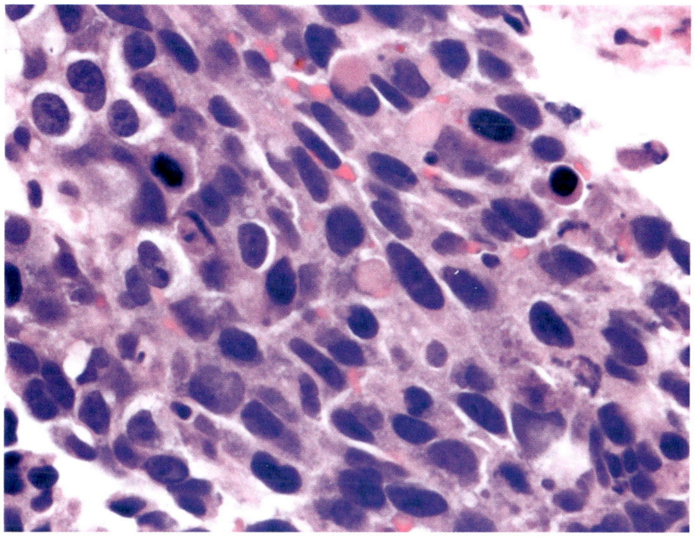

Figure 7.48a — Metastatic Urothelial Carcinoma, Biopsy [H&E Stain; High Power]. This poorly differentiated carcinoma in a patient with a history of bladder cancer has a solid growth pattern, with pleomorphic polygonal cells, a mitotic figure at the upper left, and an apoptotic cell at the upper right. As smoking is a risk factor for both urothelial carcinoma and squamous malignancies of the respiratory tract/head and neck, major diagnostic considerations include both squamous cell carcinoma (primary or metastatic) and metastatic urothelial carcinoma.

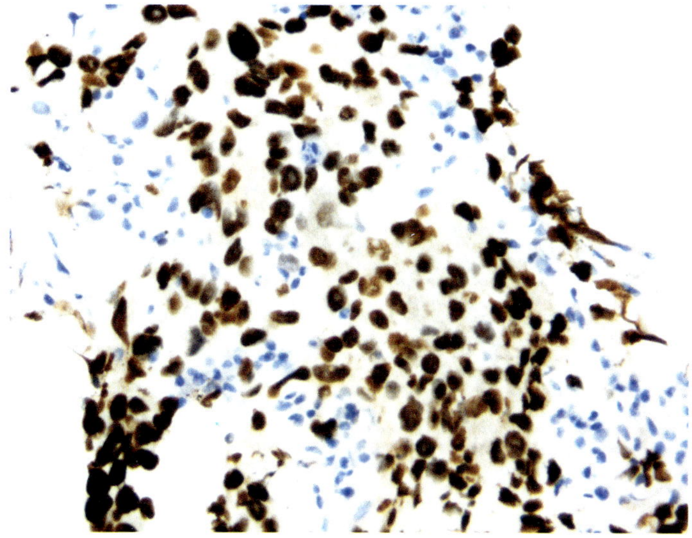

Figure 7.48b — Metastatic Urothelial Carcinoma, Biopsy [GATA-3 Immunohistochemical Stain; High Power]. The tumor cells show strong and uniform nuclear expression of GATA-3, most consistent with metastatic urothelial carcinoma. Stains for p40, p63, and CK7 were also positive. Some urothelial carcinomas also express CK20. Squamous cell carcinoma of the lung is typically positive for p40, p63, and CK5/6, and negative for GATA-3, CK7, and CK20.

Figure 7.49a — Metastatic Prostate Carcinoma, Fine Needle Aspiration [Pap Stain; High Power]. The cells in this fragment possess prominent nucleoli and are arranged in an acinar pattern. The cells have abundant, foamy cytoplasm. The nuclei are eccentrically placed. This cytomorphological pattern can also commonly be seen in renal cell carcinoma and melanoma. While prostate cancer is known to spread to bone and lymph nodes, the lung is the third common metastatic site.

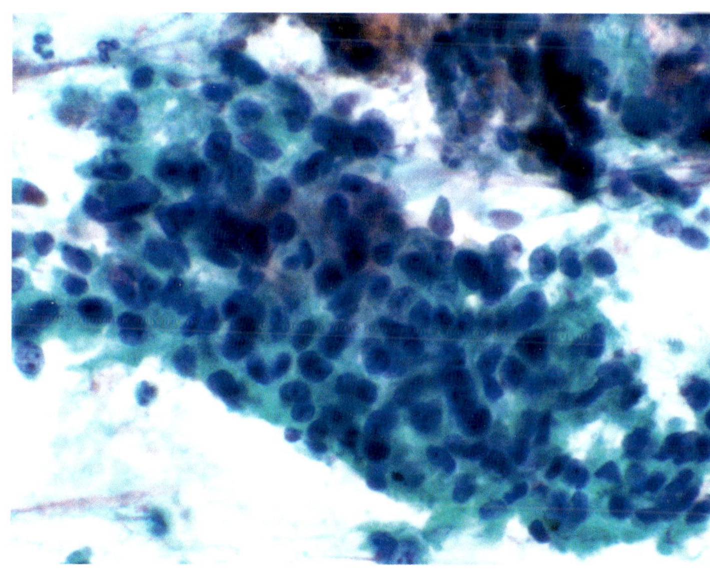

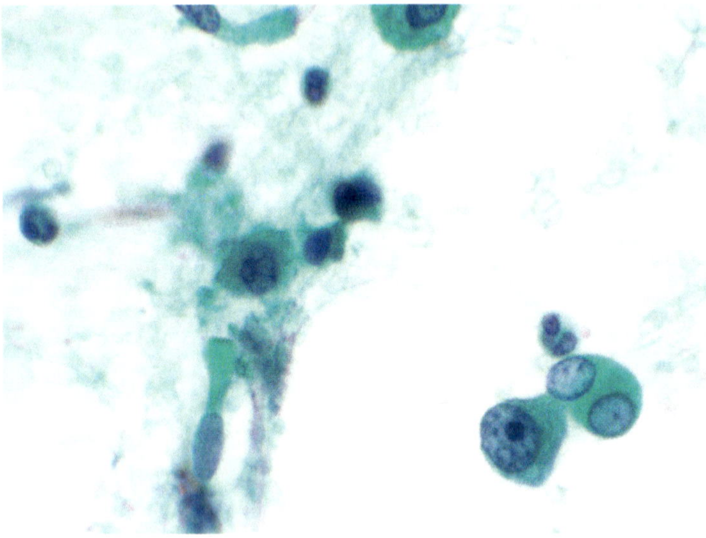

Figure 7.49b — Metastatic Prostate Carcinoma, Fine Needle Aspiration [Pap Stain; High Power]. Prostate carcinoma can look deceivingly bland, especially in instances where cytoplasm is more abundant. The foamy cytoplasm of this prostate carcinoma cell has a similar quality to that of the nearby binucleated alveolar macrophage. Both cells also contain round nuclei with regular borders, but the macronucleolus possessed by the tumor cell is difficult to ignore.

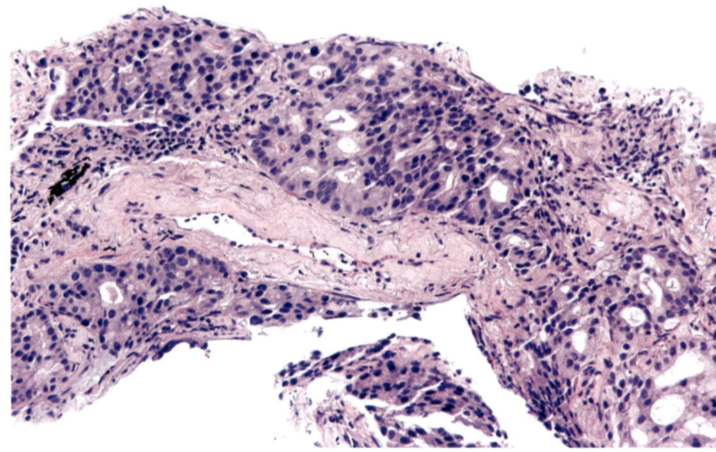

Figure 7.49c — Metastatic Prostatic Adenocarcinoma, Core Biopsy [H&E Stain; Low Power]. This core biopsy of a lung nodule shows the characteristic cribriforming and small acinar pattern of prostatic adenocarcinoma. History and serum PSA level are often helpful in establishing the diagnosis. In the absence of clinical information, a primary or metastatic neuroendocrine tumor is a consideration; neuroendocrine stains (synaptophysin, CD56, chromogranin) can address this possibility.

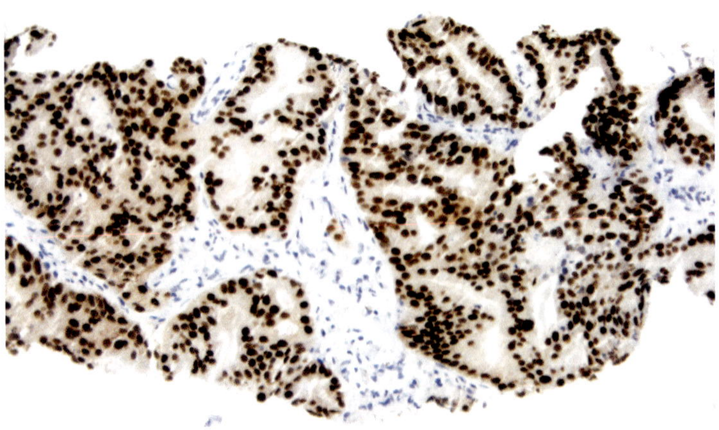

Figure 7.49d — Metastatic Prostatic Adenocarcinoma, Core Biopsy [NKX3.1 Immunohistochemical Stain; Low Power]. This lesion shows strong and diffuse nuclear expression of NKX3.1. PSA was also positive. Metastatic lesions may be less differentiated than the primary tumor, and be associated with the loss of expected markers (e.g., PSA). A panel of stains will help ensure the correct diagnosis (PSA, PSAP, NKX3.1 p501S).

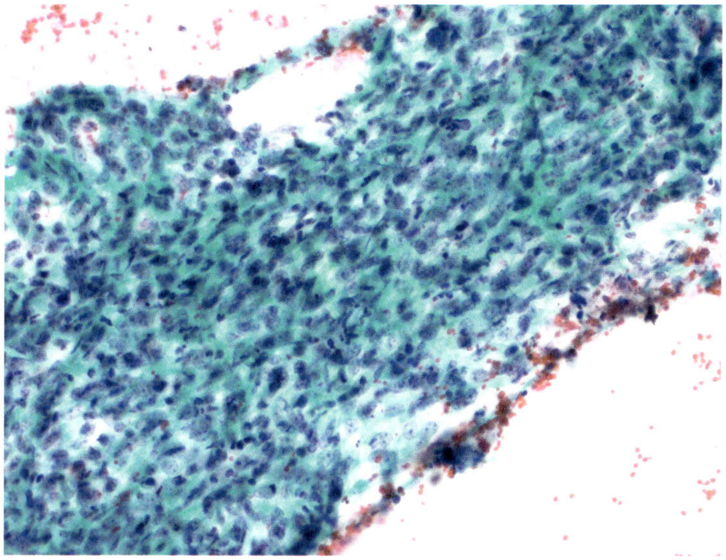

Figure 7.50a — Metastatic Sarcomatoid Prostate Carcinoma [Pap Stain; High Power]. Just as sarcomatoid carcinoma can be primary to the lung, sarcomatoid carcinoma from distant sites may metastasize to the lung. In instances where the patient has no history of malignancy, the options are numerous: Is this a primary or metastatic tumor? Is it a sarcoma or a carcinoma? Therefore, the creation of cell block material is critical, with examination of keratin expression on immunohistochemical studies often being the first step.

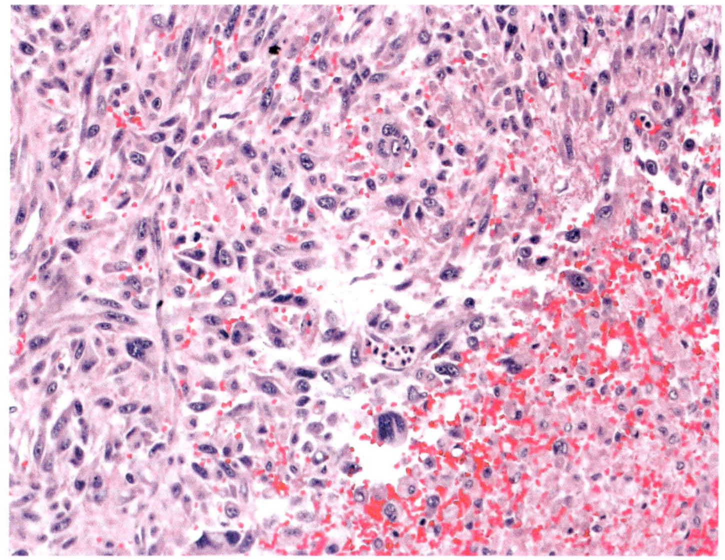

Figure 7.50b — Metastatic Sarcomatoid Prostate Carcinoma, Fine Needle Aspiration [H&E Stain; High Power]. The malignant cells are pleomorphic and spindle-shaped on the cell block preparation, providing no clue as to its origin. Because sarcomas are uncommon compared to carcinomas, malignant neoplasms with a spindled morphology are often sarcomatoid carcinomas.

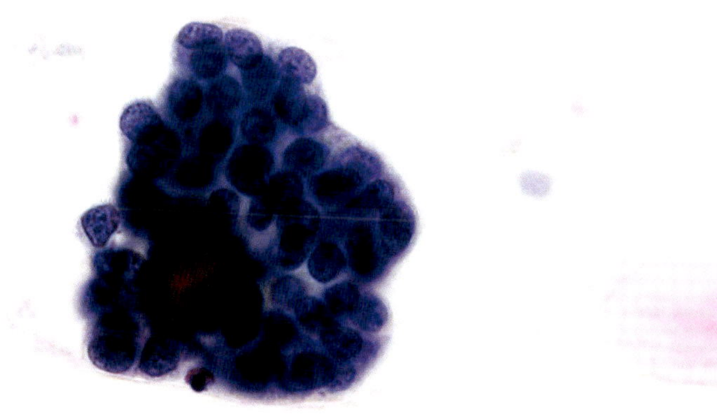

Figure 7.51a — Metastatic Endometrial Serous Carcinoma, Fine Needle Aspiration [Diff-Quik Stain; High Power]. The cells in this 3-dimensional ball are hyperchromatic and have nuclear border irregularities, coarse chromatin, and high nuclear-to-cytoplasmic ratios. The cells are centered around a red-staining and glassy-appearing psammoma body. The differential of lesions with psammoma bodies includes metastatic papillary thyroid carcinoma, metastatic papillary renal cell carcinoma, the micropapillary subtype of lung adenocarcinoma, and metastatic serous carcinoma of the ovary or endometrium.

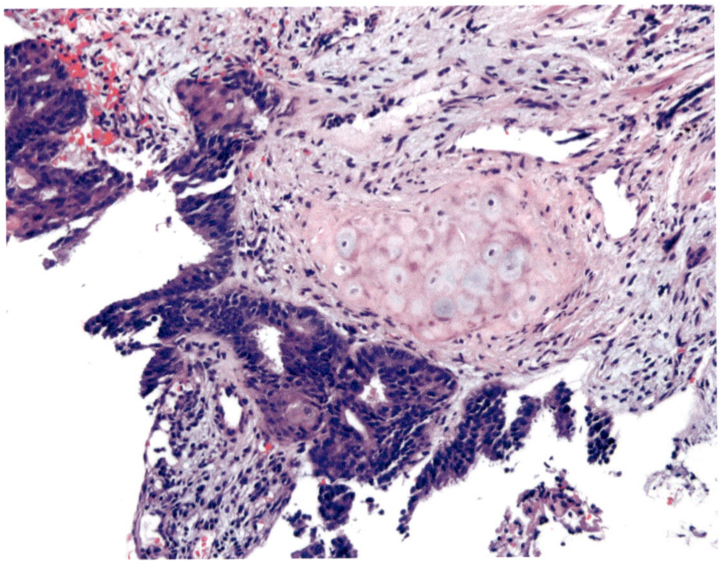

Figure 7.51b — Metastatic Endometrioid Endometrial Adenocarcinoma, Biopsy [H&E Stain; Low Power]. This transbronchial biopsy shows a cribriform adenocarcinoma invading the wall of a bronchus; two squamous morules are present. If imaging shows multiple small peripheral nodules and there is a history of endometrial adenocarcinoma, stains may not be needed. In a smoker with no history, the differential diagnosis will include adenosquamous carcinoma of the lung.

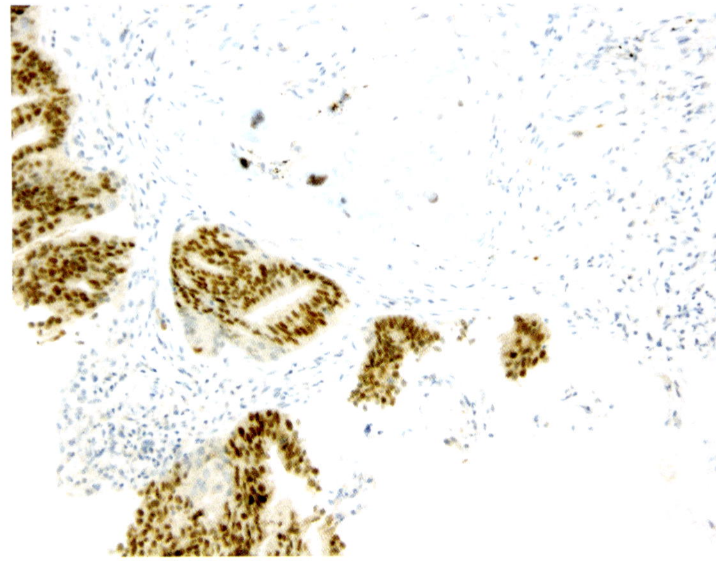

Figure 7.52 — Metastatic Endometrioid Endometrial Adenocarcinoma, Biopsy [PAX8 Immunohistochemical Stain; Low Power]. Many epithelial tumors of the gynecologic tract express PAX8, making it a useful marker in evaluating metastases in female patients. Diffuse nuclear expression is present here, and a stain for nuclear ER was also diffusely positive. TTF-1 and napsin A can be included in a panel of stains to help exclude primary lung cancer.

Figure 7.53a — Metastatic Malignant Mixed Mullerian Tumor, Fine Needle Aspiration [Diff-Quik Stain; High Power]. The cells are clearly malignant, with irregularly folded nuclei, large nucleoli which are sometimes multiple, and an erratic arrangement. Some cells appear slightly spindled as well. Malignant mixed Muellerian tumors are uncommon carcinosarcomas of the uterus and typically arise in postmenopausal women.

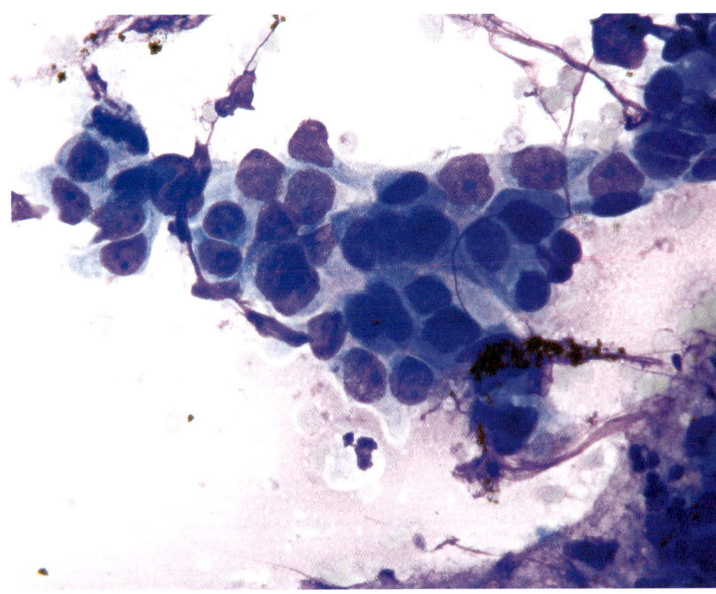

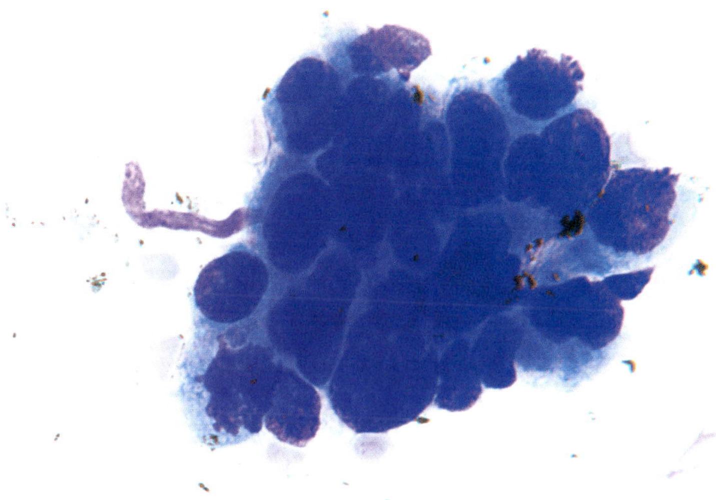

Figure 7.53b — Metastatic Malignant Mixed Mullerian Tumor, Fine Needle Aspiration [Diff-Quik Stain; High Power]. This image shows the highly pleomorphic tumor cells. The close cell-cell adherence suggests these cells are showing more carcinomatous differentiation. Malignant mixed Muellerian tumor may show heterologous differentiation, although this is not prognostically significant.

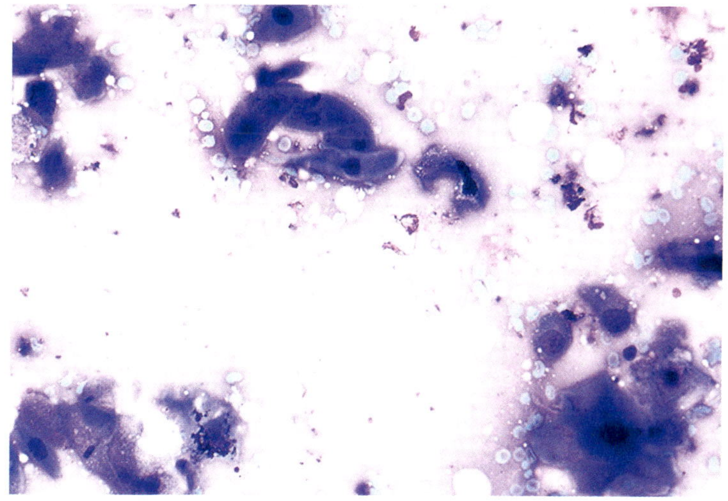

Figure 7.54 — Metastatic Cervical Squamous Cell Carcinoma, Fine Needle Aspiration [Diff-Quik Stain; High Power]. Squamous cell carcinoma may be primary to the lung, but also may be a metastasis from the head and neck region or the cervix. In this case, the carcinoma metastasized from the patient's known cervical carcinoma, an uncommon event. Because most lung squamous cell carcinomas are not human papillomavirus related, diffuse expression of p16 by immunohistochemistry or the demonstration of human papillomavirus by ancillary studies, such as in situ hybridization, indicates a metastasis to the lung from either the gynecologic tract or the head and neck region.

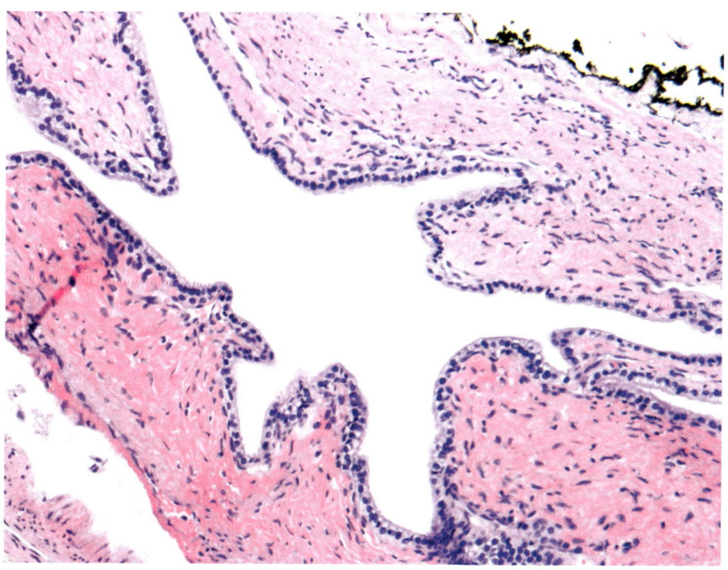

Figure 7.55 — Metastatic Teratoma, Resection [H&E Stain; Low Power]. While germ cell tumors from a variety of primary sites metastasize to the lung with some frequency, mature teratoma is the pattern most often encountered in surgical lung specimens. Other components of metastatic mixed germ cell tumors typically respond to chemotherapy, often leaving only the mature teratoma component to be surgically resected. Teratoma is grossly and microscopically multicystic with fibrous walls, as seen here. This nonciliated columnar epithelium has features of gastric or biliary origin, and is bland and orderly.

Index